REVIEW GUIDE FOR

RN Pre-Entrance EXAM

NLN | Assessment and Evaluation Division

REVIEW GUIDE FOR
RN Pre-Entrance EXAM

Edited by
Mary McDonald

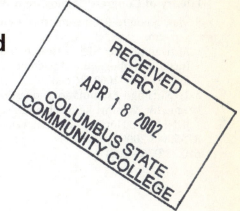

Jones and Bartlett Publishers
Sudbury, Massachusetts
Boston • London • Toronto • Singapore

World Headquarters
Jones and Bartlett Publishers
40 Tall Pine Drive
Sudbury, MA 01776
978-443-5000
info@jbpub.com
www.jbpub.com

Jones and Bartlett Publishers Canada
2100 Bloor Street West
Suite 6-272
Toronto, ON M6S 5A5
CANADA

Jones and Bartlett Publishers International
Barb House, Barb Mews
London W6 7PA
UK

Senior Acquisitions Editor: Greg Vis
Production Editor: Linda DeBruyn
Associate Editor: John Danielowich
Editorial/Production Assistant: Christine Tridente
Manufacturing Buyer: Kristen Guevara
Editorial, Design, and Production Service: Modern Graphics
Cover Design: Anne Spencer
Typesetting: Modern Graphics
Printing and Binding: Courier Westford

Library of Congress Cataloging-in-Publication Data

Review guide to RN pre-entrance exam / edited by Mary McDonald.
    p. cm.
  At head of title: NLN, Research and Evaluation Division.
  Includes bibliographical references.
  ISBN 0-7637-1062-8 (pbk)
  1. Nursing—Examinations, questions, etc.   I. McDonald, Mary, 1947–   II. National League for Nursing. Research and Evaluation Division.
  [DNLM: 1. Nursing—Examination Questions. WY 18.2 R455 2000]
RT55.R48 2000
610.73'076—dc21
                                                                99-042997
                                                                CIP

Cover photo credit: Copyright © 1999 Photodisc

Printed in the United States of America
03 02 01 00   10 9 8 7 6 5 4 3 2

Contents

Preface

If you are applying to a nursing program, you have found the book that you need to succeed. Over the past several years, an overwhelming number of requests have been received at the National League for Nursing (NLN) headquarters from nursing school applicants who were looking for a solid reference to guide them in preparing for nursing school entrance exams. This book was written in response to those requests.

Not only is this book a worthwhile preparation tool for the NLN Pre-Admission Examination, applicants who are preparing for the Psychological Corporation's entrance exam (RNEE), the Psychological Services Bureau's PSB-Nursing School Aptitude Examination, the Educational Resources Nurse Entrance Test (NET), or the Pre-Nursing Assessment Test from the Center for Nurse Education and Testing (CNET) will also find it to be an invaluable study aide. In addition, students who are seeking admission to programs in various health-related fields, such as medical technology, dental hygiene, dietician and physician's assistant programs, can use this book as a comprehensive study guide.

This book offers the most thorough and comprehensive subject matter overview that you will find in any review book. It also includes over **1000** practice questions from previous NLN exams. Although these questions are no longer used in the current exams, they are actual questions from real tests.

The **Introduction** discusses career options in nursing and describes the types of nursing programs available. Helpful advice is offered to assist you in selecting the nursing program that is right for you. The introduction also reviews the content of pre-admission exams and provides proven study strategies and test-taking skills to help you to maximize your score.

Section A provides a comprehensive review of the verbal and reading comprehension components of the test. This section offers a number of practical methods to improve your vocabulary and reading skills. A detailed analysis of a reading comprehension passage is also offered. Three verbal and reading comprehension exams (60 questions each), with answer keys, are provided for practice at the end of the section.

Section B offers an excellent overview of the math content that you will need to be familiar with for a nursing school pre-admission exam. Detailed examples are provided to help you solve the various problems and identify your strengths and weaknesses. Four math exams (40 questions each), with answer keys and detailed explanations, are provided for practice at the end of the section.

Section C reviews the science content that is included on a nursing school pre-admission exam. Clear and detailed summaries of high school biology, chemistry, and physics will guide your study in these areas. Three science exams (60 questions each), with answer keys and detailed explanations, are provided for practice at the end of the section.

Comprehensive Practice Tests are provided in the final section. Each of these exams is an actual NLN Pre-Admission Exam that is no longer in use. These tests each have 160 questions: 60 verbal, 40 math, and 60 science. Answer keys and detailed explanations follow each exam.

The *NLN Review Guide for RN Pre-Entrance Exam* provides a sound basis for successful preparation for a nursing pre-admission exam. We are certain that you will find it to be a useful tool to assist you to maximize your exam score and gain admission to the nursing program of your choice.

Mary E. McDonald, RN, MA, CS
Test Consultant
National League for Nursing

Editoral Review Board

Introduction

Career Options in Nursing

You purchased this book because you have decided that you want to be a nurse. You have made **two** wise decisions. First, the profession of nursing is a rewarding and challenging career, which will afford you the opportunity to make a meaningful difference in the lives of others. Second, this book is designed to assist you in succeeding in your initial step toward reaching your career goal—scoring your best on a nursing school entrance examination.

Despite the fact that there are more nurses employed today than ever before, there is an alarming shortage of registered nurses and nurses who have advanced degrees. The opportunities currently available in nursing are extensive, and education is the key to career advancement. It is very important that you carefully consider your professional goals before choosing a particular educational path. You should evaluate each of the three types of educational programs in nursing that are available in the United States before deciding which route you will follow.

Diploma Programs are the oldest type of educational programs for preparing registered nurses in the United States. The number of these programs is steadily declining as ADN programs have increased in popularity. State-approved diploma programs are affiliated with hospitals and last from 24–30 months, preparing their graduates to take the state licensing exam for registered nurses. In addition to nursing courses in the care of adults, children, childbearing families, and individuals who have mental illness, diploma students are required to take prerequisite science courses. General education courses are not always required because diploma programs do not grant a degree. Diploma graduates are intensively prepared to provide individualized, direct care to hospitalized patients.

Associate Degree Nursing (ADN) programs prepare their graduates to take the registered nurse state licensure examination. The majority of these programs require two academic years of study and are usually offered at community colleges. Following completion of the program, students are awarded an associate degree. Requirements include general education and basic science courses as well as nursing theory and clinical experience in the care of adults, children, childbearing families, and individuals who have mental illness. Associate degree graduates are equipped to solve problems, make decisions, and provide direct patient care.

Baccalaureate Programs are at least four years in length and are offered in colleges and universities. Baccalaureate students take the general education requirements of their college in addition to prerequisite courses in the physical, biological, and behavioral sciences. The nursing major requires clinical coursework in the care of adults, children, childbearing families, and individuals who have mental illness, with an emphasis on community health, leadership, and the role of the professional nurse as a manager. Nursing theory, professional ethics and issues, and nursing research are also included in baccalaureate curriculum. The baccalaureate nurse is eligible to take the registered nurse state licensing exam and is prepared for positions in community health. The baccalaureate degree is considered a requirement for managerial and advanced nursing positions.

Nursing education at all levels provides a basis for career development. A large number of ADN programs offer upward mobility programs for diploma graduates. Many baccalaureate programs offer a completion track for registered nurses who are graduates of diploma and ADN programs. These programs often admit students with advanced standing based on their nursing experience and also on their performance on an advanced standing exam, such as the National League for Nursing (NLN) Accelerated Completion Exam (ACE). In this way nurses are able to build on their experience to complete the requirements for the baccalaureate degree, which is required for entrance to graduate education. Graduate preparation at the Masters and Doctorate levels opens the door to even greater career opportunities in nursing, including teaching, administration, and nursing research.

Which Nursing Program is Right for You?

When selecting which nursing path you want to pursue, the first thing you should consider is your career goal. Do you want to work in a community health setting? Are you interested in providing direct patient care in a hospital? Do you envision yourself as a nursing administrator or in a nursing leadership position? Does your ultimate career goal require graduate nursing education? Should you choose a basic baccalaureate program to provide you with the foundation for an advanced nursing education? Or, should you choose another entry level program to achieve your goals through career mobility programs? Your ultimate decision should be based on a careful consideration of your own needs.

Nursing will provide you with a satisfying career, both personally and financially, at whatever educational level you choose to pursue. There are many reasons for selecting a particular program, but remember, nursing is a career that requires intelligence, self-discipline, and a life-long dedication to learning. The nursing profession will provide you with many opportunities for continuing education and career advancement. It will be up to you to take full advantage of the opportunities to grow, both as a person and a professional.

How will you finance your education?

Nursing education is expensive. There are many factors that will influence your school choice. Baccalaureate programs are the most expensive, because they require the most extensive coursework. Private colleges are more expensive than public institutions. The demands of a full-time program may prevent you from working.

Perhaps your financial situation will steer you to consider a part-time program that will allow you to continue to work. You may decide to obtain a diploma or pursue an associate degree in nursing. Each of these credentials will provide you with the ability to pursue a satisfying nursing career and will also be a stepping stone for you to advance your nursing education. Examine your own individual situation before making a decision about which avenue to pursue. Whatever program you choose, nursing is a unique profession that encourages career mobility and will provide you with the opportunity to reach your ultimate goal.

When considering your educational options, it is important to remember that financial assistance is available for all types of nursing programs. Aid is available in the form of scholarships and grants that do not need to be repaid. Educational loans, that carry a low interest rate and are repaid after graduation, are also available. The amount and type of aid you receive will depend on your need and the financial aid available at the institution you attend. The programs that you are considering applying to will provide you with specific information about financial aid opportunities. There is always competition for financial aid, so it is important for you to find out early what aid is available, what the eligibility requirements are, and what the application procedure involves. Applying early to several programs that meet your criteria will provide you with the best opportunities both for admission and for receiving the financial aid package you need.

Which programs do you qualify for?

Before you submit an application to a nursing program you must make an honest evaluation of your credentials. Acceptance is dependent on several factors, including your grade point average (GPA), standardized test scores, references, extracurricular activities, interview, work experience, and writing ability. Admission is competitive and schools establish their own criteria standards for admission. Nursing programs are very rigorous.They are all looking for motivated students who will succeed. Coursework requires long hours of intense study. In addition, nursing students are often scheduled for 8 to 18 hours a week of clinical practice. The number of admissions to each program is limited and schools will accept the most qualified students who apply. Therefore, it is always a good idea to apply to several programs.

As a general rule, the higher the educational level of the program, the higher the standards for admission. Your high school or community college grades are very important. The higher your GPA the better, although schools will consider the level of difficulty of the coursework you have taken. A school may require a certain GPA for admission, but it is important to note that your GPA will neither guarantee nor exclude your admission to a program. This is why your personal references and interview are so important. References from qualified teachers and employers can provide a school with a more complete picture of you. If a school offers you an interview, be sure to make the most of the opportunity; arrive early and dress professionally. Your personal interview will give you the opportunity to present yourself as a motivated and qualified applicant, as well as allow you the chance to explain any weakness in your application.

Selecting a Program to Meet Your Needs

Once you have sorted out your career goals and identified the educational path that best suits you, the next step is to identify several schools that fit your criteria. In addition to financial aid availability and admission requirements, it is essential for you to evaluate the quality of the programs you are interested in. There are several questions that you will want to ask.

Is the program approved by the state?

Each state's Board of Nurse Examiners grants permission for nursing graduates to take the National Council Licensure Exam (NCLEX). Nursing graduates who successfully pass this exam apply directly to their state to obtain licensure to practice as a registered nurse. For information on your state's licensing procedure, visit the National Council on State Boards of Nursing's web site at www.ncsbn.org.

Is the program accredited by the National League for Nursing Accrediting Commission?

Accreditation assures you of the quality of the educational program. If you plan to continue your education many nursing programs will only accept your credentials for advanced placement or graduate work if your nursing program is accredited by the National League for Nursing Accrediting Commission (NLNAC). For information visit the NLN's web site at www.nln.org.

What is the NCLEX pass rate for the graduates of the program over the last five years?

Determine how successful the school's graduates have been with passing the licensure exam. If the pass rate has been high over several years, it indicates that the graduates are well prepared to take the NCLEX exam.

What is the reputation of the graduates of the school?

Are the graduates well respected in the health care community? If the new graduate employment rate is high, it indicates that the program is preparing its students well for the work environment.

Is the environment of the school comfortable for you?

Some people prefer to attend a large institution which offers many extracurricular activities. Others prefer the close community atmosphere of a small institution. Are you interested in dormitory life or would you prefer to commute to school? Examine the social experience that each school offers and decide if you are comfortable with it.

It is important for you to look seriously at all the options that are available. Once you identify the schools that meet your needs, you will probably find that these schools will consider you to be an attractive candidate. Admission to a nursing program is not dependent on one factor. Schools will consider you as a whole package. Maximize your profile and be an informed applicant. Remember, there are many routes to your ultimate career goal in nursing.

Nursing School Entrance Examinations

Most nursing programs require that you take an admissions test, such as the National League for Nursing (NLN) Pre-Admission Examination, the Psychological Corporation's Entrance Exam (RNEE), the Psychological Services Bureau's PSB-Nursing School Aptitude Examination, Educational Resources' Nurse Entrance Test (NET), or the Center for Nursing Education and Testings' Pre-Nursing Assessment Test. Whatever test you are required to take, you will find this book to be an invaluable tool. The book contains actual questions from previous NLN exams. The questions thoroughly cover the areas that are tested on all nursing school admission exams.

The schools that you are applying to will provide you with the necessary information and application forms for the required exam. While each school determines for themselves how these scores will be used for admission, the higher your exam score the better your chance for nursing school admission. Find out exactly how the scores are used at the school to which you are applying, then use this book to maximize your nursing admission exam score.

Content of the Pre-Admission Exams

The purpose of an entrance exam is to evaluate academic ability in order to identify the most qualified applicants. Nursing entrance exams are carefully designed to measure an individual's ability in areas that provide a basis for nursing education. The exams provide schools of nursing with a common basis for evaluating the academic abilities of applicants to assist faculty in making admission decisions. All of the nursing pre-admission tests use four-option multiple-choice questions to assess an applicant's verbal ability, reading comprehension, mathematic ability, and knowledge of physical and life sciences.

The pre-admission exams that are included in this book consist of actual questions that were used in previously administered NLN Pre-Admission examinations. These exams will provide you with an actual pre-admission exam experience. Answer keys and rationales for every question will give you important feedback to guide your future test preparation.

The 60 question **verbal** test measures your word knowledge ability and reading comprehension. Word knowledge questions require you to identify the meaning of a word as it is used in a sentence. The reading comprehension section focuses on your reasoning and critical thinking ability. Five short passages in each test require you to analyze and interpret the material presented. These questions assess your ability to determine the main ideas and supporting details, draw conclusions, make inferences, and apply information to new situations.

The 40 question **mathematics** test consists of straight calculations and word problems that cover basic operations (integers, decimals, fractions, and percents), algebra, geometry, conversions, graphs, and concepts. Data interpretation, applied mathematics, and scientific notation are also included.

The 60 question **science** test measures high-school level knowledge of science. Questions are included on general biology, chemistry, physics, and earth science.

Use This Book to Maximize Your Score

Step one for success on an exam is to keep your anxiety to a minimum. Being well prepared is the best antidote for test anxiety. This book is designed to help you maximize your test score with thorough preparation. The guidelines are all here; it is up to you to commit the time necessary for your own success.

This book is divided into three review sections—verbal, math, and science. Each section begins with a comprehensive overview that summarizes the important facts and concepts of the subject. The review is meant to be a "refresher" for what you have already learned, it is not an introduction to the subject. If you have not completed a high school course in a subject, these reviews will not provide you with the knowledge that you need to be successful on a nursing entrance examination.

It is important for you to carefully plan your study strategy. Start early, set a study schedule, and stick to it. Plan to finish your test preparation 3–4 days before the test. Cramming right before the test will not be as helpful as a planned approach over time. Use each review section as a study guide to carefully review the content summary for each subject before you answer the practice questions. Study one section at a time. Then, follow the test-taking tips outlined in the next section to answer the practice questions at the end of each section. Check your answers with the key, and review the rationales to identify your strengths and weakness. Use your score as a guide for further study. Refer to the bibliography at the end of each section for study references to improve your knowledge in the areas where you are weak.

After you have completed the verbal, math, and science sections following the above guidelines, take the three comprehensive Practice Tests at the end of the book. Time yourself carefully and use the answer sheet provided on pages 11–12 to "bubble in" one of the exams. Be very careful to fill in the circle that corresponds to your answer choice. This will help to familiarize you with the actual format used on the tests. Score your exams and carefully focus on the rationales provided for each question. For each answer that you missed ask yourself, "Why did I get this question wrong?" Did you misread the question or were you unfamiliar with the content? Your analysis of your weaknesses will guide your review preparation. Decide which areas you need to focus on for your final review. Carefully following these guidelines to complete your review will help boost the confidence that you need to succeed on any of the nursing pre-admission exams.

Score Report

The report on page 10 is a sample of the report that you will receive after taking a Pre-Admission exam. This particular report is an NLN Pre-Admission performance report. Your test results are sent to you and to whichever schools you choose. You will notice that a *Guide for Interpretation of the Test Report* is part of the test report. Read the guide carefully, it explains how to interpret your scores. The guide also shows you how to determine where you rank among all the applicants who have taken the test. Find out how the nursing programs to which you are applying use these scores for making admission decisions. Remember, an informed applicant is a successful applicant. (See sample score report on page 10, Figure 1.)

Test-Taking Strategies

Nothing is more important to successful test-taking than studying. A thorough understanding of the test material is essential to your success. While test-taking strategies are not a substitute for good study habits, these skills will enhance your overall performance on a test, as long as you have a good grasp of the knowledge being measured. Follow the study plan guidelines discussed above and use these hints to increase your probability of choosing the correct answer. Remember, the right answer is right there in front of you. Have confidence in yourself.

Plan ahead

The night before the test is no time for cramming. Review the test-taking strategies below and put your books away. Relax and get a good night's sleep. Plan to wear comfortable clothes. It is hard to predict the climate variations of most testing sites, so dress in layers and bring a sweater. Avoid confusion on the day of the test by being well prepared. Have your admission ticket, your photo identification, a watch, and several #2 pencils ready. Make sure you are familiar with the trip to the testing site and allow yourself plenty of time. Arrive early and choose a seat where you feel comfortable. A little bit of anxiety is a positive force and planning ahead will help to keep your anxiety at this positive level. Relaxation techniques such as breathing or imaging will help you to feel calm and unhurried when the test begins.

Listen to directions

Once the testing session begins, the proctor will give directions about filling in your identifying information and answer sheet. Pay close attention to the proctor and read the written directions carefully. Completeness and neatness are important. Incorrect or stray marks on your answer sheet can cause your score to be delayed, or worse, penalize your final score. The proctor will tell you how much time you have for each section and when breaks will be allowed. When the proctor tells you to begin the test, note what time it will be when you will still have ten minutes left to review your work.

Read each question carefully

Read the question all the way through. Pay attention to detail; every word counts. Be alert for key words. Word such as "only," "never," "first," "last," "always," "except," "never" are strong words that limit the choice of the correct answer. Ask yourself, "What is this question asking?" Consider the question as it is written—do not read anything into it. No one is trying to trick you. Rephrase and answer the question in your own words.

Read each answer choice carefully

Even if the first or second answer choice looks good to you, it is a mistake to think that you don't need to read the others. Sometimes another choice provides a more precise answer or makes you realize that you misunderstood the question. Under the stress of taking a test, you may be tempted to select the first answer that looks right. Resist the temptation. Careful examination may reveal that your first choice does not answer the question at all. Eliminate the obviously incorrect options quickly and compare the plausible options for similarities or conflicts. Since there is only one correct answer to each question, options that are similar must both be wrong. If two options are opposite, one of them is frequently correct. Eliminate wrong answer choices one by one. This process of elimination will be completed quickly for simple recall questions, while it may take longer for more complex questions. Although this method sounds time consuming, it will assist you in clarifying the question and selecting more correct answers. Practicing this method of eliminating answers on the sample tests included in this book will help you to develop the speed you will need in the real exam.

Re-read the question and the answer choices

Choose your answer from your remaining choices based on the re-reading. Spend time considering the plausible choices. Have confidence in your selection, but if you are unable to answer the question after eliminating the obviously wrong choices, move on to the next question. Don't get bogged down on any one question. Spending too much time on a difficult question could compromise your final test score. If you skip a question, remember to skip the corresponding number on the answer sheet. Check frequently to make sure that you are filling in the correct "bubble" on the answer sheet. Go through the whole test this way, answering only those questions that you are sure of.

Stay focused

Keep yourself focused. Think only about the question in front of you. If stray thoughts distract you, or you find yourself wandering back to a previous question, turn your focus back to the question at hand. Congratulate yourself for being in control of the situation.

Pace yourself

Don't puzzle more than a few seconds over any question. On the other hand, don't race through the test so fast that you make careless errors. Pace yourself. Answer all the questions that you are sure of first, and then go back to the more difficult ones. Your objective is to be able to consider all questions at least once, and some more than once. If there are sixty questions on a test and you want ten minutes for review, you should be half way through the test in 25 minutes. Therefore you would allow yourself 45–50 seconds per question. Plan your timing strategy in advance. Your application materials will tell you how many questions are in each section of the test you are scheduled to take and how much time is allowed. Use the practice tests in this book to practice pacing yourself. Be sure to use all the allotted time. Rushing to finish a test will not benefit your score. Do not be distracted by other students who leave the testing room before you do. Everyone works at a different pace, and paying attention to what others are doing takes time away from your test. Use every minute of the allotted time to maximize your final score.

Take an educated guess

Read all the material that is provided when you apply to take a test. Be sure that you know whether there is a penalty for guessing. If there is a penalty for guessing, your score will be reduced by the number of incorrect responses indicated. If your score is equal to the total number of correct answers, there is no penalty for guessing. Wild guessing should be always be avoided, but even with a penalty for guessing, a guessing strategy can improve your score. Your chance of guessing the correct answer increases with every option that you can eliminate. You will probably be able to spot one or two wrong choices in even the most difficult questions. If you eliminate these wrong options and make an educated guess from the choices that remain, you are bound to pick up some extra points on the test.

Obviously, the most effective way to eliminate wrong choices, or choose the correct one, is to base your decision on your knowledge of the subject. You should guess only after you have tried your best to answer the question. However, there are some tips that will help you to make an educated guess when you are unable to pick the correct answer. Remember that test developers are very aware of these tips and attempt to eliminate them from their exams. In addition, there are exceptions to every rule, so answer with caution and never let a hunch or a tip overrule an answer that you have decided on based on your knowledge. Have confidence in yourself, because the best chance for successfully answering a question is to have a thorough understanding of the subject.

Watch for grammatical inconsistencies. If an answer is inconsistent with the question it probably is an incorrect response.

When a word is used in both the stem and one option it is a clue that the option is the correct choice.

There can only be one correct answer. When two answers are very similar, neither one is correct.

Definitive words such as "always," "never," "only," or "all" in an option usually mean that the that option is incorrect.

Avoid looking for an answer pattern. It is not unusual for several consecutive questions to have the same answer letter.

Do not assume that one letter is favored as the answer. Test developers are very cautious to equally distribute answers across all four letter options, one letter is not chosen over another. Some experts say that "C" is most often the correct choice. However, because an effort is made to equally distribute the answers randomly, each letter has an equal choice of being the correct response. Choose a letter. If you have absolutely no idea of the correct answer and you have decided to guess, choose a letter and pick that letter consistently. You will have a 25% chance of guessing correctly.

Many times the correct answer is the longest one. Test developers are very cautious about keeping the choices of equal length, but if you are in doubt, you may decide to choose the longest option as the correct one.

Recall clues from other questions. Sometimes information in one question will give away the answer to another question.

Stay with your first answer unless you have a very specific reason to make a change. Do not change your answer on a whim, but you should be willing to change your answer for a good reason. When you score your practice tests note if your changed answers helped or hurt your score. If it helped you have a tendency to improve your score by changing answers. If you discover on the practice tests that you consistently change your answers to an incorrect choice, stop changing your answers.

Positive Attitude

Having a positive attitude about yourself and your test-taking ability is fundamental to success on any exam. Getting down on yourself can rob you of your confidence. It is important to think positive thoughts that will keep your confidence up. You took the first step toward developing a positive attitude when you purchased this book. Follow the guidelines outlined in this chapter and you will be well on your way to sharpening your positive attitude.

Remember to keep the admission test in perspective. The test is only one factor in nursing school admission. Your grades, recommendations, and interview will all play an important part in the admission decision. In addition, schools often allow you to repeat the test if you do not do as well as you wanted to.

You will increase self-confidence by studying effectively, and maximize your test-taking ability by utilizing the skills that have been outlined in this book. Follow the guidelines and practice your skills on the sample exams that accompany this book and you will find that you have the positive attitude that you need for success on a nursing school pre-admission examination.

NLN ASSESSMENT AND EVALUATION   61 BROADWAY   NEW YORK, NY 10006

Site #   **NATIONAL LEAGUE FOR NURSING**   Form   45
                                    REPORT OF PERFORMANCE ON
                                   Pre-Admission Examination -   RN
Applicant Name   **Identification Number**   Test Date   Report Date
                                                              04/03/99   04/12/99
                                        Program Code

		Percentile Norms*		
Test	Score	DI	AD	All
Verbal Ability	40	82	69	73
Mathematics	31	94	94	94
Science	34	79	72	74
Composite	121	87	82	83

		INDIV.	PROG.	STATES	
*PERCENTILE NORMS ARE BASED ON PERFORMANCE OF:					
APPLICANTS TO DIPLOMA PROGRAMS ------------		641	39	13	1983
APPLICANTS TO ASSOCIATE DEGREE PROGRAMS----		1897	33	20	1983
ALL APPLICANTS TO BASIC NURSING PROGRAMS----		2615	75	25	1983

SCORES ON THIS EXAMINATION FORM WERE UPDATED USING A
PRE-EQUATING SAMPLE OF 22.962 EXAMINEES TESTED IN 1993-94.

A copy of this report was sent to:

GUIDE FOR THE INTERPRETATION OF THE TEST REPORT

SCORES The individual tests included in the examination are identified in the left-hand column of the report. Immediately to the right, in the column labeled "Score" is the **raw score** earned. This score is the number of test items you answered correctly. Each test contains some additional items that were included for test development purposes only. These items were not used to calculate the scores. The highest possible raw score in each test is as follows: Verbal Ability - 60; Mathematics - 40; Science - 60.

THE COMPOSITE SCORE is based on your performance on the total examination, but is not the sum of the items answered correctly. It is a standard score, i.e., a weighted combination of the scores on the individual tests. Composite scores may range from 0 to 200. The average is 100, and the standard deviation, a measure of variability around this average score, is 20. Most scores range between 50 and 150.

A PERCENTILE SCORE for each test and for the composite score is reported in the column labeled "Percentile Norms." Percentiles, which range from 0-99, indicate what portion of a reference group of applicants to similar nursing programs earned raw scores lower than yours. For example, if the report shows a percentile score of 84 for a raw score of 049 on the Verbal Ability test, it means that 84% of the norms group received a raw score of 49 or less. The percentile scores do NOT indicate the percentage of items that were answered correctly.

NORMS GROUP Each norms group used in preparing this report is identified at the top of the column labeled "Percentile Norms." For the Pre-Admission Examination-PN the norms group is comprised of all applicants to practical nursing programs who took this test during the period identified at the bottom of the report. For the Pre-Admission Examination-RN three sets of norms are provided: "DI" refers to applicants to diploma programs; "AD" refers to applicants to associate degree programs; and "ALL" refers to all applicants to any of the three types of programs preparing students for registered nurse practice. The most appropriate norms group to use is the group which matches or includes the type of program to which you are applying. This allows comparisons with other applicants to similar programs. Each norms group is described in the section following the test scores.

INTERPRETING THE SCORES Percentiles substantially above the 50th percentile indicate better than average performance, percentiles ranging from about 40-60 average, and those substantially below the 50th percentile poorer than average. Areas of strength or weakness may be identified by noting those parts of the examination for which the percentiles are high or low. It should be noted that equal differences in percentiles do not indicate equal differences in ability since examinees' test scores tend to group around the average score. The further one is from the average, in either direction, the greater is the degree of ability represented by each additional percentage point. The difference between percentiles of 80 and 89 is far greater in terms of ability than the difference between 50 and 59; similarly, the difference between percentiles 10 and 19 is greater that the difference between 50 and 59.

While no test score is an exact measure, the score should provide a very good estimate of your ability and achievement level at the time the examination was taken. The scores reported here are one source of information that can be used along with other information about an applicant, by nursing education programs when making admission decisions.

Figure 1. Sample Score Report

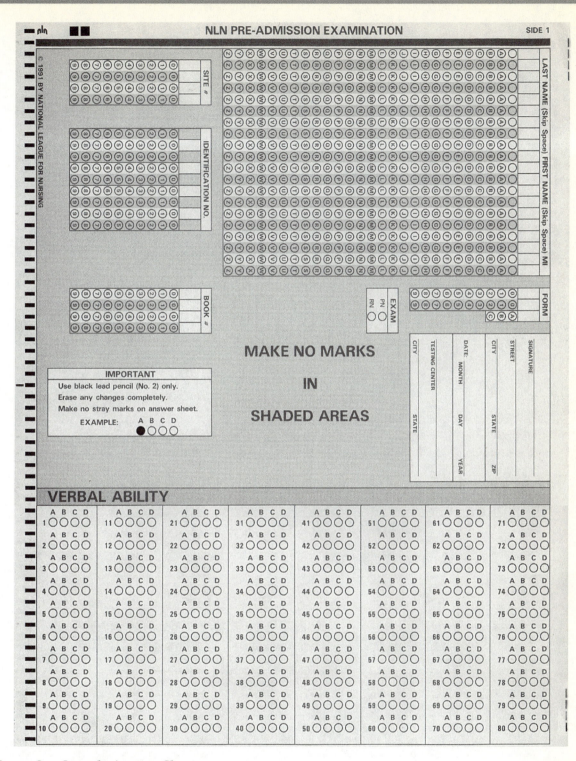

Figure 2a. Sample Answer Sheet

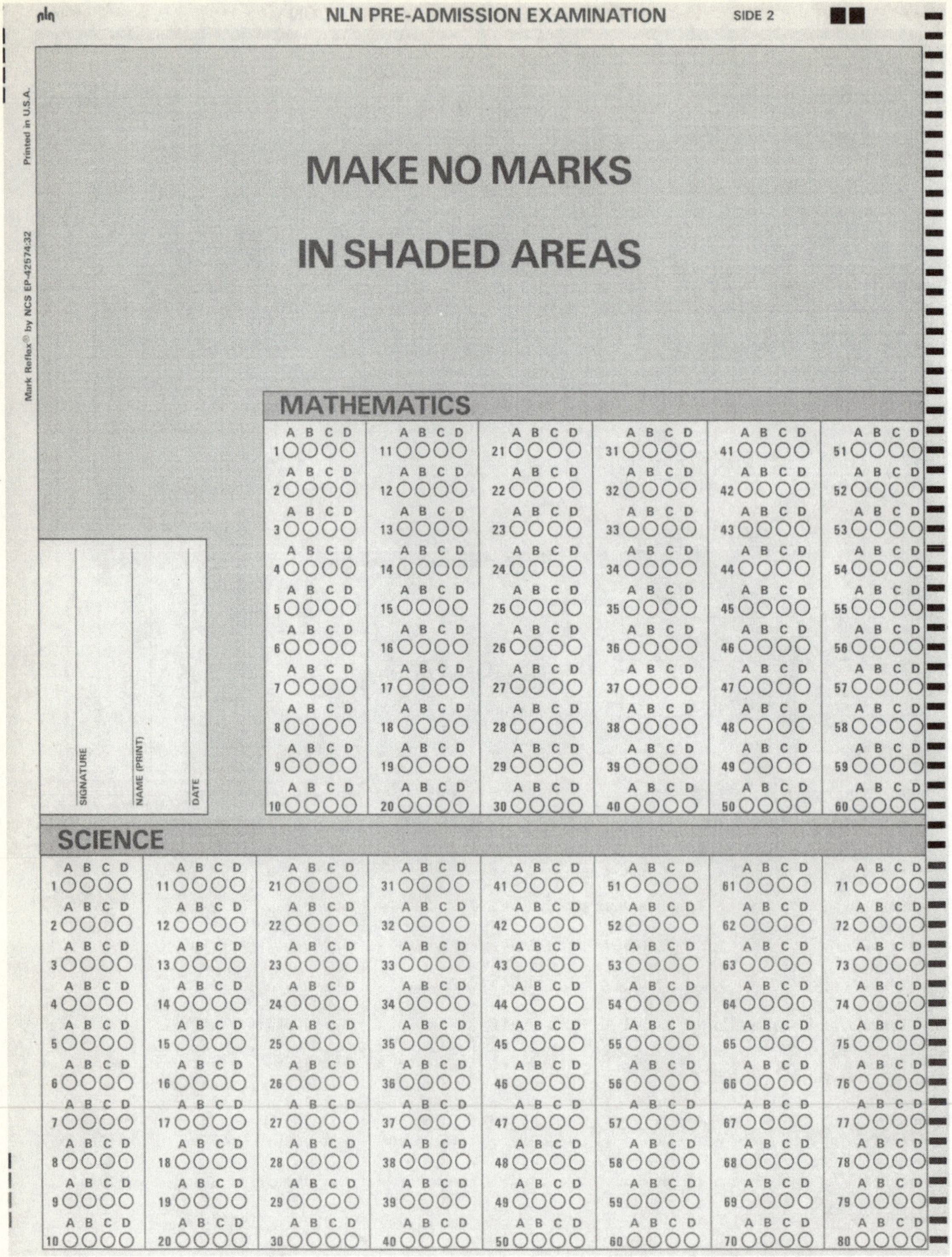
NLN PRE-ADMISSION EXAMINATION
SIDE 2
Printed in U.S.A.
Mark Reflex® by NCS EP-42574:32
MAKE NO MARKS
IN SHADED AREAS
SIGNATURE
NAME (PRINT)
DATE
MATHEMATICS
SCIENCE

Figure 2b. Sample Answer Sheet

Verbal Content Review

Many people who are smart and articulate still have trouble when they are asked to take a test on verbal skills. There are, fortunately, some proven methods to help people overcome some of their test-taking problems and to maximize their performance on standardized tests. Some of these are long-term programs used by students to develop their verbal skills; some are very simple techniques that can be used when answering specific test questions.

In this guide you will find methods you can use to improve both your basic reading skills and your test-taking ability.

Ways to Develop Your Reading Skills

Building Your Vocabulary

You have probably noticed that almost every test of reading skills includes two types of questions: (1) those that ask you about details, main ideas, and implications in reading passages, and (2) those that ask you the meaning of words. The vocabulary questions are included because you cannot be a good reader—or a good writer, or even a truly good thinker—if you don't know a great number of words.

Take this sentence, for instance:

Sandra grimaced when she tasted the brackish water.

The reader who knows the words *grimaced* and *brackish* will have a much better understanding of what Sandra did (made a sour face) and why she did it (because the water was slightly salty) than the reader who knew only one of those words or who knew neither of them. One of your long-term goals, then, should be to improve your vocabulary, not just to score well on tests but to become a better reader and a more effective communicator.

There are five things you can do to build your word power:

1. Make vocabulary study fun
2. Read as much as possible
3. Use a dictionary often
4. Make word lists
5. Break words down into roots and affixes

Make Vocabulary Study Fun

No vocabulary program is likely to succeed if you don't get involved with words and have fun pursuing their meanings. Play word games, do crossword puzzles, and listen to effective speakers for new words that intrigue you; words that you want to make yours.

Help yourself remember new words by using memory devices that are fun and fanciful. If you want to remember the meaning of *brackish,* for example, you might play with the word and make a sentence: "Brrrr! . . . Ack! . . . Ish! It's salty!" Sometimes the sillier the association, the better the chance that you'll remember the word.

Read As Much As Possible

When you converse with friends, go to movies, or watch television, you are exposed to many words—but not nearly so many as when you read. This can sometimes be daunting, so many new words that you don't know where to begin. But by using the context that a word is used in, it is often possible to get a general indication of a word's meaning. Someone, for example, who knew the meaning of the word *grimaced* in the sentence above but didn't know *brackish* could still be quite sure that *brackish* describes a negative quality.

Stop when you hit a new word and see if you can work out its meaning from the context, and look up words that are unclear. If you are reading a book that would require you to look up words all the time, be reasonable and patient, looking up only the words that seem crucial to the meaning of a passage or that you find interesting. Don't assign yourself impossible numbers of words to learn from your reading or you will be likely to give up your program before it really gets started. With time, you'll find yourself needing to check fewer and fewer words.

Use a Dictionary

When you read, you should have a dictionary nearby so that you can look up the meanings of words that you don't know or know only vaguely. A word that is hazy in your mind, that you recognize but couldn't really define, is probably the most important to look up, for that research may provide just the refresher you need to retain the word clearly and permanently. (Most of us have a hard time remembering the meaning of a brand new word that we've only looked up once.)

Make sure your dictionary is large enough to give full definitions, pronunciation keys, and word origins. By checking the pronunciation of a word, and saying it aloud, you put the memory of that word into different parts of your brain. And the origin of a word—*grimace,* for example, is related to the Old English word *grima,* a *mask*—can also help you understand it and retain its meaning.

Make Word Lists

Of course you can't always have a dictionary with you, but if you are in school or watching an educational program, you can have a pen and paper handy to jot down words that are new and interesting. (If you have time, it is best to write them in their context, in the phrase or sentence that the speaker has used, since English words often have several meanings.) You can look these words up later, and then you should try to use them in sentences of your own in order to make them more memorable.

A second and more important list is one that you keep in a notebook for study. After looking up a word, write it on your list with a short definition. The writing process itself helps you remember the word by putting it into still another area of your brain. Go over your list from time to time, testing yourself on your words, always saying them aloud to help retention. Then see if you can find ways to work your new words into conversations or writing.

Break Words Down into Roots and Affixes

One shortcut to vocabulary development is to learn the meanings of word roots and of the affixes that we add on to those roots. The **root** of a word (sometimes called its **stem**) is its main part, its core meaning. The root of *brackish* is *brack-,* derived from the Dutch word *brac,* which means *salty.*

An **affix** is a letter combination that we add to a root to modify its meaning—a **prefix** is added on before a root and a **suffix** after it. To the root *brack-* we add *-ish,* a suffix that means *like, somewhat,* and we get *brackish, somewhat salty.*

By learning word roots and knowing the meanings of common English affixes you can learn whole groups of words more easily. If you know, for example, that the root *fract* means *break,* then it is much easier to learn and remember words like *fracture* (*a break*), *fraction* (*portion—i.e., a breaking of the whole*), *refract* (*to break up*), and *fractious* (*unruly, irritable—i.e., breaking from propriety*).

Another reason for you to look up the etymology of a word when you check it in the dictionary is to find the word from which it is derived, often a Latin, Greek, or German word, and see if you can think of other words that are derived from that same root. Later when you hit a new word, it is likely that you will be able to spot its root and, by putting it together with its context, you can then formulate a very close approximation of its definition without even consulting a dictionary.

Below is a sample list of roots and affixes and some common words made up from them. You can also find many vocabulary study books, some listed in the bibliography at the end of this section, that have sections devoted to roots and affixes.

Prefix	Meaning	Examples (Short Definition)
ante-	before	antecedent (preceding event or word)
anti-	against	antidote (something that acts against poison)
bene-	good, well	beneficent (producing good like charitable acts)
intra-	within	intravenous (within the veins)
mal-	ill, evil	malady (illness); malevolent (wishing evil)
mis-	incorrect	misconduct (incorrect behavior)
omni-	all	omnipotent (all powerful)
sub-	under	subcutaneous (under the skin)
trans-	across	transgress (go beyond the limits; violate)

Root	Meaning	Examples (Short Definition)
aqua	water	aquatic (living in or pertaining to water)
clude, clus	shut, close	preclude (shut beforehand; prevent)
cog, cogn	know, knowledge	cognizant (knowledgeable about; aware)
duce, duct	lead	induce (lead to; bring about)
fact, fect, fict	make, do	factory (place where things are made)
graph, gram	write, record, picture	graphic (creating a strong image)
hydr, hydro	water	dehydrate (remove water from)
ject, jac	throw, cast	interject (throw in between)

Root	Meaning	Examples (Short Definition)
logue, logy	speech; science	eulogy (speech of praise); zoology (animal science)
man; manu	hand; by hand	manual (handbook)
meter	measure	thermometer (instrument to measure heat)
ped, pod	foot	podiatrist (foot doctor)
pend, pense	hang, weigh	impend (menace, as in "hanging overhead")
scribe, script	write	inscribe (write on, autograph)
sec, sect	cut	bisect (cut in half)
spire, spirat	breath, breathe	expire (die, as in "breathe your last breath")
tract	draw, drag	extract (draw out)
vene, vent	come	convene (come together)
vocat, voke	call	vocation (profession, as in your "calling")
volve, volu	roll, turn	evolve (develop, as in "roll forward")

Suffix	Meaning	Examples (Short Definition)
-able, ible	capable or worthy of	defensible (capable of being defended)
-ance, -ence	relating to, state of	despondence (state of being dejected; depression)
-ic	pertaining to	dramatic (pertaining to drama); aquatic (*see above*)
-ish	like, somewhat	mulish (like a mule); greenish (somewhat green)
-less	without	childless (without a child)
-ment	result; action	deferment (act of delaying)
-ness	condition, quality of	happiness (condition of being happy)

Becoming a Better Reader

Increase Your Reading Speed

Some people think that slower readers must be better readers, but slow reading can actually hurt your overall comprehension, especially your understanding of main ideas. It is much harder to get "the big picture" if you get stalled on every little detail along the way. Furthermore, slow readers are more likely to let their minds wander from the text. There are courses and books that teach "speed reading," but on your own you can practice a few simple techniques to make reading a quicker and more enjoyable process.

First, you must learn to **avoid regression**, which is what we do when we have to go back and reread a sentence—or a whole paragraph or more—because even though our eyes have been traveling over the words on the page, our minds have been elsewhere. By letting your mind wander when you read, you not only cut down your speed dramatically because of the need to read some things twice, you also make it harder to connect ideas, to see that "bigger picture."

Regression can be a difficult habit to break, but there are several ways to combat it. Learn, first of all, to read with a purpose. If you are just having fun with a story or if you want to stop and reread some deep idea or beautiful sentence, fine—don't worry about regressing. But if you are reading a piece of which you really must have excellent comprehension, or if you want to get the main idea of a piece in a hurry, then tell yourself before you start that you are not going to let yourself look back, that you're going to get all the main ideas the first time. As a mechanical aid you can take a postcard or a piece of paper and hold it above the line you are reading, dragging it down the page as you go so that it blocks out the text that you have just read. The more you employ that "no regression policy," practicing at first for short durations and gradually extending your commitment, the easier it will be to make your reading more efficient.

A second technique to increase your reading speed is quite simple and obvious: **practice pushing yourself.** You'll be surprised how just by trying to read faster, by telling yourself that you're going to concentrate and increase your speed for a short while, you can do it. And unless you've chosen a Shakespeare play, a tax instruction manual, or some other inappropriate text, you'll be surprised to find that you've understood the reading just as well as if you had read at your normal speed.

One of the things that makes people read more slowly is the fear of not catching every idea. Speed reading courses try to break through this anxiety by asking for only about eighty percent comprehension when they ask questions about reading passages. But if you know that you are more likely to grasp main ideas if you push yourself, and if you eliminate regression, you can read considerably faster and achieve very high comprehension levels.

Finally, **avoid vocalization.** People who vocalize when they read are sometimes called "lip readers" because they move their lips or pronounce the words to themselves even though they are not reading aloud. Your eyes can dart across a line of print much more quickly than you can say the words. Make sure that you are just taking ideas into your mind, not using your throat muscles even if your lips are still, not even hearing the words spoken in your head.

Find Main Ideas Efficiently

Whether you are reading a passage on a test or reading a newspaper article, one of your main goals is always to determine the main ideas of the writing. In newspapers main ideas are usually easy to spot since editors have distilled them into headlines, and reporters try to include most of their key points in the first few lines of their articles. But in most of your reading, it is up to you to cull out crucial ideas and controlling themes. Below are a few techniques that good readers use to find main ideas.

1. Scan Before Reading

If you decide to drive to a new vacation spot, you don't get right into your car and begin driving. First, you consult a map. And when you look at the map, you don't start tracing your path until you have located your destination and have an overall idea of the kinds of roads you are going to take and the areas you'll be passing through.

Readers who fail to get an overall impression of the reading journey that they are about to embark on face the same problems as travelers who start without consulting a map. Since they don't really know where they are going, they are probably going to encounter unwanted surprises, and they are likely to get lost and need to retrace their steps, i.e., reread whole sections to find out where they are and why they are there. To make your reading journey fast and efficient, then, you need to do some preliminary "map reading" by using a technique that is called **scanning.**

Scanning is really no more than looking over your reading material quickly before setting out to read it. For a book or long article, look at the title, at the subtitle if there is one, at the table of contents, and then very quickly thumb through it. Are there photos, illustrations, charts, maps? Has the work been divided into sections? Read a sample sentence here and there to prepare yourself for the author's style.

For a short article or for test questions, first glance over the whole piece to see how it has been divided into paragraphs. Then very quickly read the first sentence of the piece, one or two of the sentences that begin paragraphs in the middle, and the last sentence. Get a feel for the author's style and tone and develop some expectations. Does the author intend to amuse you with a personal anecdote? Instruct you about a new scientific discovery? Convince you about the importance of a historical event? Now when you read the material, you already have an idea of where you are going and the way the author is going to take you there.

2. Be Aware of Topic Sentences

When you were asked to write essays in school, it is likely that your teachers asked you to state the thesis of your essay in your first paragraph. Or maybe they called it your theme or your purpose statement. However they expressed it, they were asking you to put the main idea of your writing into the opening paragraph, more often than not as the very first line. *Most writers follow this procedure in their writing, not just stating the main idea of their whole book or article at the beginning of the work, but starting each paragraph with the main idea of that paragraph.*

Sentences that state the main ideas of paragraphs are called **topic sentences**, *and they often appear at the beginning of the paragraph.* Sometimes, though, writers organize their paragraphs by building up to the main idea with a series of details or examples. In that case the topic sentence will come at the end of the paragraph. Or, as in this very paragraph, in addition to a topic sentence at the opening of the paragraph, there may be a "clincher sentence" at the end that provides a summary of the main idea. *As a reader you should, then, pay special attention to the beginnings and endings of paragraphs.*

*Warning: there is not always a topic sentence in every paragraph—or a thesis statement in every article or book—*for the author may have found no need to state the main idea blatantly if it is already apparent in the details of the discussion. *Still, you will discover main ideas much faster if you look for and pay attention to topic sentences.*

Note: To illustrate the idea of topic sentences—and the fact that they usually but don't always appear at the beginning of a paragraph or a discussion—the topic sentences in this section have been put into italics. Notice that the second and third paragraphs stated new topics and then summarized the main ideas with "clincher sentences." And the clincher sentence at the end of the last paragraph contained the main idea of the entire discussion: Be aware of topic sentences because they will help you find main ideas more efficiently.

3. Separate Main Ideas from Supporting Material

Before you begin a reading comprehension test, you already know one of the questions that you are going to be asked after every reading selection: What is the main idea of this passage? It may not be phrased just that way. Perhaps you'll be asked for the best title for the passage, or maybe the question will start something like this: "It is the author's belief that. . ." But since every author's purpose is to impart particular ideas, then reading tests are always going to check to see if you grasped those key points.

As the prior section on topic sentences mentioned, the main idea of an essay, an article, or even a book is very often found at the beginning of the piece. Sometimes, however, writers will open with a provocative fact or incident and then, once they've caught your interest, move from the specific to the general, letting the main idea grow out of the example. It is important, then, that you always have an idea of the type of material that you are reading. Is it supporting material that is there to illustrate or prove a main idea, or is it the main idea itself?

To return to the metaphor used before of reading as a kind of journey, the main idea should be seen as your destination. The supporting ideas, explanations, and examples are the roads that you must take to get there. As you read, then, you should keep track of what road you're on—a main highway that is hurrying you to your goal by providing key ideas and crucial facts, or a byway that is offering interesting scenery but is not really essential to reaching your destination.

4. Be Aware of Tone

"You look great today!" Marcia said _____.

How did Marcia say that? Spurred on by that exclamation point, you probably filled in the blank in your mind, not even knowing that you did so, by supplying the word *enthusiastically* or *admiringly*. But Marcia may not have used one of those tones. What if the word in the blank actually was *sarcastically?* In that case she meant just the opposite of what her words said. Without that blank filled in, we can't really know what Marcia meant. That missing word defines her **tone.**

Fiction writers can indicate a speaker's tone by telling us just how a speaker communicated—sarcastically, morosely, earnestly, sadly. But all writing has a tone, even if the writer, as is usually the case, never identifies it for us. We can't communicate without, in some subtle way, indicating our underlying attitude—either our attitude about what we are saying or our attitude towards the person who is hearing or reading what we are saying. In writing, tone is the author's attitude that you "hear" when you read. Is she being ironic? Is he being sentimental? Is the material objectively stated, passionately argued, cautiously optimistic, or quite nostalgic? To understand a person fully we must hear not just what they say but how they say it.

When you try to identify an author's tone, you must be careful not to confuse your own response with the tone of the writing. A piece that you find funny—and that the author fully intends to be funny—probably does not have a humorous tone. In fact, comedians often make us laugh because of the disparity between the ridiculous things they are saying and the mock serious tone that they are using. And a story that moves you to tears may well be written in a very understated, controlled tone.

5. Be Objective

You probably can remember occasions when parents or friends haven't understood you because they were hearing what they thought you were saying rather than what you really said. Probably they had already decided what you were going to say before you ever opened your mouth and then didn't really listen to you. Readers can be just as deaf to an author's ideas if they let their prior expectations influence their reading experience.

Subjective misunderstandings are also caused by entrenched attitudes about a topic. In our desire to have our own ideas or values confirmed, we distort what a writer is actually saying. You don't have to always agree with everything you read, but you should try to understand clearly and fairly the ideas that are on the page. Although it is probably impossible to eliminate subjectivity completely, you should make it a goal to approach texts with an open mind and a desire to be objective.

Ways to Become a Better Test Taker

There are two types of questions on these tests, ones that test your **word knowledge** and ones that test your **reading comprehension.** In this section you can find explanations of these questions and techniques to help you answer them correctly.

The Word Knowledge Test

Sample Questions

Vocabulary tests are not all alike. Some ask you to find synonyms, some ask you to choose antonyms, and some ask you to complete sentences where words have been omitted, testing both reading comprehension and vocabulary at the same time. Still another approach is the one used on the NLN tests whereby you are asked to determine the meaning of words used in sentences, allowing you to see them in context.

Here are three sample questions of the type you will find on the NLN tests.

1.   The athlete was famished after her long workout.
     Famished means
     a.   exhausted.
     b.   strained.
     c.   hungry.
     d.   well known.

2.   Dr. Stone showed great animosity toward his colleagues. He treated them with
     a.   gratitude
     b.   respect.
     c.   discernment.
     d.   hatred.

3.   To say that William Shakespeare typed his plays is an
     a.   affinity.
     b.   antithesis.
     c.   anachronism.
     d.   atrophy.

Before you check your answers below, take a moment to look at the questions themselves. Notice that the three questions are essentially alike because they all provide full sentences to give you a definition or a context. But notice also that in the second sample the word in question—*animosity*—has not been underlined or singled out in any way for you. And the third question does not even provide a synonym but asks you to complete a whole thought with the appropriate word.

Analysis of the Answers
Question 1   Answer: C

In Number 1 you might—unwisely—have tried to take a shortcut by looking only at the last part of the question: "**Famished** means. . . ." And if you knew the meaning of **famished**, you probably were able to get the question right. When questions of this type get difficult, you make it much more likely that you will choose an incorrect answer if you don't give yourself the benefit of seeing the word used correctly in a sentence. Also, you should read all of the answer choices. If you jump at the first answer that sounds "about right," you may miss the right one that sounds even better—or that makes you realize that you were confusing the word with another word that is similar. By not reading the opening sentence and all the answers in this type of question you may save yourself a second or two, but those saved seconds will be totally negated if you answer the question wrong when you could have answered it correctly.

Notice that all of the answer choices could conceivably fit into the context of the sentence. You are not, for example, given an answer choice like *cold* that would be easy to pick out as wrong. But even if the sentence that you are given does not give away the answer, it can still help you determine the correct choice by stimulating your memory about the kind of situation where you might hear that word used. Even if you didn't know that *famished* means *hungry*, you might get a feeling that it's a negative sort of word, ruling out answer D, *well known*.

The "feeling" of a word—whether it has a positive or a negative aura—is its **connotation**; its regular dictionary definition is its **denotation**. The synonyms *fat* and *chubby* both mean *overweight*, but *chubby* has a more positive connotation. Often when we aren't sure of a word's denotation, we know, from having heard the word before, that it has a positive or negative connotation. On word knowledge questions you should "check your feelings" even when you aren't sure of a word's literal meaning, for they can often lead you to the right answer.

Question 2   Answer: D

In this question you could not have known what word you were trying to define without reading the first sentence. Yes, it was *animosity,* but it might also have been *colleagues*. In this type of question you must first be sure to ascertain what word or idea you are being asked to define.

This question illustrates one of the pitfalls to be avoided when you see the word in context. Like most people, you probably have positive feelings about doctors, and thus you were likely to have suspected Dr. Stone to be a fine fellow. If you didn't know the meaning of *animosity* and took a guess, you would have been likely to have chosen a positive word like *respect.* On the other hand, if you didn't know the exact meaning of animosity but knew that it was a negative word, you would have guessed right because the other three choices all have positive connotations.

Question 3   Answer: C

In this third type of question there is no synonym provided at all. The question itself provides a definition or, in this case, a situation that can be defined by one of the right words in the answers.

Notice in this question that you are given no help by the last word of the opening line *an,* a signal that the right answer will begin with a vowel, because all of the answers start with the letter *a*. You could get some help, however, if you have a knowledge of word roots. *Anachronism* has at its heart the root - *chron-*, which means *time,* and the question indicates a situation where something is out of its proper place in time, just the meaning of the word *anachronism.*

The Reading Comprehension Test and Analysis of the Answers

Like all reading tests, this test asks you to read several short passages and determine the main ideas, pick out important details, draw conclusions, and infer ideas that are implied but not specifically stated. Since there are only six questions about each passage, you will not have to do all of these things for every passage, but you can be sure that you will be asked each time for the main idea and for key details.

Below is a sample reading comprehension passage followed by an analysis of the questions and the answers.

Sample Reading Comprehension Test

Titles frequently fall into three different categories. It's your decision as the writer to choose the one that suits your purpose.

Summary titles are those that provide the most general information. By giving facts without details they lure the reader into the paper if she or he would like to know more. Newspaper headlines are frequently good examples of these kinds of titles: "Hurricane Hits Florida Coast," "Sunset Concert Series Starts Saturday," and "*Star Wars* Breaks Box Office Records."

Preview or *Give-a-Glimpse titles* aim to create reader curiosity. They introduce the subject by attempting to grab a reader's attention with a question or thought-provoking statement like "If Shakespeare Were Alive Today," "Why Won't Disco Disappear?" or "Where Will You Be in 2001?"

Teasing or *Whimsical titles* leave your reader guessing about what's to come. They usually refer to the subject indirectly and make readers curious enough to read on. These titles can be fun for both the writer and the reader, although you might want to include a subtitle under the teaser to avoid any confusion. How about something like "Good Morning, Sunshine" (subtitled "Solar Energy in Our Town") or "Boiling Water and Opening Cans" (subtitled "My Turn to Cook").

A striking title, whatever the type, can only work in your favor. Just be certain that it is not misleading. A good title should *honestly* lure the reader into the rest of the paper and not promise more than it will actually deliver. (Several newspapers and magazines are noted for sensational-type headlines. This practice of selling a product by exaggerating what's in the copy only serves to anger and alienate readers and is *not* a recommended example to follow.) Here are some things to keep in mind when you're trying to think of a good title:

1. *Consider the material.* The title should be related to the central idea or thesis of your paper.

2. *Consider the audience.* Will your readers understand a serious, technical title? Will they appreciate a humorous or clever title?

3. *Consider the words* carefully, thinking of how they sound as well as what they mean.

(Copyright © 1980 by Diane Rubins. Reprinted by permission of Scholastic Books Service, a division of Scholastic, Inc.)

1. The best title for this selection is
   a. "Three Categories of Writing"
   b. "Choosing a Good Title"
   c. "Leading and Misleading Titles"
   d. "Gaining the Reader's Attention"

Question 1

This is a question that asks you to formulate the main idea of the passage. A frequent way to pose this question is to ask for a good title for the piece, although there are several other ways that main idea questions are worded: What is the main topic of the passage? The author's primary focus is. . . What is the main idea of the selection?

The key to answering main idea questions correctly is to find the choice that is neither too broad nor too specific. Answer D is too broad because the article focuses on only one aspect of gaining the reader's attention, namely, by choosing a good title. Answer C is too narrow because, while this idea is mentioned in the fifth paragraph, it is not the main idea of the whole article. Answer A does not mention titles and is a distortion of the idea presented in the opening sentence.

Answer: B

2.   The end result of using the three types of titles mentioned in the passage is
    a.   arousing the reader's curiosity.
    b.   providing general information.
    c.   amusing the writer and reader.
    d.   selling a product.

Question 2
        This question asks you to generalize information found in the passage and to draw conclusions. Nowhere in the article is it precisely stated that one purpose of each kind of title is to arouse reader curiosity. Each of the three discussions of title types does mention this idea, however: ". . . lure the reader into the paper . . ." in the second paragraph, ". . . create reader curiosity . . ." in the third paragraph, and ". . . leave your reader guessing about what is to come . . ." in the fourth paragraph.
        Answers B and C state functions of some titles, but neither of them is true for all three kinds of titles mentioned in the passage. Be sure that your answer fits all of the requirements of the question.

        Answer: A

3.   For an article on the frustrations of losing weight, the title "Don't Be a Sore Loser" would be considered a
    a.   sensational-type title.
    b.   give-a-glimpse title.
    c.   summary title.
    d.   teasing title.

Question 3
        Sometimes questions ask you to take what is stated in a passage and apply it to a new situation. In this question you had to see that the pun in the answer "Don't Be a Sore Loser" put it into the category of teasing or whimsical titles, like the ones mentioned as examples at the end of the fourth paragraph—e.g., "Good Morning Sunshine" for an article on solar energy.
        When you are asked about situations similar to, but not exactly the same as, what is in a reading passage, you need to make sure that they fit the main idea of the piece and that they seem similar to details or examples stated in the passage.

        Answer: D

4.   Subtitles are recommended in order to
    a.   provide additional details.
    b.   amuse the reader.
    c.   provoke thought.
    d.   avoid confusion.

Question 4
        In this question you are asked to pick out a correct supporting idea based on the statements and details of the passage. In the fourth paragraph this idea points to the right answer: ". . . you might want to include a subtitle under the teaser to avoid any confusion."

Be careful about answer choices that state ideas that are mentioned in the passage but that are not the idea of that particular question. Answer B—*amuse the reader*—states a purpose of *teasing titles* but not of the *subtitles* added to these teasers. Answer A—*provide additional details*—illustrates another possible pitfall. It completes a statement that is surely true for many subtitles, but that idea, even if correct, is not the one that this author stresses. Be sure that you base your answers on what the particular passage states, not on ideas that you think are right or have learned from other sources.

Answer: D

5.   The author warns against titles that promise more than they deliver because they
a.   are dishonest.
b.   may make a reader angry.
c.   grab a reader's attention.
d.   lead to reader disappointment.

Question 5
This type of question asks you to be accurate in finding details in the passage. In the fifth paragraph the author states: "This practice of . . . exaggerating what's in the copy only serves to anger and alienate the reader."

Be careful about answer choices that are close to what is mentioned in the passage but not precisely the same. Although the fifth paragraph says that titles "should *honestly* lure the reader into the rest of the paper," it does not single out dishonesty, like answer A, as the reason for avoiding exaggeration. Also watch out for examples of ideas that are not actually stated in the passage, as in answer D—*lead to reader disappointment*. Disappointment might truly be a result of an exaggerated title, but this reaction was never stated in the passage.

Answer: B

6.   The writer's intended audience was probably
a.   newspaper reporters.
b.   business executives.
c.   student writers.
d.   magazine editors.

Question 6
This question asks you to be an observant, thorough reader and to infer ideas from the passage as a whole. The author addresses writers in the opening paragraph: "It's your decision as the writer . . . ," suggesting that her intended audience is probably not business executives or magazine editors, ruling out answers B and D. The tone and style of the writing also sound as if they were meant for students, not professional reporters, making answer C more likely than answer A. Finally, the citation at the end of the article reads in part: "Reprinted by permission of Scholastic Books Service, a division of Scholastic, Inc.," and Scholastic is a publisher mainly for students and teachers.

When you read passages on comprehension tests, don't skip over any material that tells you about the source of the article or its publication history. Often, as in this question, these explanations can give you clues about the author's tone and purpose.

Answer: C

A Final Word

When you take reading comprehension tests—or any test, for that matter—it is crucial that you maintain your focus and, especially, that you avoid panic attacks that muddle your thinking and slow you to a standstill. It doesn't hurt to be nervous before a test as long as that nervous energy gets converted into positive energy and focus once the test is underway.

The best way to avoid the kind of nervousness that destroys concentration is to practice taking the tests beforehand. If you feel positive about your skills and know what you are going to find on the day of the real test, you are much more likely to do well. Build up your confidence by doing lots of practice questions, at first without timing yourself. Work out the answers carefully. Later, if you wish, you can make your practice sessions more like the real thing by timing yourself.

On test day if you find questions that are very difficult, don't let them rattle you. Skip over them—making sure that you keep track of where you are on your answer sheet—and come back to them after you feel that you have answered several questions correctly and are working efficiently with reestablished focus.

The best test-takers are usually people who have fun taking tests. You may not be one of those lucky individuals, but with preparation, practice, and reasonable goals you can at least take tests with confidence, knowing that your score will truly reflect your ability.

I. Verbal Ability
Word Knowledge And Reading Comprehension

60 Minutes

WORD KNOWLEDGE: Read each sentence carefully. Then, *on the basis of what is stated in the sentence,* select the best completion of the incomplete statement. The correct answers will be found at the end of this section.

DIRECTIONS

The Verbal Ability Test in this book contains three tests with two sections each, Word Knowledge and Reading Comprehension. You should be able to answer all the questions in 60 minutes per test.

Each test question consists of an incomplete sentence or a question followed by four choices. Read each question carefully, then decide which choice is the best answer.

Your score will be the total number of correct answers. You may answer a question even if you are not completely sure of the correct answer. Do not spend too much time on any one question. If you cannot answer a question, go on to the next question.

If you finish the Verbal Ability test before the 60 minutes are up, go back and check your work.

1. Although the argument among the aides was noisy, it was of little importance. The argument was
   a. superior.
   b. restrained.
   c. petty.
   d. persistent.

2. The nursing student was absent for 9 days in a row. She had missed the whole instructional unit because her absences were
   a. collective.
   b. consecutive.
   c. obsolete.
   d. deleted.

3. The surgeon's instructions were very clearly stated. In other words, they were
   a. callous.
   b. detailed.
   c. explicit.
   d. legible.

4. The senator strongly supported one side of the issue. He was
   a. partisan.
   b. arrogant.
   c. impertinent.
   d. ambitious.

5. The patient was going through a long period during which the symptoms of his disease disappeared. His disease was in a state of
    a. inertia.
    b. remission.
    c. limbo.
    d. suspense.

6. An employee who pretends to be ill in order to avoid work is guilty of
    a. fantasizing.
    b. abducting.
    c. succumbing.
    d. malingering.

7. There was great ill will between the two physicians. It was hard to ignore their
    a. allocation.
    b. animosity.
    c. admonition.
    d. veneration.

8. The aide was given work regarded as low or degrading. These tasks could be considered
    a. menial.
    b. obscure.
    c. contemptible.
    d. nominal.

9. The mayor's comments were always honest and open. For this reason, reporters felt that his interviews were
    a. cynical.
    b. eloquent.
    c. candid.
    d. casual.

10. The medical and nursing staffs participated in the conference organized to discuss hospital policy. They took part in a
    a. continuum.
    b. momentum.
    c. symposium.
    d. pandemonium.

11. The animal ate both meat and plants. It was
    a. carnivorous.
    b. omnivorous.
    c. amphibious.
    d. herbivorous.

12. The story "The Turn of the Screw" can be interpreted in several ways. The story is
    a. presumptuous.
    b. bogus.
    c. expansive.
    d. ambiguous.

13. John couldn't decide between the red truck and the green one. He _____ between them.
    a. vacillated
    b. facilitated

    c. transgressed

    d. agitated

14.   A scientist who leads an ascetic life is

    a. self-denying.

    b. hygienic.

    c. sterile.

    d. indulgent.

15.   One small group agitated against the proposal to change health administrators. The group was

    a. incongruous.

    b. antiquated.

    c. nondescript.

    d. dissident.

16.   The patient's leisurely walk could be termed a

    a. lope.

    b. canter.

    c. saunter.

    d. falter.

17.   In the phrase "combine together," the word "together" is

    a. precise.

    b. concise.

    c. tentative.

    d. redundant.

18.   The comedian caused laughter because of his ridiculous conduct. His behavior was

    a. ludicrous.

    b. pretentious.

    c. obnoxious.

    d. notorious.

19.   It was difficult to get the patient's history because he did not like to talk. The patient was

    a. taciturn.

    b. immobile.

    c. devious.

    d. voluble.

20.   The nurse's aide was culpable. She deserved the

    a. praise.

    b. assignment.

    c. promotion.

    d. blame.

21.   Many of us are concerned with the mundane aspects of life. Our interest is in the

    a. unessential.

    b. material.

    c. melancholy.

    d. commonplace.

22.   During their service, the personnel were concerned only with money. They were

    a. scrupulous.

    b. mercenary.

c. disdainful.
d. contraband.

23. The library program in the hospital was praiseworthy. It was
    a. laudable.
    b. glorified.
    c. notorious.
    d. materialistic.

24. The warehouse was unsanitary because of long neglect. It was
    a. stagnant.
    b. depraved.
    c. squalid.
    d. dogged.

25. The moment she was promoted, the nurse became aloof and scornful of those who worked with her. Her manner was
    a. solicitous.
    b. supercilious.
    c. unscrupulous.
    d. vociferous.

26. You can only obfuscate the issue by using arguments that are
    a. convincing.
    b. obvious.
    c. confusing.
    d. logical.

27. The newspaper reported the lurid happenings of the day.
    Lurid means
    a. lucrative.
    b. sensational.
    c. ludicrous.
    d. significant.

28. The boy's conduct was cowardly. It was
    a. impetuous.
    b. pusillanimous.
    c. quiescent.
    d. callous.

29. The plot of the book was one that aroused sympathy and a sense of pity. The story was filled with
    a. tranquility.
    b. melodrama.
    c. pathos.
    d. suspense.

30. The agreement contained provisions that were not expressed openly but were implied. The provisions were
    a. illicit.
    b. elicit.
    c. explicit.
    d. tacit.

READING: There are five reading passages in this section. Read each passage carefully. Then, ***on the basis of what you have read in the passage***, select the best answer for each question.

I

A placebo may be nothing more than a sugar pill, but in certain situations it can relieve acute or chronic pain, promote healing of ulcers and warts and even bring on such drug side effects as drowsiness, nausea, headache and dryness in the mouth. Its power is undeniably real, yet most people still think of the placebo as something to snicker at, play medicine that helps only imaginary ills.

The placebo's widest use in modern science—as the bench mark against which new treatments are judged—aggravates this lowly image. A drug or therapy that produces no benefit beyond the "placebo effect" is deemed worthless.

Literally, "placebo" is something that pleases. The "placebo effect" describes an inexplicable improvement in a person's condition brought on by something that should not have intrinsic power to cause such an improvement. It is this nonspecificity of action that has kept the placebo from serious appreciation in modern medical practice.

Recent discoveries, however, indicate that the placebo may indeed work in a specific fashion, tapping a previously unknown reservoir of chemicals in the brain. The body produces its own pain relievers—"endorphins" or "the morphine within"—that are released spontaneously or in response to a placebo.

A 1978 study of dental patients reported in *The Lancet,* a British medical journal, helped verify this placebo-endorphin link. Researchers Jon. D. Levine, Newton C. Gordon and Howard L. Fields of the University of California at San Francisco found that patients given placebos reported reduced pain after tooth extraction. They concluded that endorphins actually provided the relief.

The same study showed that patients who responded to the placebo began to ache again when given a drug that ordinarily counters the effects of morphine, and thus endorphins.

With a possible mechanism by which placebos may aid pain relief thus demonstrated, scientists are eager to learn more about the physiology of the placebo effect. Other, still undiscovered brain chemicals or physiological reactions may account for placebo effects not related to pain.

Dr. Herbert Benson of Harvard Medical School, for example, has shown that the relaxation response brought on by certain forms of meditation or prayer, is really an innate body response. Practices such as Transcendental Meditation, the telling of rosary beads and the traditional rocking and chanting during Hebrew prayers can cause the body to relax.

The body's relaxing involves decreased respiratory rate, heart rate and blood pressure, among other changes. Dr. Benson recognized this as the physiological opposite of the so-called "fight-or-flight" response that prepares an animal for emergency action.

31.   According to the passage, a placebo
    a.   helps only imaginary ailments.
    b.   counters the effects of endorphins.
    c.   releases pain relievers.
    d.   induces pain after tooth extraction.

32.   Most people think that in the treatment of true pain, the placebo effect is
    a.   negative.
    b.   worthless.
    c.   real.
    d.   underestimated.

33.   The effect of the placebo may be similar to that of medication in calling forth
    a.   drug-like side effects.
    b.   elevated blood pressure.
    c.   physiological emergency reactions.
    d.   an inborn body response.

34.   In medical experiments, the placebo is typically used as a
    a.   control condition.
    b.   pain reliever.
    c.   specific treatment.
    d.   body stimulant.

35.   The typical lay person considers the placebo
    a.   "a fight-or-flight response."
    b.   "play medicine."
    c.   "the morphine within."
    d.   "the relaxation response."

36.   The "nonspecificity" of placebo action referred to in the passage means that
    a.   placebos have the same side effects as some drugs.
    b.   endorphins and morphine have the same effect as placebo.
    c.   placebos have an effect on both pain and relaxation.
    d.   the reason for the change in a patient's condition is not understood.

II

Proper treatment of any condition depends on a knowledge of its causes. The process of finding out the cause of a condition is called diagnosis. Most conditions have not only immediate causes but also contributing causes. A man may have a broken arm from getting hit by a motorcar; perhaps he was blind in one eye and would not have been hit by the car had he been able to see it. A person gets tuberculosis when invaded by the germ of tuberculosis if his body is such as to be unable to overcome the germ. His body may have been weakened by undernutrition and exposure to cold and damp. Moreover, his germs may have come in overwhelming numbers from a boarder who had the disease, and who lived closely crowded with the family and did not know how to dispose properly of his sputum.

One of the first steps in making a diagnosis of a disease is to get a record of the patient's life and environment related to his trouble. This the doctors call a "history." Some remote fact in the patient's past may carry the chief responsibility for his condition. If a prospective mother has German measles during the first three months of pregnancy, the child when born may be damaged in the eyes, the hearing or the heart. A difficult childbirth may be responsible for cerebral palsy in the child. A man may get ulcers in the nose from inhaling chromium substances at his work. A woman may have a swollen eye because she touched it with a finger contaminated by some substance to which she is especially sensitive. A baby may have eczema because of sensitivity to milk. An executive may have high blood pressure because he is constantly at war with his employees and the board of directors. These are contributing causes with direct manifestations in body disturbances. Sometimes, however, the causes are remote. The mind seems to play a part in affecting the part of the body that may succumb to disease.

(Excerpt from *The Handy Home Medical Advisor* by Morris Fishbein. Copyright © 1953 by Doubleday & Company, Inc. Reprinted by permission of the publisher.)

37.　The best title for this passage is
　　a.　"How to Make a Physical Diagnosis"
　　b.　"Proper Treatment of Disease"
　　c.　"Searching for Causes of Disease"
　　d.　"The Mind's Effect on Disease"

38.　Diagnosis is primarily concerned with
　　a.　discovering causes.
　　b.　planning treatment.
　　c.　identifying sensitive substances.
　　d.　describing the patient's past.

39.　The immediate cause of tuberculosis is
　　a.　sputum.
　　b.　a germ.
　　c.　exposure to cold and damp.
　　d.　overcrowding.

40.　The condition mentioned in the passage that most likely illustrates the part that the mind plays in disease is
　　a.　eczema.
　　b.　cerebral palsy.
　　c.　nose ulcers.
　　d.　high blood pressure.

41.　The conditions mentioned in the passage that are probably most closely related in cause are
　　a.　swollen eyes and eczema.
　　b.　German measles and cerebral palsy.
　　c.　nose ulcers and high blood pressure.
　　d.　damaged hearing and difficult childbirth.

42.　Of the following, the factor most likely to be considered a remote cause is
　　a.　contact with a boarder who had tuberculosis.
　　b.　feeding the baby milk to which she is sensitive.
　　c.　the role of the mind in affecting the part of the body that becomes diseased.
　　d.　a difficult childbirth resulting in cerebral palsy in the child.

III

Whatever happened to the fine old art of political insult? Maybe it's because they've been squeezed through too many TV tubes, but don't modern politicians seem a bit bland?

With no polls, PR wizards or slick video ads to rely on, candidates used to go into combat armed with razor wits and luxuriant vocabularies. Maledictions sizzled through the air like rockets. And a sharpened slur could be lethal.

For instance: the eloquent John Randolph, of Virginia, was not fond of his fellow Congressman, Henry Clay, of Kentucky. One day, brimming with bile, Randolph shot off this description of Clay: "This being, so brilliant yet so corrupt, which, like a rotten mackerel by moonlight, shines and stunk."

Slapped with a sentence like that, a man might forever smell faintly of fish. That sort of invective led one foreign observer of our political style to note that Americans were the only people he knew to pass from barbarism to decadence without experiencing civilization.

Disgusted with a campaigner who was trampling all over the facts, a reporter told fellow newsman Heywood Broun, "He's murdering the truth!" "Don't worry," Broun replied. "He'll never get close enough to do it any harm." New York attorney Roscoe Conkling, asked to campaign for Presidential candidate James G. Blaine, replied, "I do not engage in criminal practice."

It was Theodore Roosevelt who inspired one of the neatest political barbs. Teddy had just left on a much-publicized lion-hunting safari in Africa when the following notice appeared on a wall at the New York Stock Exchange: "Wall Street expects every lion to do his duty."

Politicians weren't the only ones with sharp tongues. Hecklers, too, knew the potency *of a booby-trapped sentence, as William Jennings Bryan discovered. During a political speech he unleashed his famous oratorical ability, crying, "I wish I had the wings of a bird to fly to every village and hamlet in America to tell the people about this silver question." Cried a voice from the audience, "You'd be shot for a goose before you've flown a mile."*

(Reprinted with permission from *Smithsonian Magazine*, June 1980, by Richard Wolkomir.)

---

43.   The best title for this selection is
  a.   "Political Campaigns of Yesteryear"
  b.   "The Fine Art of Political Insult"
  c.   "From Barbarism to Decadence"
  d.   "Murdering the Truth"

44.   The passage contrasts
  a.   political styles of yesterday and today.
  b.   candidates and reporters.
  c.   barbarism and decadence.
  d.   politicians and hecklers.

45. It can be inferred from the passage that "brimming with bile" refers to John Randolph's
    a. brilliance.
    b. eloquence.
    c. anger.
    d. impatience.

46. The person correctly paired with his position is
    a. Theodore Roosevelt—financier.
    b. John Randolph—congressman.
    c. Roscoe Conkling—presidential candidate.
    d. William Jennings Bryan—newsman.

47. Henry Clay was described as resembling
    a. bile.
    b. moonlight.
    c. a goose.
    d. a fish.

48. A person well known as a public speaker was
    a. Roscoe Conkling.
    b. Heywood Broun.
    c. William Jennings Bryan.
    d. Theodore Roosevelt.

IV

Man has lived in close contact with change since he first appeared on Earth. During every one of the thirty-six million minutes of his life, his own body alters imperceptibly as it moves from birth to maturity to death. Around him, the physical world too is in constant change, as the seasons pass: each day brings visible evidence of the annual cycle of growth, fertility and decay.

These fundamental changes have a rhythm with which mankind has become familiar over the ages. Each generation the population is replenished, each year nature is renewed, each day the sun rises and sets, and although the new plants and animals and children differ from their predecessors, they are recognizably of the same family. When a new species appears, or the constellations shift in the heavens, the change occurs over immeasurably long periods during which man can gradually adapt to it.

But the moment man first picked up a stone or a branch to use as a tool, he altered irrevocably the balance between him and his environment. From this point on, the way in which the world around him changed was different. It was no longer regular or predictable. New objects appeared that were not recognizable as a mutation of something that had existed before, and as each one emerged it altered the environment not for a season, but for ever. While the number of these tools remained small, their effect took a long time to spread and to cause change. But as they increased, so did their effects: the more tools, the faster the rate of change.

It is with that aspect of change that this book is concerned. Today the rate of change has reached a point where it is questionable whether the environment can sustain it. My purpose is to acquaint the reader with some of the forces that have caused change in the past, looking in particular at eight recent innovations which may be most influential in structuring our own futures and in causing a further increase in the rate of change to which we may have to adapt. These are the atomic bomb, the telephone, the computer, the production-line system of manufacturing, the aircraft, plastics, the guided rocket and television.

Each one of these is part of a family of similar devices, and is the result of a sequence of closely connected events extending from the ancient world until the present day. Each has enormous potential for man's benefit—or his destruction.

49.   This passage might best be used as
    a.   a summary.
    b.   a persuasive statement.
    c.   an introduction.
    d.   an evaluation.

50.   The "fundamental changes" referred to by the author in the second paragraph are the
    a.   small alterations continuously occurring in the life cycle.
    b.   mutations of species.
    c.   changed due to the use of tools.
    d.   eight most influential innovations.

51.   The author implies that
    a.   the greater the change, the greater the benefit to mankind.
    b.   population is increasing faster than the environment can sustain it.
    c.   man may have difficulty in adapting to rapid changes.
    d.   the atomic bomb and the guided rocket are destructive forces.

52.   Which of these topics would probably *not* be discussed by the author at some point in the book?
    a.   the effects of rapid change on the environment
    b.   the benefits of the atom bomb
    c.   the history behind the development of television
    d.   changes in the human body from birth to death

53.   The world changed in regular and predictable ways until
    a.   technology became more sophisticated.
    b.   man polluted the environment.
    c.   unrecognizable new objects began to appear.
    d.   man first started using tools.

54.   The author believes that mankind has adjusted gradually to all these changes *EXCEPT* the
    a.   telephone.
    b.   mutation of species.
    c.   shifts in the physical world.
    d.   cycle from birth to maturity to death.

V

To err is part of the human condition. Our assertive right to make errors *and be responsible for them* simply describes part of the reality of being human. However, we are susceptible to manipulation by other people for their own ends if we do not recognize that errors are simply that; just errors. We allow manipulation of our behavior and emotions if we believe that errors are somehow "wrong" and "should" not be made. Many of us feel that since errors are "wrongdoing," they must be atoned for and somehow a "right" behavior must be engaged in to make up for the error. This demand for atonement of errors which other people tack onto the tail end of our mistakes is the basis on which they manipulate our future behavior through our past mistakes. The childish belief underlying this manipulation is approximately as follows: *You must not make errors. Errors are wrong and cause problems to other people. If you make errors, you should feel guilty. You are likely to make more errors and problems and therefore you cannot cope properly or make proper decisions. Other people should control your behavior and decisions so you will not cause problems; in this way you can make up for the wrong you have done to them.* Again, as with our other childish beliefs, you can see this one expressed in our everyday behavior. As a result of this belief, husbands and wives, for instance, commonly try to control behavior in each other that is totally unrelated to their errors. This is done by implying that the mistakes of the spouse are "wrong" and therefore must somehow be atoned for (usually by doing something else the "offended" party wants done). For example, while balancing the family checkbook, a nonassertive husband may tell his wife with some emotion that she again forgot to write down the information on a check she wrote last month. Instead of coming right out assertively and saying, "I don't like it and want you to be more careful," the husband implies with his emotional tone that his wife did something "wrong" and she owes him something because of it—perhaps at that moment only some visceral squirming as a token of guilty feelings to be made up for later on!

If the wife is nonassertive enough to let her husband make judgments about her behavior for her, she is likely to (1) deny the error; (2) give reasons why she could not make the entry; (3) pooh-pooh the importance of the error, forcing her husband either to suppress his feelings about her error, thereby resenting her, or to escalate the conflict into a fight to express his nonassertive angry feelings; or (4) apologize for making an error that inconvenienced him and feel resentfully obligated to make it up to him. If, on the other hand, his wife is assertive enough to make her own judgment about her errors, she would likely reply to his raising of the issue by saying: "You're right. That was a dumb thing for me to do again and cause you all that extra work." It's a brief comment, raises no future problems, and says a lot: I did make a mistake, the mistake made trouble for you, I'm not afraid to admit it. Like everyone else, I make mistakes too.

(From *When I Say No, I Feel Guilty* by Manuel J. Smith, PhD. Copyright © 1975 by Manuel J. Smith. Used by permission of THE DIAL PRESS.)

55. The best title for this selection is:
    a. "Right and Wrong Behaviors"
    b. "You Have a Right to Make Mistakes"
    c. "Assertive and Nonassertive Husbands and Wives"
    d. "Atoning for Human Error"

56. The writer disapproves of
    a. atoning for errors.
    b. admitting one's mistakes.
    c. the right to make errors.
    d. decisions not to repeat errors.

57. The author maintains that past errors are often used to
    a. eradicate childish beliefs.
    b. teach people to be assertive.
    c. help people learn to cope properly.
    d. control the behavior of others.

58. According to the author, the wife in the example given in the passage should
    a. apologize for the error.
    b. explain why the error was made.
    c. minimize the importance of the error.
    d. admit to making the error.

59. According to the author, the husband should tell his wife that he
    a. feels that she did something wrong.
    b. is unhappy about her error.
    c. wants her to make up for her mistake.
    d. expects her to feel guilty.

60. The author believes that being human means being
    a. manipulative.
    b. assertive.
    c. imperfect.
    d. guilty.

II. Verbal Ability
Word Knowledge And Reading Comprehension

60 Minutes

WORD KNOWLEDGE: Read each sentence carefully. Then, ***on the basis of what is stated in the sentence,*** select the correct completion of the incomplete statement. The correct answers will be found at the end of section A.

1. Any extreme misfortune that brings great loss and sorrow is considered a
    a. calamity.
    b. climax.
    c. commotion.
    d. conversion.

2. A person who is inclined to do things suddenly and with little thought is
    a. impassioned.
    b. impertinent.
    c. impetuous.
    d. impressionable.

3. Someone who is always blamed for the mistakes of others is
    a. a martyr.
    b. a scapegoat.
    c. an interloper.
    d. a stereotype.

4. She showed an indomitable spirit in facing her illness.
    Indomitable means
    a. cheerful.
    b. resigned.
    c. unconquerable.
    d. unquestioning.

5. A person who has been reproved has been given
    a. a reprimand.
    b. a second chance.
    c. an award.
    d. an order.

6. A person who is *conversant* with the details of a case is
    a. at odds with them.
    b. ignorant of them.
    c. familiar with them.
    d. skeptical of them.

7. The receptionist was frequently *gauche* when dealing with clients. She was
    a. abrupt.
    b. helpful.
    c. hurried.
    d. tactless.

8. A person who is sly and cunning when dealing with others displays
    a. guile.
    b. integrity.
    c. naivete.
    d. arrogance.

9. The staff inferred from the administrator's remarks that she was satisfied with their work.
    To *infer* means to make
    a. an allusion.
    b. an error.
    c. a proposal.
    d. a deduction.

10. The businesswoman was at the *apex* of her career. Her career was
    a. at its lowest point.
    b. at its highest point.
    c. beginning.
    d. ending.

11. Scuba, a word formed from the first letters of *s*elf-*c*ontained *u*nderwater *b*reathing *a*pparatus,
    is an example of
    a. an acronym.
    b. an antonym.
    c. a synonym.
    d. a pseudonym.

12. A person who cannot believe what he is told is
    a. ecstatic.
    b. gullible.
    c. incredulous.
    d. stupefied.

13. The movements of the intruder were *furtive*. His movements were
    a. jerky.
    b. noisy.
    c. unpredictable.
    d. sneaky.

14. A person who feels helpless and powerless feels
    a. impartial.
    b. impotent.
    c. impoverished.
    d. inconsolable.

15. A person who eats and drinks sparingly is
    a. stoical.
    b. self-effacing.
    c. esthetic.
    d. abstemious.

16. There was bedlam when the team won the close game.
    Bedlam means
    a. uproar and confusion.
    b. surprise and relief.

c. disappointment and anger.
d. laughter and rejoicing.

17. Statements that contain coarse and abusive language are
    a. apathetic.
    b. sinister.
    c. scurrilous.
    d. convivial.

18. The attendant was *sedulous* in her efforts to make the patient comfortable. She was
    a. diligent.
    b. neglectful.
    c. sparing.
    d. sloppy.

19. A *florid* complexion is
    a. blemished.
    b. reddish.
    c. pallid.
    d. yellowish.

20. Rights that may not be taken away are said to be
    a. irrepressible.
    b. indelible.
    c. inevitable.
    d. inalienable.

21. The unpredictable changes that keep taking place in life are called life's
    a. vicissitudes.
    b. enticements.
    c. infractions.
    d. accolades.

22. As she considered the problems that faced her, she became pensive.
    Pensive means
    a. goal directed.
    b. pessimistic.
    c. optimistic.
    d. thoughtful.

23. The doctor challenged the veracity of the laboratory study.
    Veracity means
    a. methodology.
    b. thoroughness.
    c. truthfulness.
    d. appropriateness.

24. The indolent worker needed constant supervision.
    Indolent means
    a. awkward.
    b. lazy.
    c. inexperienced.
    d. incompetent.

25. The nursing organization held its *biennial* meeting. It met
    a. once every 2 years.
    b. twice in 2 years.
    c. twice a year.
    d. once every 2 months.

26. This week's paycheck contained an *increment.* It contained
    a. a deduction.
    b. an error.
    c. a larger amount.
    d. a penalty.

27. When denied his request, the worker became surly.
    Surly means
    a. bitter.
    b. disappointed.
    c. violent.
    d. bad tempered.

28. The *nomenclature* of a profession's field of study is its
    a. specific procedures.
    b. set of words and phrases.
    c. rules and regulations.
    d. code of ethics.

29. The wound began to form and discharge pus. The wound had
    a. eructated.
    b. nictitated.
    c. triturated.
    d. suppurated.

30. A substance that causes sweating is
    a. perspicacious.
    b. sudorific.
    c. pernicious.
    d. ubiquitous.

READING: There are five reading passages in this section. Read each passage carefully. Then, *on the basis of what you have read in the passage,* select the best answer for each question.

I

It has been estimated that 15 to 25 percent of the population in the United States is above desirable body weight because of overeating. Overeating has been observed to relieve anxiety while those who are at average or below average weight tend to eat simply to satisfy hunger. Also, obese as well as underweight persons tend to eat more in the presence of boredom. In such instances, eating gives people something to do. While endocrine and genetic factors may often play a role, psychosocial factors certainly are important in determining one's weight also.

A great variety of diets to lose or gain weight are described in the layperson's literature. Many are eccentric and nutritionally unsound, especially those for persons who wish to lose weight. Weight loss after crash dieting is very often temporary since the person usually returns to the same eating habits that brought obesity in the first place. There are no reducing or weight-gaining foods but only different caloric content in various foods. For many people, the problem of obesity or thinness might well be mostly a problem of arithmetic and lack of knowledge concerning the body's caloric needs. This can be validated with relative ease by totaling the number of calories consumed each day by the obese person who states that he eats little but "it all goes to fat," or the thin person who states that he eats "well but cannot gain weight."

Obesity is no simple matter for overweight persons. It has been demonstrated rather conclusively that obesity plays an important part in premature death. In addition, it may be undesirable from the point of view of comfort and appearance.

The nurse counseling the obese person must begin by demonstrating acceptance of the individual and by recognizing that excess caloric intake can rarely be controlled without consideration of psychological as well as physical factors that contribute to the condition. The most efficient way to control obesity is through dietary discretion, exercise, and the change of eating habits. The diet should be well-balanced but limited in the amount of calories eaten. It is recommended that no person wishing to lose weight consume fewer than 1,200 calories daily without professional supervision. For many people, the will power to follow a reducing diet appears to be strengthened when people work together toward weight loss in groups.

(Passage taken from Wolff, LuVerne, Wertzel, Marlene H., and Fuerst, Elinor V. *Fundamentals of Nursing.* Philadelphia: J.B. Lippincott, 1979. Reprinted with permission.)

31.   Which of these topics is the main focus of this passage?
   a.   techniques of weight reduction
   b.   hazards of obesity
   c.   methods of regulating caloric intake
   d.   factors that influence body weight

32.   Approximately what fraction of the American population is overweight because of eating too much?
   a.   ⅕
   b.   ⅓
   c.   ⅖
   d.   ½

33.   According to this passage, which of these factors does *NOT* contribute to obesity?
   a.   lack of interesting activities
   b.   hidden hunger for vitamins
   c.   a person's hereditary makeup
   d.   lack of knowledge about calories

34.   Which of the following is identified in the passage as a disadvantage of crash diets for losing weight?
   a.   The weight loss from these diets is not maintained.
   b.   These diets require extensive arithmetical calculations.
   c.   The weight loss from these diets is frequently too drastic.
   d.   These diets require special reducing foods.

35. When a person wants to lose extra pounds, he must
    a. undergo a series of endocrine system lab tests.
    b. have professional counseling and guidance on weight reduction.
    c. learn which foods are nourishing and low in calories.
    d. join a group interested in weight reduction.

36. One might infer from this passage that
    a. Americans have become obsessed about obesity.
    b. the control of body weight is complex.
    c. Americans are more obese than people in other countries.
    d. the best foods are low in calories.

II

The Canadian Cooperative Study reported striking results concerning the use of aspirin to prevent strokes in those at risk (*New England Journal of Medicine,* July 13, 1978). In order to appreciate the recommendations resulting from their report, it is useful to review briefly the events that lead to strokes and "transient ischemic attacks":

(1) *Strokes* refer to instances of brain damage caused by decreased blood flow to the brain. Decreased blood flow can have many causes—including circulatory problems such as failure of the heart to pump blood adequately, or a sudden drop in blood pressure due to hemorrhage, reaction to a drug, etc. However, most strokes are caused by local disturbances in the blood vessels leading to or situated within the brain. The two major types of blood vessel problems are: 1) leaking or breaking of those vessels damaged by high blood pressure and "hardening of the arteries" and 2) obstruction by clots or arteriosclerotic material that have formed locally or traveled after being dislodged elsewhere (emboli).

(2) About ten per cent of strokes are preceded by "warning" events, usually described as *transient ischemic attacks* (TIA's)—meaning temporary symptoms caused by poor blood flow (ischemia) to the brain. (Another phrase—threatened stroke—was used by the authors of the Canadian study to describe these warning events, some of which resulted in less serious but permanent symptoms.) And while only a minority of those who eventually experience a full-blown stroke have such warning events, they are important because those who have them are at considerably increased risk (as much as four-to tenfold) for a stroke, compared to persons without TIA's.

The Canadian study involved the use of aspirin (four regular tablets per day—a total of 1200 mg.) *in persons who had experienced a "threatened stroke."* In other words, the effect of aspirin in persons who had not experienced warning symptoms was not studied. (It is also important to point out that persons with ulcers were excluded from the study and that coated aspirin was not tried.) Five hundred eighty-three persons who had experienced at least one threatened stroke during the previous three months were given either a placebo, aspirin, sulfinpyrazone (another anti-platelet drug), or sulfinpyrazone and aspirin together. No reduced risk for subsequent stroke could be attributed to sulfinpyrazone, but *males taking four aspirin per day—during an average follow-up period of 26 months—demonstrated a reduced risk for stroke or death of 48% as compared to males not receiving aspirin. There was no substantial benefit for females.*

(Excerpted from the October, 1978 issue of *The Harvard Medical School Health Letter.* © 1978, President & Fellows of Harvard College. Used with permission.)

37.   The major topic of this passage is
      a.   aspirin and stroke prevention.
      b.   reduced risk of stroke.
      c.   transient ischemic attacks.
      d.   "warning" events.

38.   Strokes result in
      a.   failure of the heart to pump blood adequately.
      b.   sudden drop in blood pressure throughout the body.
      c.   damage to the brain.
      d.   a hardening of arteries throughout the body.

39.   Most strokes are caused by
      a.   transient ischemic attacks.
      b.   circulatory problems throughout the body.
      c.   interruptions in the brain's circulation.
      d.   sudden drops in blood pressure.

40.   How many different treatment groups were involved in the study?
      a.   four
      b.   three
      c.   two
      d.   one

41.   Which of these groups were *NOT* included in the Canadian study?
      a.   women
      b.   persons having a high risk of strokes
      c.   persons who had experienced warning symptoms
      d.   over 90% of the population who might suffer strokes

42.   Which of the following statements is a conclusion reached by the study?
      a.   Anti-platelet drugs help reduce the risk of stroke.
      b.   Aspirin helps men who have had threatened strokes.
      c.   Men can reduce their risk of stroke by taking sulfinpyrazone.
      d.   Aspirin alone was less effective than in combination with sulfinpyrazone.

III

Although comparing an individual child with the norms for his age group is a useful screening technique, those averages must not be accepted as absolute standards, and variations from the norms must not be considered defective ipso facto. An awareness of the process by which norms are derived is helpful in preventing their misuse.

The quality of interest—say, height at age 4—is measured on a large number of 4-year-olds. Statistical computations are then performed to find the height that is most representative of the group. The statistic most frequently used is the median (also called the 50th percentile), which is the midpoint of the group; 50 percent of the children are taller than that height, and 50 percent are shorter. The median height of any group of typical 4-year-olds in the United States is around 103 cm (40 in). The median of 103 cm does not mean that *any* of the children in the group were actually 103 cm tall, only that half the children were taller than that and half were shorter. More important, the median does not in any way indicate that a 4-year-old *must* be 103 cm tall, that it is more advantageous to be 103 cm than another height, or that a 4-year-old who *is* 103 cm tall is in good health.

Normative charts or tables are more useful if they also show how much the members of the group varied from the average. A height table for 4-year-olds, for example, might include the information that only 10 percent of the children measured less than 99 cm (39 in) and only 10 percent were taller than 109 cm (43 in). The fact that 80 percent of the group were somewhat between 99 and 109 cm tells more about that group of children than the median value alone. The nurse or other person referring to the norms can now ascertain whether a particular child is like or different from an 80 percent majority of the reference group. However, it is not possible to say on the basis of how well the child conforms to the norms whether that child is well and growing properly.

Every child has his own unique qualities and consequently is likely to differ in several ways from the norms. Even newborns differ from one another and from a hypothetical "average" baby in length and weight, degree of physiologic stability, assertiveness, feeding behavior, and so forth. Especially as children grow older and varieties in their experience increase, they reflect their individual enrichments or deprivations in addition to their unique inborn traits, and considerable difference is to be expected from child to child.

(Reprinted from Scipien, Gladys M., et al. *Comprehensive Pediatric Nursing.* New York: McGraw Hill, 1979.)

43.   This passage contains information about how to
      a.   predict norms for growing children.
      b.   determine how well children are developing.
      c.   identify children who are not healthy.
      d.   obtain and use norms.

44.   Median is defined as
      a.   the average of all heights in the group.
      b.   that point that divides the group into two equal halves.
      c.   the range that identifies the middle 50% of the group.
      d.   the height occurring most frequently among the group of children.

45.   Understanding the process of deriving norms can help to
      a.   identify the correct height for healthy children.
      b.   define the height that is best for children of different ages.
      c.   promote the correct use of norms for height.
      d.   identify the qualities that should be measured in children

46.   According to the passage, a 110-cm (43-in) tall 4-year-old child is taller than what percentage of 4-year-old children?
      a.   10%
      b.   50%
      c.   80%
      d.   90%

47.   The term "individual enrichments" in the last paragraph most likely refers to
      a.   experiences that help a child grow and develop.
      b.   genetically determined differences between children.
      c.   the child's special capabilities.
      d.   unique physiologic characteristics.

48.   The term "hypothetical" in the fourth paragraph refers to a baby who
      a. has been selected because he or she conforms to all the norms.
      b. has a moderately enriched environment.
      c. has unique inborn traits.
      d. doesn't really exist but represents the typical baby in many ways.

IV

Emotional problems and conflicts, especially depression and anxiety, are by far the most common causes of prolonged fatigue. Fatigue may represent a defense mechanism that prevents you from having to face the true cause of your depression, such as the fact that you hate your job. It is also your body's safety valve for expressing repressed emotional conflicts, such as feeling trapped in an ungratifying role or an unhappy marriage.

When such feelings are not expressed openly, they often come out as physical symptoms, with fatigue as one of the most common manifestations. "Many people who are extremely fatigued don't even know they're depressed," Dr. Bulette says. "They're so busy distracting themselves or just worrying about being tired that they don't recognize their depression."

One of these situations is so common it's been given a name—tired housewife syndrome. The victims are commonly young mothers who day in and day out face the predictable tedium of caring for a home and small children, fixing meals, dealing with repairmen, and generally having no one interesting to talk to and nothing enjoyable to look forward to at the end of their boring and unrewarding day. The tired housewife may be inwardly resentful, envious of her husband's job, and guilty about her feelings. But rather than face them head on, she becomes extremely fatigued.

Today, with nearly half the mothers of young children working outside the home, the tired housewife syndrome has taken on a new twist—that of conflicting roles and responsibilities and guilt over leaving the children, often with an overlay of genuine physical exhaustion from trying to be all things to all people.

Compounding emotionally induced fatigue may be the problem of sleep disturbance that results from the underlying psychological conflict. A person may develop insomnia, or may sleep the requisite number of hours but fitfully, tossing and turning all night, having disturbing dreams and awakening . . . feeling as if she had "been run over by a truck."

Understanding the underlying emotional problem is the crucial first step toward curing psychological fatigue, and by itself often results in considerable lessening of the tiredness. Professional psychological help or career or marriage counseling may be needed. But there is also a great deal you can do on your own to deal with both severe prolonged fatigue and periodic "washed-out" feelings.

Vitamins and tranquilizers are almost never the right answer, sleeping pills and alcohol are counterproductive, and caffeine is at best a temporary solution that can backfire with abuse and cause life-disrupting symptoms of anxiety.

49.   Which of these topics is the *primary* focus of this passage?
      a.   combatting "washed-out" feelings
      b.   the emotional basis for fatigue
      c.   sleep disturbance as a cause of fatigue
      d.   variations of the tired housewife syndrome

50.   The writer implies that fatigue frequently results when people
      a.   are not understood.
      b.   attempt to do too much.
      c.   fail to face their true feelings.
      d.   seek temporary solutions.

51.   According to the writer, one of the actions that a person should take to combat fatigue is to
      a.   seek counseling.
      b.   drink coffee.
      c.   keep busy.
      d.   obtain adequate medication.

52.   Which of these factors adds to the tired housewife syndrome often felt by today's young mothers?
      a.   a successful husband
      b.   an unhappy marriage
      c.   role conflict
      d.   daily routine

53.   According to the passage, people suffering from fatigue
      a.   have no defense mechanisms.
      b.   fail to use the body's safety valve.
      c.   require an unusual amount of sleep.
      d.   often do not know its cause.

54.   According to the passage, both fatigue and sleep disturbances
      a.   cause psychological conflict.
      b.   may have the same cause.
      c.   are helped by sleeping pills.
      d.   result in disturbing dreams.

V

Transactions within groups satisfy a person's need for establishing and maintaining his interdependency within the social, cultural and economic environments. As we have advanced in our technological development so too have our interdependent needs expanded within these environs. History reveals, with each era, shifts in the priorities of needs that affect interpersonal relationships—to man, with one or several others and with our environment. The twentieth century is an era of complex interdependent relationships. This complexity is manifested through the types of group relationships that individuals form.

Group relationships are divided into three major categories—primary, secondary and tertiary. The rationale for this categorization is based on the individual's need to set priorities in his search for fulfillment.

A *primary* group can be defined as a unit composed of close-knit, mutually interdependent and reciprocal memberships. In other words, the primary group is any small group to which an individual belongs because of a vested interest, specialized activity or fulfillment of need gratification. Familial, peer or religious groups are examples of primary groups. It is in conjunction with the primary group that the individual establishes the norms and mores for his particular position in life. It is through his continuous involvement with this type of group relationship that the individual finds validation for his ideas, thoughts, actions and feelings. This type of group relationship provides the members with group security and a means of identity, establishes role expectations and functionings and contributes a sense of belonging and acceptance.

Secondary groups are those formed for the purpose of enrichment and refinement of the individual's total living experience. The kinds of interdependent relationships formed within this category manifest a moderate degree of intimacy. The individual retains freedom to move in and out of secondary groups as his priorities change. This freedom of movement is unique to secondary groups and is another characteristic that distinguishes it from the primary group. A work group, a social club, an art class, or a professional organization exemplifies this secondary group category. Secondary group memberships are formed because they serve as a necessary and significant vehicle for the individual to meet his social, cultural and financial needs.

Tertiary groups are those in which there exists between members a limited degree of intimacy and involvement. Membership is based on the necessity for gratifying immediate needs. The relationships formed within the group are not designed to be continuous. They are based on priorities which, most likely but not exclusively, have been established by the individual within his primary or secondary groups. Participating in a fund raising campaign, becoming a member of a committee, joining a vacation tour group or taking part in a community action group is identified as a tertiary type of interpersonal group relationship.

(Kreigh & Perko, *Psychiatric and Mental Health Nursing: Commitment to Care and Concern*, 1979, pgs. 58-59. Reprinted with permission of Reston Publishing Co., a Prentice-Hall Co., 11480 Sunset Hills Road, Reston, Va. 22090.)

55.   The major subject of this passage is
   a.   the rules governing social behavior in three types of groups.
   b.   the differences between group relationships of the present and those of earlier times.
   c.   the distinctive characteristics of different types of groups.
   d.   the changes made by technological advances on the nature of group participation.

56.   The three kinds of groups discussed in this passage differ from each other primarily by
   a.   the emotional closeness of the members of the group.
   b.   the success with which the members' needs are met by the group.
   c.   the variety of activities carried out by the group.
   d.   the status that the community gives to the group.

57.   Which of these statements describes a characteristic of any interdependent relationship?
   a.   Participants in the relationship have equal status.
   b.   Participants in the relationship satisfy each other's needs.
   c.   The relationship is essential to the participants' well-being.
   d.   The relationship is based on priorities established in adulthood.

58.   The term "validation," as it is used in the third paragraph, can best be defined as
   a.   a sense of individuality.
   b.   an acceptable explanation.

    c. consistent satisfaction.

    d. sound support.

59.   One might infer from this passage that
    a. primary groups have the greatest influence on an individual's personality development.
    b. people are attracted to a particular category of group according to their personalities.
    c. group relationships fulfill only those needs that cannot be fulfilled by one-to-one relationships.
    d. tertiary groups are characterized by a similarity in the members' educational backgrounds.

60.   This passage implies that the purpose of studying groups is to help a person
    a. participate more effectively in groups.
    b. understand human behavior.
    c. select those groups that are most suited to his needs.
    d. understand the quest for self-identity.

III. Verbal Ability
Word Knowledge and Reading Comprehension

60 Minutes

WORD KNOWLEDGE: Read each sentence carefully. Then, ***on the basis of what is stated in the sentence,*** select the correct completion of the incomplete statement. The correct answers will be found at the end of section A.

1. The ancient Romans looked to several deities for support.
    Deities means
    a. gods.
    b. plants.
    c. neighbors.
    d. groups.

2. When the child fell from the bicycle, she received several cuts and abrasions.
    Abrasions means
    a. scrapes.
    b. bruises.
    c. wounds.
    d. marks.

3. The planets and the stars are celestial bodies.
    Celestial means
    a. gaseous.
    b. heavenly.
    c. distant.
    d. gigantic.

4. The essence of the argument is that the leader disapproves of the group's activities.
    Essence means
    a. cause.
    b. end.
    c. nature.
    d. direction.

5. Even at a young age, the teenager manages a successful child care business; that teenager is a real
    a. entrepreneur.
    b. altruist.
    c. bigot.
    d. charlatan.

6. The leader treated her cabinet members more as adversaries than supporters.
    Adversaries means
    a. opponents.
    b. partners.
    c. servants.
    d. consultants.

7. A society that is based on farm production is described as
   a. agrarian.
   b. cooperative.
   c. familial.
   d. utilitarian.

8. After having surgery, I stayed with my family. This period of recovery was known as my
   a. convalescence.
   b. intervention.
   c. restoration.
   d. adjustment.

9. East Indian society was divided into distinct social classes known as
   a. peers.
   b. castes.
   c. aristocracies.
   d. degrees.

10. The buyers were unable to close the deal on the property because of the presence of a
    a. designation.
    b. tenant.
    c. lien.
    d. misdemeanor.

11. Most people feel that in a political race the advantage is held by the one already in office. This person is the
    a. resident.
    b. opponent.
    c. candidate.
    d. incumbent.

12. As soon as the ship touched the mine, the mine
    a. dissipated.
    b. deteriorated.
    c. digressed.
    d. detonated.

13. After several additions were made to the building, its corridors formed a labyrinth. *Labyrinth* means
    a. tunnel.
    b. rectangle.
    c. maze.
    d. pattern.

14. The farmer did not plant one of his fields this year; he left it
    a. fallow.
    b. organic.
    c. rejuvenated.
    d. passive.

15. The animals never stopped caterwauling. *Caterwauling* means
    a. running.
    b. rooting.

   c. howling.
   d. fighting.

16. The state representative recommended building a residence for indigent people. ***Indigent*** means
   a. impoverished.
   b. elderly.
   c. handicapped.
   d. illiterate.

17. When asked about his domicile, Peter claimed that he did not have one. ***Domicile*** means
   a. opinion.
   b. spouse.
   c. income.
   d. residence.

18. A chart that shows how a company is organized shows its
   a. posture.
   b. policy.
   c. finances.
   d. hierarchy.

19. The father apologized for his son's inexplicable behavior. ***Inexplicable*** means
   a. unalterable.
   b. undependable.
   c. uninterpretable.
   d. unsurpassable.

20. The speaker's remarks made light of a serious topic. The remarks were
   a. sarcastic.
   b. flippant.
   c. intellectual.
   d. optimistic.

21. The president of the company was so aggravated that he was almost impossible to placate. ***Placate*** means
   a. convince.
   b. inform.
   c. appease.
   d. console.

22. The students practicing in the music building produce a cacophonous sound. ***Cacophonous*** means
   a. melodic.
   b. harsh.
   c. harmonious.
   d. rhythmic.

23. Susan's vitriolic comments were meant to hurt her opponent. ***Vitriolic*** means
   a. improbable.
   b. adamant.

c. chaste.

d. caustic.

24. The movement failed to progress even though the zealots pushed with all their might. **Zealots** means
    a. practitioners.
    b. fanatics.
    c. characters.
    d. rebels.

25. Many early Americans commissioned stock portraits by itinerant painters. **Itinerant** means
    a. skilled.
    b. migrant.
    c. numerous.
    d. foreign.

26. The hypothesis must be tested
    a. figuratively.
    b. empirically.
    c. rhetorically.
    d. deciduously.

27. Paul refuses to soften his position; he's being very
    a. flaccid.
    b. pernicious.
    c. intemperate.
    d. obdurate.

28. James is so idealistic and impractical that he could be described as
    a. neurotic.
    b. quixotic.
    c. impertinent.
    d. solicitous.

29. The sorcerer is a practitioner of
    a. astrology.
    b. masochism.
    c. necromancy.
    d. philology.

30. The child refused again and again to listen to her parents; she was being
    a. oblivious.
    b. obsequious.
    c. obstreperous.
    d. obsolescent.

READING: There are five reading passages in this section. Read each passage carefully. Then, *on the basis of what you have read in the passage,* select the best answer for each question.

I

Of all its many survival techniques, the one most responsible for keeping the possum on the scene for so long is almost certainly its prodigious birthrate. Breeding takes place twice a year, and each litter may include as many as 20 offspring. The young are born anytime from December to February in the South, later in other sections, with the second litter arriving in late spring or early summer.

The possum's gestation period—just 13 days—is the shortest among mammals. Thus its young are born smaller than honey bees, looking more like embryos than tiny replicas of the mother, with no eyes or ears and only fleshy buds for hind legs and clawed stubs for front legs. After the mother has licked the fetal fluid from them, the newborn must, unaided, crawl through a forest of coarse hair to get to her warm, furry pouch and to life. The pouch usually has 13 teats, and only the first 13 to reach them survive.

At ten weeks the young are able to leave the pouch and the mother, but they almost always scamper up on her back when she leaves the den. One of the weirdest sights in nature is a female possum with 13 offspring atop her back. This backpacking continues until the young are rat-size, at about 14 weeks, and weaned.

From this point, the young are on their own. Although the possum is phenomenally long-lived as a species, individuals have a relatively short life-span, probably topping at five years, with most not making it much beyond two.

One thing is certain: This living fossil is as much a survival wonder as those architectural relics that mankind holds in such awe—the Acropolis in Greece, the Colosseum in Italy, Egypt's pyramids.

The possum also is older. And in much better shape.

(Excerpt from "Possums Play for Keeps" by Jack Denton Scott, *Reader's Digest,* September 1979. Condensation of an article published in *Outdoor Life,* May 1979.)

31.   The main topic of this passage is
    a.   the food supply of possums.
    b.   how possums carry their young.
    c.   the social behavior of possums.
    d.   how possums continue to live on.

32.   The hind legs of a baby possum can best be described as
    a.   short and fat.
    b.   soft and sprout-like.
    c.   thin and clawed.
    d.   small and furry.

33.   According to the passage, which of these facts about possums makes them unique among mammals?
    a.   They have incomplete organs of sight and hearing at birth.
    b.   The newborns grow in their mother's pouch.
    c.   The length of their pregnancy is 13 days.
    d.   The mortality rate of newborns is high.

34. The reason that possums have survived so long as a species is that
    a. they have a very high birthrate.
    b. they have a short gestation period.
    c. they live for many years.
    d. they are very active in infancy.

35. The author makes the analogy between possums and
    a. tiny insects.
    b. foreign countries.
    c. aging individuals.
    d. ancient buildings.

36. Which of the following inferences can be drawn from this passage?
    a. As a species, the possum has been around for thousands of years.
    b. At ten weeks of age, possums can survive without their mothers.
    c. Possums are found in only a few geographic areas of the world.
    d. Few young possums live to reach adulthood.

II

Erosion of America's farmland by wind and water has been a problem since settlers first broke the virgin prairies in the 19th century. But it wasn't until after the Dust Bowl days of the 1930s when wind and water savaged 282 million acres of American farmland, that erosion forced itself into the national consciousness.

In 1935, a shocked nation enacted new laws to protect the soil, as President Franklin D. Roosevelt created the U.S. Soil Conservation Service. Government agents instructed farmers in how to hold on to their soil, and billions of dollars were eventually spent building terraces, planting trees as windbreaks, trying new methods of strip-cropping, plowing and crop rotation.

The experiment worked. Erosion slowed down, and ravaged farmlands became lush and productive once more. Soon government began paying farmers to keep land idle as a way of preventing surpluses.

But by the early 1970s, with a huge new market for grain in Russia and a growing world demand, the United States stopped these subsidies.

To boost harvest volumes and meet escalating production costs, land never before touched by the plow—much of it previously thought too fragile or not fertile enough— was hastily planted or dug out to accommodate giant irrigation systems. The old terraces and tree rows, in the way of gigantic modern farm machinery, were ripped out and the land seeded. As a result, after 40 years of conservation efforts, soil erosion is *worse* today than in Dust Bowl days.

Although few dust storms are now sweeping across the Plains states, some experts see signs of their return. In 1980, 5.1 million acres of Great Plains land were damaged by routine wind erosion, almost double that of the previous year.

Nationally, water erosion is taking an even greater toll. Because marginal, hilly land has been planted, and because farmers no longer alternate grain crops with soil-conserving grasses, rain and melting snow annually strip billions of tons of soil from the land.

(Excerpt from "Where Has All Our Soil Gone?" by James Risser, in *Reader's Digest,* July, 1981, a condensation of an article published in *Smithsonian Magazine,* March, 1981. Copyright by James Risser.)

37. Which of the following titles is best for this passage?
     a. "The Problem of Soil Erosion"
     b. "The Dust Bowl"
     c. "America's Farmlands"
     d. "The U.S. Soil Conservation Service"

38. To prevent soil erosion, farmers should
     a. seed new land.
     b. plant hilly land.
     c. rotate crops.
     d. rip out terraces.

39. One of the causes of soil erosion is
     a. windbreaks.
     b. use of marginal land.
     c. farm subsidies.
     d. strip-cropping.

40. The word "subsidies," as used in the fourth paragraph, refers to
     a. payments to farmers for not planting crops.
     b. instructions to farmers in modern agricultural methods.
     c. demonstration of soil conservation by government agencies.
     d. investments in model farms by government agencies.

41. It can be concluded from the passage that soil erosion
     a. is unavoidable.
     b. is on the decline.
     c. could be slowed.
     d. has developed only in recent years.

42. The passage implies that
     a. subsidies will be resumed.
     b. conservation will be accelerated.
     c. not enough grain will be produced.
     d. erosion by water will increase.

III

Sunless, devoid of plants, cool and silent as the surrounding stone, a cave seems the very antithesis of life, a rockbound realm suitable only for the creatures that dwell in the human imagination. The idea of a cave as a habitat or ecosystem, as the home of a community of animals, seems a violation of what we think of as a law of nature. No light means essentially no vegetation, and no vegetation means an absence of the primary nourishment that rests at the base of the food web in any ecosystem. The uncompromising blackness of the cave's eternal night also means that the struggle for survival underground is a battle of the blind; eyesight, and thus the whole range of visual signals and clues that guide surface-dwelling species to their sustenance, is useless here.

Yet the astonishing fact is that many caverns bustle with life. Almost everyone who has ventured beyond a cave entrance knows that bats are often in residence. The most visible cave-dwelling animals, bats are part-time occupants who use caves as bedrooms where they rest between nocturnal hunting forays or while hibernating in the winter. Bears, too, once commonly spent the winter in caves, and European scientists have found so many fossil remains of one large and now-extinct species in underground refuges that they named it *Ursus spelaeus,* the cave bear. Two kinds of tropical birds, one a Western Hemisphere native and the other from Asia, nest in caves and possess remarkable equipment for navigating in the dark similar to that of bats. But few people know that literally thousands of other species of fish, salamanders, beetles, spiders, millipedes, snails, worms, shrimps and others have successfully adapted to the sunless and food-scarce conditions.

Underground creatures confront a uniquely demanding set of circumstances. Because no food is produced in the cave itself (with the exception of certain bacteria which derive energy from cave minerals), the stuff of life must come from outside. The principal sources are streams and flood waters which wash organic material such as mud, leaves and aquatic micro-organisms into the cave, and the guano, or wastes, deposited by part-time cave residents such as bats, birds and crickets. With this material at the base, the food web spreads out to include bacteria, fungi, worms, beetles, crickets and spiders, on up to crayfish and the fish and colorless salamanders at the top.

(From *Smithsonian Magazine,* November, 1982, by Donald Dale Jackson. Reprinted with permission of author.)

43. Which of the following titles is best for this passage?
    a. "Bats and Bears"
    b. "Cave Minerals"
    c. "Life in Surprising Places"
    d. "The Effect of Sunlight"

44. According to the passage, one of the principle sources of food in an ecosystem is
    a. guano.
    b. water.
    c. protein.
    d. plant life.

45. *Ursus spelaeus* got its name because the scientists, who were exploring the caves, found its
    a. nests.
    b. fossils.
    c. prints.
    d. cubs.

46. All of the following are mentioned as having been found in the caves *EXCEPT*
    a. bears.
    b. insects.
    c. caterpillars.
    d. shellfish.

47. It can be inferred that the environment in the cave has an effect on some animals'
    a. life span.
    b. mating habits.
    c. energy levels.
    d. feeding practices.

48.   It can be inferred from the passage that most of the animals in caves cannot
    a. swim.
    b. run.
    c. see.
    d. hear.

IV

Psychologists who write about laughter usually make the subject about as cheery as patricide, with ponderous treatises on "covariation of variables in the humor stimulus." In short order humor lies on the dissecting table like a dead frog, its innards "discouraging to any but the pure scientific mind," as E.B. White put it. Now a few scientists are leaving the nature of humor well enough alone and are asking instead what happens when people laugh. They have already shown that laughter is good medicine, primarily for relieving stress; they also suspect that it can cure headaches, fight infections and alleviate hypertension.

Medieval physicians told their patients jokes, but mirth was not widely welcome in the modern examining room until editor Norman Cousins wrote in 1976 that he had laughed his way to recovery from a degenerative spinal condition. While many doctors disparaged Cousins's claim, pointing out that the disease sometimes goes into spontaneous remission, others began taking a serious look at the biology of laughter. Dozens of scientists presented papers at a symposium on humor last month in Washington, and a two-volume "Handbook of Humor Research" is due next year. Most of the research is heavy on theory and light on data, but there are some encouraging anecdotes. Patients at a gerontology center at the University of Southern California, for instance, became more sociable and more active when volunteers reawakened their sense of humor.

A hearty laugh produces well-documented physical effects, many of them akin to moderate exercise. Muscles in the abdomen, chest, shoulders and elsewhere contract; heart rate and blood pressure increase. In a paroxysm of laughter, the pulse can double from 60 to 120, and systolic blood pressure can shoot from a norm of 120 to a very excited 200. Dr. William Fry of Stanford University describes laughter as a kind of "stationary jogging." Like other exercise, it may produce lasting benefits. Once the laughing stops, muscles are more relaxed than before it started, which could relieve some kinds of headaches. Heartbeat and blood pressure also dip below normal, a sign of reduced stress. "It is not too far-fetched" wrote psychologist Jeffrey Goldstein of Temple University in The Sciences, that "laughter is related in several ways to longevity"—mainly through the reduction of stress and hypertension.

The chemical effects of laughter are more elusive, mainly because people hooked to intravenous tubes that monitor chemicals in the blood have trouble laughing on command. Nevertheless, Fry reports that adrenaline in the blood increases, and other researchers suspect that similar chemicals flood the brain. Jogging increases the brain's supply of beta-endorphins, natural opiates that probably account for the "runner's high." Although there is no similar evidence for the effects of laughter, Goldstein believes that a rush of endorphins may make people feel better after laughing.

49. Which of the following titles is best for this passage?
    a. "The Evolution of Laughter"
    b. "Laughter Ensures Longevity"
    c. "The Analysis of Laughter"
    d. "Laughter Is Good Medicine"

50. According to this passage, scientists have shown that laughter
    a. lessens stress.
    b. heals infections.
    c. produces hypertension.
    d. prevents headaches.

51. All of the following subjects are mentioned in the passage. Which two subjects are compared?
    a. the use of laughter in medical practice in modern and medieval times
    b. the biological effects of jogging and laughter
    c. the ability to respond to humor among the elderly and seriously ill patients
    d. the results of scientific studies of laughter conducted on the east and west coasts of the United States

52. The passage cites a study in which older people were encouraged to laugh more often. The older people were found to
    a. live longer.
    b. be more sociable.
    c. have fewer headaches.
    d. be more withdrawn.

53. Which of the following inferences might be drawn about psychologists who write about laughter?
    a. They treat humor as if it were a laboratory specimen.
    b. They report their findings in an interesting manner.
    c. They describe the real meaning of humor.
    d. They do not laugh very often.

54. Which of the following statements can be inferred from the passage?
    a. Laughter should be used as part of the treatment of chronic illnesses.
    b. Scientists have discovered the chemicals that the brain produces during laughter.
    c. Physicians have been using humor to treat human ills since medieval times.
    d. Scientists are taking a fresh look at laughter as a potential form of medical treatment.

V

There is wide agreement that a successful physical outcome following heart surgery does not always lead to a good psychological result. An estimated 20 per cent of such patients experience long-term depression. "Surgeons will tell you they noticed a patient does well physiologically, but in the end it doesn't tend to benefit that much," said Dr. Theodore Nadelson, chief of psychiatry at the Boston Veterans Administration Hospital.

Despite the apparent success of the heart surgery and the reduction of symptoms, some patients "never feel quite natural," Nadelson said. And in other cases, patients seem to prefer their role as invalids. "Sometimes it makes people feel better when they have a disease," Nadelson said.

According to Dr. Murray Brown, a psychiatrist at the Veterans Administration Hospital in Sepulveda, Calif., an extraordinarily large number of patients become depressed after heart attacks or heart surgery. From studying recovering patients in a coronary care unit at the hospital, Brown said that 80 percent typically experience depression, while about 20 percent remain depressed.

In some cases, time takes care of problems. Dr. Dwight Harken, a professor emeritus at Harvard University and a pioneer in modern cardiac surgery, pointed to a variety of short-term problems that plague patients after major surgery. Many, he said, experience vision problems. Equally nettlesome are a variety of other problems that frequently occur in the days immediately following surgery. For example, a decade ago, surgeons and psychiatrists were reporting that a large number of patients became delirious a few days after heart surgery. The delirium—marked by confusion, hallucinations and, sometimes, the feeling that the hospital staff was trying to kill the patient—usually resolved itself within a few days. Some patients became so agitated that they ripped out the various tubes and wires attached to their bodies.

Researchers attributed the disturbing symptoms to several causes, including the disorienting conditions of typically windowless intensive-care units, where lights are kept on 24 hours a day. Boston's Nadelson and others reported that the symptoms could be treated in many cases by helping to orient the patient—installing clocks and calendars, making sure the patients have windows, and removing noisy and upsetting monitoring equipment.

As many as 2 percent of cardiac surgery patients experience some level of brain damage, according to Dr. Anthony Breuer, a neurologist at the Cleveland Clinic, where about 3,000 heart operations are performed every year. A larger number of patients, 11 percent, experience confusion after surgery, Breuer said, but in most of the cases, the effect disappears.

"It's no longer a question of whether the heart surgery patient will live," said Jeremy Katz, a psychologist at the Medical College of Wisconsin in Milwaukee. "Ninety-nine percent of them do. The question is the quality of life."

(Copyright 1982, the *Los Angeles Times.* Reprinted by permission. "Surgery: The Mind Also Is Affected" by Paul Jacobs, Published July 8, 1982.)

55. Which of the following subjects is the main theme of this passage?
    a. the occurrence of depression in coronary care units
    b. the psychiatric treatment of heart surgery patients
    c. the reduced risks associated with heart surgery
    d. the psychological effects of heart surgery

56. Based on the material in the passage, how are those patients who seem to feel more comfortable in the role of invalid likely to respond to heart surgery?
    a. They will show no physiological improvement.
    b. They will become accustomed to their altered condition.
    c. They will think of themselves as not well.
    d. They will have a greater risk of brain damage.

57. In the fourth paragraph of the passage, the word *nettlesome* means
    a. unanticipated.
    b. critical.

c. irritating.

d. transitory.

58. Most likely, the author's purpose in writing this passage was to
    a. recommend a course of action.
    b. provide the reader with information.
    c. appeal to the reader's emotions.
    d. express an opinion about an issue.

59. It can be inferred from the passage that a possible cause for confusion in patients who have just had major heart surgery is
    a. a lack of fresh air.
    b. an absence of time cues.
    c. the patient's need to maintain the role of invalid.
    d. the patient's suspiciousness about hospital staff.

60. On the basis of the material presented, which of the following inferences can be drawn?
    a. Improved methods of treatment have accounted for a marked decrease in the number of patients who become depressed following heart surgery.
    b. The more severe the physical symptoms before heart surgery, the greater will be the sense of well-being experienced by the patient afterward.
    c. Eliminating the risk of brain damage removes a significant cause of psychological problems associated with heart surgery.
    d. Medical science has been less successful in treating the psychological problems than in treating the physical problems of heart surgery patients.

Answers

I. Verbal Ability: Word Knowledge and Reading Comprehension

1.	c		31.	c
2.	b		32.	b
3.	c		33.	d
4.	a		34.	a
5.	b		35.	b
6.	d		36.	d
7.	b		37.	c
8.	a		38.	a
9.	c		39.	b
10.	c		40.	d
11.	b		41.	a
12.	c		42.	c
13.	a		43.	b
14.	a		44.	a
15.	d		45.	c
16.	c		46.	b
17.	d		47.	d
18.	a		48.	c
19.	a		49.	c
20.	d		50.	a
21.	d		51.	b
22.	b		52.	b
23.	a		53.	b
24.	c		54.	a
25.	b		55.	b
26.	c		56.	a
27.	b		57.	d
28.	b		58.	d
29.	c		59.	b
30.	d		60.	c

II. Verbal Ability: Word Knowledge and Reading Comprehension

1.	a		9.	d
2.	c		10.	b
3.	a		11.	a
4.	c		12.	c
5.	a		13.	d
6.	c		14.	b
7.	d		15.	d
8.	a		16.	a

17.	c		39.	c
18.	a		40.	a
19.	b		41.	d
20.	d		42.	b
21.	a		43.	d
22.	d		44.	b
23.	c		45.	c
24.	b		46.	d
25.	a		47.	a
26.	c		48.	d
27.	d		49.	b
28.	b		50.	c
29.	d		51.	a
30.	b		52.	c
31.	d		53.	d
32.	a		54.	b
33.	b		55.	c
34.	a		56.	a
35.	c		57.	b
36.	b		58.	d
37.	a		59.	a
38.	c		60.	b

III. Verbal Ability: Word Knowledge and Reading Comprehension

1.	a		25.	b
2.	a		26.	b
3.	b		27.	d
4.	c		28.	b
5.	a		29.	c
6.	a		30.	a
7.	a		31.	d
8.	a		32.	b
9.	b		33.	c
10.	b		34.	a
11.	d		35.	a
12.	d		36.	a
13.	c		37.	a
14.	a		38.	c
15.	c		39.	b
16.	a		40.	a
17.	d		41.	c
18.	d		42.	d
19.	c		43.	c
20.	b		44.	a
21.	c		45.	b
22.	b		46.	c
23.	d		47.	d
24.	b		48.	c

49.	d		55.	d
50.	a		56.	c
51.	b		57.	c
52.	b		58.	b
53.	a		59.	b
54.	d		60.	d

Bibliography

Vocabulary Study

Levine, Harold. *Vocabulary for the College-Bound Student.* New York: Amsco, 1994.

Miller, Ward S. *Word Wealth.* New York: Holt, Rinehart and Winston, 1978.

Reading Study

Coman, Marcia J. and Heavers, Kathy L. *Improving Reading Comprehension and Speed, Skimming and Scanning, Reading for Pleasure.* New York: NTC, 1997.

Kump, Peter. *Breakthrough: Rapid Reading.* Englewood Cliffs: Prentice Hall, 1979.

McWhorter, Kathleen T. *Effective and Flexible Reading.* New York: Longman, 1998.

Mathematics Review

This mathematics review is intended to give you a basic overview of the math required for this exam. The topics included in this review are whole numbers, integers, fractions, decimals, percents, converting between fractions, decimals, and percents, converting between different types of measurements, basic algebra, basic geometry, and various mathematical concepts.

CONCEPTS

Basic Vocabulary

Any mathematics review should begin with vocabulary. Here are a few terms with which you should be familiar:

addend	two or more numbers you add together
sum	the answer to an addition problem
minuend	the number you subtract from in a subtraction problem
subtrahend	the number you subtract in a subtraction problem
difference	the answer to a subtraction problem
factor	a number that is multiplied by another number
product	the answer to a multiplication problem
divisor	the number that divides into another number
dividend	the number that is divided up by the divisor
quotient	the answer to a division problem

Place Value

Our counting system is based on *place value*. Each of the digits that make up a number has a value based on units of ten. Use the following example to review some of the place values. The pattern shown below continues.

EX: 1,234,567
7 = ones (or units) place $\rightarrow 7 \cdot 1 = 7$
6 = tens place $\rightarrow 6 \cdot 10 = 60$
5 = hundreds place $\rightarrow 5 \cdot 100 = 500$
4 = thousands place   etc . . .
3 = ten-thousands place
2 = hundred-thousands place
1 = millions place

This number is read: One million, two hundred thirty-four thousand, five hundred sixty-seven.

When you add or subtract, be sure to line up the digits according to their place value:

EX: 23,345
    + 368
    23,713

EX: 3,875
    − 905
    2,970

Rounding

Sometimes the answer to a problem must be rounded off to a whole number, or to some other specified place value. No matter if you are rounding whole numbers or rational numbers (numbers that can expressed as fractions), the rules are the same.

1. Underline the place value to which you are rounding.
2. Examine the number immediately to the right of the underlined number.
3. If the number to the right is 5 or greater, round the underlined number up one.
4. If the number to the right is less than 5, leave the underlined number unchanged.

EX: Round to the nearest one: 84.71 = 84.71 = 85   123.38 = 123.38 = 123
EX: Round to the nearest hundred: 8,245 = 8275 = 8,300   3,729 = 3,729 = 3700
EX: Round to the nearest tenth: 458.296 = 458.296 = 458.3

Prime Numbers

Prime numbers are *whole numbers that have exactly two whole number factors: 1 and the number itself.* The first 10 prime numbers are: 2, 3, 5, 7, 11, 13, 17, 19, 23, 29. 2 is the only even prime number (all other even numbers have 2 as a factor, and therefore have more than two factors). The opposite of a prime number is a composite number: *a whole number (other than 0) with more than two factors.* 0 and 1 are neither prime nor composite.

Divisibility Rules

These rules help you determine if a given number is evenly divisible by another.

- *If the last digit of the number is 0, 2, 4, 6, 8, or 0, then it is divisible by 2.*
- *If the sum of the digits of the number is a multiple of 3, then it is divisible by 3.*

- *If the last digit of the number is 5 or 0, then it is divisible by 5.*
- *If the number is divisible by 2 **and** 3, then it is divisible by 6.*
- *If the sum of the digits of the number is a multiple of 9, then it is divisible by 9.*
- *If the last digit of the number is 0, then it is divisible by 10.*
- *If the number is a multiple of 3 **and** 4, then it is divisible by 12.*

Average

The average of a group of numbers is *the sum of the numbers, divided by the number of numbers added together.*

EX: The average of 5, 9, and 10 is: $\dfrac{5 + 9 + 10}{3} = \dfrac{24}{3} = 8$

Exponents

An exponent *tells you how many times to multiply the base by itself.*

EX: 5^2 2 is the *exponent* (or *power*) and 5 is the *base*. $5^2 = 5 \cdot 5 = 25$.

EX: $x^4 = x \cdot x \cdot x \cdot x$ 4 is the exponent, and x is the base.

EX: $6^{-3} = \dfrac{1}{6^3} = \dfrac{1}{6 \cdot 6 \cdot 6} = \dfrac{1}{216}$ -3 is the exponent, 6 is the base.

When the exponent is 2, the expression is called a *square,* or *perfect square.* 4^2 can be read as "four squared." 16 is the square of 4. When the exponent is 3, the expression is called a *cube,* or *perfect cube.* 4^3 can be read as "four cubed." 64 is the cube of 4. Below is a table of common squares and cubes with which you should be familiar.

$1^2 =$	1	$1^3 =$	1
$2^2 =$	4	$2^3 =$	8
$3^2 =$	9	$3^3 =$	27
$4^2 =$	16	$4^3 =$	64
$5^2 =$	25	$5^3 =$	125
$6^2 =$	36	$6^3 =$	216
$7^2 =$	49	$7^3 =$	343
$8^2 =$	64	$8^3 =$	512
$9^2 =$	81	$9^3 =$	729
$10^2 =$	100	$10^3 =$	1000

Square Roots & Cube Roots

16 is the square of 4. Conversely, 4 is called the *square root* ($\sqrt{}$) of 16. A square root is *the number that is multiplied by itself to obtain another number.* For example, $\sqrt{16} = 4$, because $4 \cdot 4 = 16$. The symbol used is called the *radical,* and the number underneath the symbol is called the *radicand.*

EX: In the equation $\sqrt{36} = 6$, $\sqrt{}$ = radical, 36 = radicand, 6 = square root

Similarly, 4 is called the cube root ($\sqrt[3]{}$) of 64 because 64 is the cube of 4. A cube root is *the number that is multiplied by itself three times to obtain another number.* For example, $\sqrt[3]{8} = 2$, because $2 \cdot 2 \cdot 2 = 8$.

EX: In the equation $\sqrt[3]{64} = 4$, $\sqrt[3]{}$ = radical, 64 = radicand, 4 = cube root

Radicals work in a similar fashion for fourth roots, fifth roots, etc.

Here are two rules that apply to multiplying and dividing *radical expressions* (expressions containing square roots, cube roots, etc.).

1. $\sqrt{AB} = \sqrt{A} \cdot \sqrt{B}$

EX: $\sqrt{81} = \sqrt{9 \cdot 9} = \sqrt{9} \cdot \sqrt{9} = 3 \cdot 3 = 9$

EX: $\sqrt{12} = \sqrt{4 \cdot 3} = \sqrt{4} \cdot \sqrt{3} = 2 \cdot \sqrt{3} = 2\sqrt{3}$

This rule also works in reverse:

$\sqrt{A} \cdot \sqrt{B} = \sqrt{AB}$

EX: $\sqrt{3} \cdot \sqrt{5} = \sqrt{15}$

EX: $\sqrt[3]{2} \cdot \sqrt[3]{4} = \sqrt[3]{8} = 2$

2. $\sqrt{\dfrac{A}{B}} = \dfrac{\sqrt{A}}{\sqrt{B}}$

EX: $\sqrt{\dfrac{9}{25}} = \dfrac{\sqrt{9}}{\sqrt{25}} = \dfrac{3}{5}$

EX: $\sqrt{\dfrac{27}{16}} = \dfrac{\sqrt{27}}{\sqrt{16}} = \dfrac{3}{4}$

This rule also works in reverse:

$\dfrac{\sqrt{A}}{\sqrt{B}} = \sqrt{\dfrac{A}{B}}$

EX: $\dfrac{\sqrt{48}}{\sqrt{12}} = \sqrt{\dfrac{48}{12}} = \sqrt{4} = 2$

You may add or subtract radical expressions only if:

- *the radicands are the same*
- *they are the same type of radical (square root, cube root, fourth root, etc.)*

EX: These may all be combined:

$2\sqrt{5} + 4\sqrt{5} = 6\sqrt{5}$

$9\sqrt{7} - 2\sqrt{7} = 7\sqrt{7}$

$2\sqrt[4]{8} + 3\sqrt[4]{8} = 5\sqrt[4]{8}$

None of these may be combined:

$5\sqrt{3} + 8\sqrt{11}$

$4\sqrt{7} - 12\sqrt{15}$

$\sqrt{5} + \sqrt[3]{7}$

You may need to simplify the radical expressions before you can combine them.

EX: $\sqrt{60} + 3\sqrt{15} =$
$\sqrt{4 \cdot 15} + 3\sqrt{15} =$
$2\sqrt{15} + 3\sqrt{15} = 5\sqrt{15}$

EX: $7\sqrt{3} + 5\sqrt{12}$
$7\sqrt{3} + 5(\sqrt{4} \cdot \sqrt{3}) =$
$7\sqrt{3} + 5(2\sqrt{3}) =$
$7\sqrt{3} + 10\sqrt{3} = 17\sqrt{3}$

INTEGERS

An integer is *any positive whole number, negative whole number, or zero.* Some examples of integers are 6, −12, 0, 234, −87. Integers may not contain fractions or decimals. The set of integers is just one set of numbers we use. Below is a table relating the major number sets we use. Each set of numbers contains all of the numbers in the set beneath it.

Real Numbers	*all numbers on the number line*
Rational Numbers	*numbers that can be expressed as fractions*
Integers	*{ . . . −3, −2, −1, 0, 1, 2, 3 . . .}*
Whole Numbers	*{0, 1, 2, 3, 4 . . .}*
Counting (or Natural) Numbers	*{1, 2, 3, 4 . . .}*

According to the table, the set of integers includes all whole numbers and counting numbers. In the same way, the set of real numbers contains all of the numbers in the sets beneath it.

Adding Integers

When the signs are the same, adding two (or more) integers works just like you might remember:

positive + positive = positive
negative + negative = negative

EX: $^{+}12 + {}^{+}17 = 29$ The positive (plus) sign is usually omitted.
EX: $^{-}12 + {}^{-}17 = {}^{-}29$ The negative (minus) sign may or may not be raised, but it means the same thing: a negative number.

When the signs are different, adding integers is a tad trickier, but not too much more.

1. Ignore the signs until the end of your work.
2. Subtract the smaller number from the larger number.
3. Give your answer the same sign as the larger number from step 2.

EX: $-7 + 24 \rightarrow 24 - 7 \rightarrow 17$

Now put the correct sign in: $+17$
Why a positive sign? Without the signs, "24" is the larger number.
Therefore, $-7 + 24 = 17$.

EX: $-25 + 4 \rightarrow 25 - 4 \rightarrow 21$

Now put the correct sign in: -21
Why a negative sign? Without the signs, "25" is the larger number.
Therefore, $4 + -25 = -21$.

Subtracting Integers

One of the easiest ways to subtract integers is to turn subtraction into addition.

Subtracting a positive is the same as adding a negative:

EX: $+15 - {}^{+}5 = +15 + -5 = 10$ EX: $-20 - {}^{+}5 = -20 + -5 = -25$

Subtracting a negative is the same as adding a positive:

EX: $+15 - -5 = +15 + {}^{+}5 = 20$ EX: $-20 - -5 = -20 + {}^{+}5 = -15$

Multiplying Integers

An even number of negative numbers will give you a positive product.

EX: $2 \cdot -5 \cdot -3 \cdot 4 = 120$

An odd number of negative numbers will give you a negative product.

EX: $-2 \cdot -5 \cdot -3 \cdot 4 = -120$

Dividing Integers

positive ÷ positive = positive   EX: $20 \div 5 = 4$
negative ÷ negative = positive   EX: $-20 \div -5 = 4$
positive ÷ negative = negative   EX: $20 \div -5 = -4$

FRACTIONS

A fraction is *any number that can be written in the form $\frac{A}{B}$ where A and B are integers, and B is not zero.* A is called the *numerator,* B is called the *denominator.* It may also help to think of a fraction as part of something, or a piece of something. Just be careful: a fraction can represent less than the whole thing, the whole thing, or more than the whole thing.

proper fraction	A fraction in which A is less than B; EX: $\frac{4}{5}$ and $\frac{25}{100}$. A fraction is another way of writing a division problem: $\frac{4}{5} = 4 \div 5 = 5\overline{)4}$. You may turn any whole number into a fraction by giving the whole number a denominator of 1. $5 = \frac{5}{1}$ because $5 \div 1 = 5$, and $12 = \frac{12}{1}$ because $12 \div 1 = 12$. Fractions may not have a denominator of zero, because it is not possible to divide by zero.
improper fraction	A fraction in which A is greater than or equal to B; EX: $\frac{9}{5}$ and $\frac{12}{12}$. When A = B, the fraction is equal to 1 whole (because $12 \div 12 = 1$). When adding or subtracting fractions, it is often useful to rewrite 1 whole as a fraction.
mixed number	A mixed number is the *sum* of a whole number and a fraction; or just another way of writing an improper fraction; EX: $1\frac{4}{5}$ really means $1 + \frac{4}{5}$.
unit fraction	In the fraction $\frac{A}{B}$, where A = 1.
complex fraction	In the fraction $\frac{A}{B}$, where A and/or B are fractions.
equivalent fractions	Two equal fractions
greatest common factor	The largest number that divides evenly into two or more numbers
least common multiple	The smallest number that two or more numbers divide into evenly
relatively prime	Two or more numbers whose greatest common factor is 1
lowest terms	In a fraction $\frac{A}{B}$, when A and B are relatively prime
least common denominator	The smallest denominator that two or more fractions have in common
reciprocal	The reciprocal of $\frac{A}{B}$ is $\frac{B}{A}$. *The fraction $\frac{0}{B}$ has no reciprocal.*

To convert *improper fractions* to mixed numbers: EX: $\frac{9}{5} = 1\frac{4}{5}$

1. Divide the denominator into the numerator, $9 \div 5$.
2. The answer becomes the whole number part of the mixed number, in this case: 1.

3. The remainder becomes the numerator part of the mixed number, in this case: 4.
4. The original denominator becomes the denominator part of the mixed number, in this case: 5.

To convert a *mixed number* into an improper fraction: EX: $1\frac{4}{5} = \frac{9}{5}$

1. Multiply the denominator by the whole number, and add this to the numerator.
   $(5 \cdot 1) + 4$.
2. The answer becomes the numerator of the improper fraction, in this case: 9.
3. The denominator of the original mixed number becomes the denominator of the improper fraction, in this case: 5.

Reducing Fractions

Reducing fractions to their lowest terms is always a good idea. To reduce a fraction, *divide its numerator and denominator by the **largest** number that divides evenly into both.*

EX: to reduce $\frac{5}{10}$, divide both the numerator and denominator by 5.

$$\frac{5}{10} = \frac{5 \div 5}{10 \div 5} = \frac{1}{2}$$

EX: to reduce $\frac{18}{30}$, divide both the numerator and denominator by 6.

$$\frac{18}{30} = \frac{18 \div 6}{30 \div 6} = \frac{3}{5}$$

Multiplying Fractions

Multiply the numerators together and multiply the denominators together.

EX: $\frac{4}{5} \cdot \frac{2}{3} = \frac{8}{15}$

If you are multiplying mixed numbers, convert them to improper fractions and then multiply.

EX: $1\frac{2}{3} \cdot 3\frac{1}{2}$ becomes $\frac{5}{3} \cdot \frac{7}{2}$ and $\frac{5}{3} \cdot \frac{7}{2} = \frac{35}{6}$ or $5\frac{5}{6}$

Remember, you may need to reduce your final answer.

Dividing Fractions

Invert the second fraction, and then multiply the two together.

EX: $\frac{1}{5} \div \frac{2}{3} = \frac{1}{5} \cdot \frac{3}{2} = \frac{3}{10}$ EX: $15 \div \frac{2}{3} = \frac{15}{1} \cdot \frac{3}{2} = \frac{45}{2}$ or $22\frac{1}{2}$

Adding and Subtracting Fractions

All of the fractions in the problem must have the same (or common) denominator.

common denominator   Add or subtract the numerators. DO NOT add or subtract the denominators.

EX: $\frac{4}{15} + \frac{8}{15} = \frac{12}{15} = \frac{4}{5}$

different denominator   Convert the fractions into equivalent fractions with common denominators. In other words, you must make sure that all of the fractions in the problem have the same denominator. To do this, determine the lowest common denominator (LCD). The LCD is the smallest number that divides evenly into all denominators in the problem.

EX: $\dfrac{1}{4} + \dfrac{5}{6}$

Determine the smallest number that 4 and 6 go into.

4 and 6 both go into 12, so **12** is the LCD. Convert the original fractions into equivalent fractions with a common denominator. Multiply the numerator and denominator by the same number. Choose a number that will give each original fraction the LCD.

EX: $\dfrac{1}{4} = \dfrac{1 \cdot 3}{4 \cdot 3} = \dfrac{3}{12}$ and $\dfrac{5}{6} = \dfrac{5 \cdot 2}{6 \cdot 2} = \dfrac{10}{12}$

So, $\dfrac{1}{4} + \dfrac{5}{6} = \dfrac{3}{12} + \dfrac{10}{12} = \dfrac{13}{12} = 1\dfrac{1}{12}$

EX: $\dfrac{5}{8} - \dfrac{1}{5} = \dfrac{25}{40} - \dfrac{8}{40} = \dfrac{17}{40}$

DECIMALS

Like fractions, decimals allow you to represent part of a whole, the entire whole, or more than the whole. To represent these different amounts, decimals use place value to the *right* of the decimal point. Fractions use different denominators to do the same thing. So, it seems that decimals are really a type of fraction! Use the following example to review some of the place values used in decimals. The pattern shown below continues.

EX: 78.123456   1 = tenths place
                 2 = hundredths place
                 3 = thousandths place
                 4 = ten-thousandths place
                 5 = hundred-thousandths place
                 6 = millionths place

EX: 0.78 is read: 78 hundredths

EX: 2.305 is read: two and three hundred-five thousandths

To make the connection between decimals and fractions a little clearer, consider the factions with denominators of 10, 100, 1,000, etc.

EX: $0.1 = \dfrac{1}{10}$ $0.23 = \dfrac{23}{100}$ $2.75 = 2\dfrac{75}{100}$

Converting Between Fractions and Decimals

To convert a fraction into a decimal, *divide the denominator into the numerator.*

EX: $\dfrac{2}{5}$ = 2 divided by 5 = 0.4   EX: $2\dfrac{3}{4}$ = 2 + (3 divided by 4) = 2.75

To convert a decimal into a fraction, *you must know the name of the decimal. The name will tell you what the denominator of your fraction will be.*

EX: 0.86 = 86 hundredths   This means your denominator should be 100.

Therefore, $0.86 = \dfrac{86}{100} = \dfrac{43}{50}$

EX: $0.235 = \dfrac{235}{1000}$

Adding and Subtracting Decimals

The only difference between adding or subtracting decimals and whole numbers is the decimal point. To add or subtract decimals, remember to line up the decimal point (and, more importantly, the place values). Lining up the decimal point should ensure that you add tenths to tenths, hundredths to hundredths, and so on. It's not hard, you just have to be careful!

EX: 2.34 + 8.56 = $\begin{array}{r} 2.34 \\ +\ 8.56 \\ \hline 11.90 \end{array}$ EX: 23.8 − 7.09 = $\begin{array}{r} 23.80 \\ -\ 7.09 \\ \hline 30.71 \end{array}$ (it's ok to add a 0 after the decimal point.)

Multiplying Decimals

You don't have to line up the decimal points when you are multiplying decimals. In fact, you don't have to worry about the decimal points until the very end of the problem.

1. Multiply the numbers together as you would normally.
2. Count the number of decimal places in each number you are multiplying and add them together.
3. Starting from the right end in your product, count to the left the same number of places as your answer in step 2.

Don't panic—this sounds complicated, but it's really not. Follow this example:

Step #1: $\begin{array}{r} 23.74 \\ \times\ 16.5 \\ \hline 39171 \end{array}$ *Notice the decimals are not lined up.*
Multiply the numbers together as you would normally
Your answer has no decimal yet, and it's ok!

Step #2:   23.74 has 2 decimal places →   *Count the number of decimal places in*
16.5 has 1 decimal place   *each number you are multiplying and*
Total decimal places = 3   *add them together.*

Step #3:   39.171 →   *Starting from the right end in your product, count to the left the same number of places as your answer in step 2.*

EX: 42.3   A total of 2 decimal places up here . . .
$\underline{\times\ 1.6}$
67.68   So, a total of 2 decimal places down here!

Multiplying decimals by powers of 10

There is a very useful shortcut worth knowing when it comes to *multiplying* decimals by powers of 10 (10, 100, 1000, etc.).

EX: 45.67 · 100

*Move the decimal point to the **right** the same number of places as there are zeros in the power of 10—in this case 2.* Therefore, 45.67 · 100 = 4567

EX: 123.456 · 1000 = 123,456

Dividing Decimals

You only need to learn one simple trick to make dividing decimals as simple as dividing whole numbers.

EX: 0.25)0.625   *Multiply the divisor by the appropriate power of 10 to make it a whole number.*

25)62.5   *In this example, multiply the divisor by 100 to turn 0.25 into 25. You must also multiply the dividend by the same power of 10. In this example, 0.625 becomes 62.5. Now you may divide normally.*

2.5
25)62.5   *Remember to bring the decimal point up to the top of the box: place it directly over the decimal in the dividend.*

EX: 1.3)1.56   *Multiply both the divisor and the dividend by 10.*

13)15.6   *Now you may divide normally. Just remember to place the decimal in the quotient.*

1.2
13)15.6   *The decimal in the quotient is directly over the decimal in the dividend.*

Dividing decimals by powers of 10

There is a very useful shortcut worth knowing when it comes to *dividing* decimals by powers of 10 (10, 100, 1000, etc.).

EX: 45.67 ÷ 100

*Move the decimal point to the **left** the same number of places as there are zeros in the power of 10—in this case 2.* Therefore, 45.67 ÷ 100 = 0.4567

EX: 23.45 ÷ 1000 = 0.02345

PERCENT

A percent is really *a fraction with a denominator of 100*. The percent symbol, %, is another way of writing a denominator of 100. In other words, 25% is really $\frac{25}{100}$, and 3% is really $\frac{3}{100}$. If you think about percents in this way, you can readily see how percents less than 100% are really fractions less than 1 whole, and percents greater than 100% are really fractions greater than 1 whole.

EX: $10\% = \frac{10}{100}$, both of which are less than 1 whole.

EX: $150\% = \frac{150}{100}$, both of which are greater than 1 whole.

Converting between decimals, fractions, and percents.

To convert a decimal to a percent, *multiply by 100.*

EX: $0.426 = 0.426 \cdot 100 = 42.6\%$ EX: 55 or $55.0 = 55.0 \cdot 100 = 5500\%$

To convert a percent to a decimal, *divide by 100.*

EX: $45\% = 45\% \div 100 = 0.45$ EX: $12.5\% = 12.5\% \div 100 = 0.125$

To convert a fraction to a percent:

1. change the fraction to a decimal
2. change the decimal to a percent

EX: $\frac{2}{5} = 0.4 = 40\%$ EX: $\frac{9}{2} = 4.5 = 450\%$

To convert a percent to a fraction:

1. change the percent to a fraction
2. reduce the fraction

EX: $35\% = \frac{35}{100} = \frac{7}{20}$ EX: $6\% = \frac{6}{100} = \frac{3}{50}$

You should be familiar with the common fractional-decimal equivalents listed below. If you learn these, you can convert quickly between many fractions, decimals, and percents.

The bar over a digit (or digits) means that digit (or those digits) repeat to infinity.

Fraction	Decimal	Percent
$\frac{1}{4}$	0.25	25%
$\frac{2}{4} = \frac{1}{2}$	0.5	50%
$\frac{3}{4}$	0.75	75%
$\frac{1}{3}$	$0.\overline{3}$	$33.\overline{3}\%$
$\frac{2}{3}$	$0.\overline{6}$	$66.\overline{6}\%$

$\frac{1}{5}$	0.2	20%
$\frac{2}{5}$	0.4	40%
$\frac{3}{5}$	0.6	60%
$\frac{4}{5}$	0.8	80%
$\frac{1}{8}$	0.125	12.5%
$\frac{3}{8}$	0.375	37.5%
$\frac{5}{8}$	0.625	62.5%
$\frac{7}{8}$	0.875	87.5%

Basic percentage problems have 3 components:

EX: 25% of 200 is 50   "25%" = the percent
                         "200" = the base
                         "50" = the percentage

It often helps to turn a percent problem into an equation, and you usually need to turn the percent into a decimal (divide it by 100).

EX: 25% of 200 is 50   "of" means to multiply; "is" means "="
$0.25 \cdot 200 = 50$

Basic Percent Problems:

Find the percent of a given number.

EX: What is 10% of 50?
$x = 0.1 \cdot 50$
$x = 5$

Find the base when you know the percent and the percentage.

EX: 10% of what number is 5?
$0.1 \cdot x = 5$
$0.1x = 5$ Divide both sides by 0.1 to solve for x.
$x = 50$ This is your answer.

Find the percent when you know the base and the percentage.

EX: What percent of 50 is 5?
$x\% \cdot 50 = 5$ Deal with "x" being a percent at the end of
                           the problem.
$50x = 5$ Divide both sides by 50.
$x = 0.1$ Turn 0.1 into a percent by multiplying by 100.
10% is your answer.

Percent Discount / Tax Increase

To find the amount of discount or increase when the percent is known, *change the percent to a decimal (or fraction), multiply by the original cost, and add or subtract accordingly.*

EX: A $250 stereo is discounted 18%. Find the new sale price.

1. Convert 18% to a decimal by dividing by 100: $18\% \div 100 = 0.18$.
2. Calculate 18% of $250 by multiplying: $0.18 \cdot 250 = 45$.
3. Subtract $45 (the 18% decrease) from $250 (the original cost) to find the new cost: $250 − $45 = $205.

Percentage Increase and Decrease

Often times the problem asks you to determine the percentage of increase or decrease. This type of problem is easily solved by making a fraction out of the information. Write the *amount of increase or decrease* as the numerator, and write the *original amount* as the denominator. Finally, change the fraction to a percent.

EX: My little brother grew from 60 inches to 66 inches in the last year. What percent increase is this?

Solution: The amount of increase is 6 inches. Make this the numerator, and make his original height (60 inches) the denominator. Then change the fraction to a percent.

$\dfrac{6}{60} = \dfrac{1}{10} = 0.1 = 10\%$ My little brother's height increased by 10%.

RATIO AND PROPORTION

Ratio—*a comparison of two numbers, usually by division*
   EX: In a class of 15 people, there are 7 boys and 8 girls.

   The ratio of boys to girls is: 7 to 8, or 7:8, or $\dfrac{7}{8}$

Rate—*a ratio made up of two different units or amounts*
   EX: I can drive my car 50 miles on 10 gallons of gas. This relationship can be expressed

   as a ratio of miles to gallons: 50 to 10, or 50:10, or $\dfrac{50 \; miles}{10 \; gallons} = \dfrac{5}{1}$

Proportion—*an equation of two equal ratios*
EX: If my car gets 5 miles to the gallon (as in the previous example), then how many gallons will I need to drive 125 miles?
Solution: Set up a proportion to solve this problem. Make sure you align your units correctly: in this case, miles across from miles, and gallons across from gallons.

$\dfrac{5 \; miles}{1 \; gallon} = \dfrac{125 \; miles}{x}$

At this point I must state that all proportions have a special property: *cross products are equal.* In our example, this means that when you cross multiply (multiply one numerator by the other denominator, and multiply one denominator by the other numerator), the products are equal to each other.

$5x = 125$ Now divide both sides by 5 to solve for x.

$x = 25$ This is your answer in gallons.

Use proportions when converting from one form of measurement to another.

EX: If one quart equals 0.9 liters, how many liters equal 4.5 quarts?

Solution: Set up a proportion. Be sure to align the units correctly: quarts across from quarts, and liters across from liters.

$$\frac{1\ qt}{0.9\ liters} = \frac{4.5\ qt}{x}$$ Cross multiply to solve for x.

$x = 4.5 \cdot 0.9$

$x = 4.05$ This is your answer, in liters.

You may also use proportions when you are working with scaled measurements.

EX: The scale on a map is 1 cm for every 15 km. If the actual distance traveled is 78 km, how far is the same distance on the map?

Solution: Set up a proportion to solve this problem. Be sure to align the units correctly: cm across from cm, and km across from km.

$$\frac{1\ cm}{15\ km} = \frac{x}{78\ km}$$ Cross multiply.

$15\ x = 78$ Divide both sides by 15 to solve for x.

$x = 5.2$ This is your answer, in cm.

ALGEBRA

Algebra makes use of letters and symbols (called variables) as well as numbers. All of the same rules you learned for arithmetic apply in algebra. However, algebra contains many new rules you must learn. This review will present some of the basic rules.

variable	A symbol, usually a letter, that takes the place of a number. Very often you will need to substitute a number for a letter in an expression, or you will need to solve an equation for a certain variable.
algebraic expression	A collection of numbers and variables connected by addition and subtraction signs. EX: $3x$ $2y^3 + 4$ 5 $a - b$
term	An individual piece of an expression.

EX: $3x$ $2y^3 + 4$ 5 $a - b + c$
      1 term   2 terms   1 term   3 terms

In the term $3x$, "3" is the *numerical coefficient*. In other words, "3" is a number (numeral), and it is a factor ("3" and "x" are being multiplied together). In the term $2y^3 + 4$, "-2" is the numerical coefficient (or just coefficient).

like terms   Terms with the same variables **and** same exponents,

x^2 and $3x^2$ are like terms $2x$ and $4y$ are unlike terms

$2a^2b$ and $-9ba^2$ are like terms x^3 and x^2 are unlike terms

equation   Two equal expressions.

EX: $2x - 8\ y^2 - 9 = 0$ $a^2 - b^2 = c^2$

$\frac{2}{3}f + 7 = f^2 - 24$ $2(x - 4) + x^2 = 3x - 8$

Evaluating Expressions / Order of Operations

To evaluate means *to find the value of something.* When you are asked to evaluate an algebraic expression, you need to substitute a number for a variable in the expression, and then simplify the expression. You will need to follow the *order of operations.* The order of operations is simply a set of rules that guarantees that you perform operations (addition, multiplication, etc.) in the proper order.

1. Start from the inner most set of grouping symbols (parentheses, brackets, or braces) and perform the operations within. Once you've performed the operations, remove the grouping symbols.
2. Simplify all exponents or radicals.
3. Multiply or divide, moving from left to right.
4. Add or subtract, moving from left to right.

EX: Evaluate $6x^2 \cdot (4 + 3x) - 6 + (x^2 \div 2)$ when $x = 2$
$6(2)^2 \cdot (4 + 3(2)) - 6 + (2^2 \div 2) =$ *substitute 2 for x*
$6(2)^2 \cdot (4 + 6) - 6 + (4 \div 2) =$
$6(2)^2 \cdot 10 - 6 + 2 =$
$6(4) \cdot 10 - 6 + 2 =$
$24 \cdot 10 - 6 + 2 =$
$240 - 6 + 2 = 236$

Distributive Property

A key concept in algebra is the distributive property.

EX: $6(x + 3) = 6x + 18$

"6" is a factor that is distributed (multiplied) over the "x" and the "3."

EX: $-5(y - 2x) = -5y + 10x$ EX: $-(4x + 7y) = -1(4x + 7y) = -4x - 7y$

Property of Zero

Another key concept in algebra is the property of zero: *in a multiplication problem if one of the factors is zero, then the product must be zero.* Another way of stating this rule is: if $a \cdot b = 0$, then either $a = 0$ or $b = 0$. This property also works in reverse. That is, if you know that one (or more) of the factors in a multiplication problem is zero, then the product will be zero. Stated another way, if $a = 0$ or $b = 0$, than $a \cdot b = 0$. This property is essential in solving equations involving squared terms.

The heart and soul of algebra is simplifying expressions and solving equations. If you learn to master these two skills, you will be in good shape.

Simplifying Expressions

To simplify expressions, *combine (add or subtract) like terms.* You may not combine unlike terms. When you combine like terms, add their numerical coefficients together; *the exponents remain unchanged.*

EX: $6 + x^2 - 2x - 5x^2 + 6x + 9 + 5x^3$ Combine like terms
$-4x^2 + 4x + 15 + 5x^3$ This is your answer

Solving Equations

There are two essential rules you must remember whenever you are solving equations.

1. The goal is to *isolate the variable.*
2. The method is to *do the same thing to both sides of the equation, using inverse operations.*

If you remember these two rules, you will be able to solve almost any equation!

EX: Solve for x: $7x - 10 = 12$

The goal is to isolate "x," to get it by itself on one side of the equals sign.

$7x - 10 = 11$ First, add 10 (the inverse of subtraction) to both sides.
$+10\ +10$
$7x = 21$ Next, divide (inverse of multiply) both sides by 7.
$\frac{7x}{7} = \frac{21}{7}$
$x = 3$ This is your answer.

To check your answer, substitute 3 for x in the original equation, and simplify.

$7x - 10 = 11$
$7(3) - 10 = 11$
$21 - 10 = 11$
$11 = 11$ If the left side equals the right side, you've done it right!

Sometimes you may need to combine like terms on one (or both sides) of the equation before you use inverse operations.

EX: $19z - 10 + 4z = 3z - 4$ On the left side, combine $19z$ and $4z$.
$23z - 10 = 3z - 4$ Add 10 to both sides.
$23z = 3z + 6$ Subtract $3z$ from both sides.
$20z = 6$ Divide both sides by 6 to solve for z.
$z = \frac{6}{20} = \frac{3}{10}$ This is your answer.

EX: $5(x + 3) + 9 = 3(x - 2) + 6$ Distribute.
$5x + 15 + 9 = 3x - 6 + 6$ Combine like terms.
$5x + 24 = 3x$ Subtract $5x$ from both sides.
$24 = -2x$ Divide both sides by -2.
$-12 = x$ This is your answer.

Clearing Fractions

If the equation contains fractions, you can change them to whole numbers. This is called *clearing fractions.* To clear the fractions, *multiply each term in the equation by the LCD of the fractions.*

EX: $\frac{3}{5}y + 2 = \frac{1}{2}y$ The LCD is 10, because both 5 and 2 are factors of 10.

$\frac{10}{1} \cdot \frac{3}{5}y + 2 \cdot 10 = \frac{10}{1} \cdot \frac{1}{2}y$ Multiply *each term* by 10.

$\frac{30}{5}y + 20 = \frac{10}{2}y$ Reduce the fractions to get whole numbers.

$6y + 20 = 5y$ Subtract 6y from both sides.
$20 = -y$ Never leave the variable negative. Multiply by -1.
$-20 = y$ This is your answer.

Systems of Equations

A system of equations is merely two or more equations (with the same variables) worked on at the same time. Systems of equations contain two or more variables. When you solve a system of equations in two variables, you are looking for the pair of variables that makes both equations true at the same time.

EX: $x + 2y = 12$ You are looking for values of "x" and "y" that will make
$7x - 2y = 4$ both equations true (make the left side equal the right side) at the same time.

You can solve a system of equations by adding the equations together. Do this in order to eliminate either the x-terms or the y-terms. To eliminate the x-terms or y-terms, both need to have the same coefficient but be opposite in sign (ex: $2y$ and $-2y$). Add the equations together.

$x + 2y = 12$
$\underline{+\ 7x - 2y = 4}$
$8x = 16$ Divide both sides by 8 to solve for x.
$x = 2$

Now substitute 2 for x into either of the original equations to solve for y.

$x + 2y = 12$
$2 + 2y = 12$ Subtract 2 from both sides.
$2y = 12$ Divide both sides by 2.
$y = 6$
$(x = 2, y = 6)$ This pair of values makes both equations true.

If the equations do not already have terms with the same coefficients but opposite signs, you must multiply the equations by the appropriate number. Make sure to multiply *each term* in the equation by the number you choose.

EX: $5x - 2y = -25$
$3x + y = -4$

Multiply both sides of the second equation by 2.

$2 \cdot (3x + y) = 2 \cdot -4 \rightarrow$ $6x + 2y = -8$ Now the equations can be added together.
First equation $\rightarrow$ $\underline{5x - 2y = -25}$ This will eliminate the y-terms.
        $11x = -33$ Divide both sides by 11.
        $x = -3$

Now substitute -3 for x into either of the original equations to solve for y:

$$3x + y = -4$$
$$3(-3) + y = -4 \quad \text{Simplify.}$$
$$-9 + y = -4 \quad \text{Add 9 to both sides.}$$
$$y = 5$$
$$(x = -3, y = 5) \quad \text{This pair of values makes both equations true.}$$

Word Problems

Word problems are often described as everyone's least favorite topic in algebra, and yet solving word problems is the area in which algebra is most useful. It is also true that of all the parts of solving word problems, people find it most difficult to translate the words into equations. Once this is done, however, the rest is just algebra! Here are a few tips to help you solve word problems:

- *Express the unknown quantity as a variable (or variables).*
- *"increased by," "more than," and "total" all indicate addition.*
- *"decreased by," "less than," "less," indicate subtraction.*
- *"is" means "="*
- *"of" usually indicates multiplication (ex: one-fourth of 12 $\rightarrow \frac{1}{4} \cdot 12$).*
- *Recall the vocabulary words sum, difference, product, and quotient.*

A note about "difference." If the word problem says: "The difference of a number and 3 is 2," you may assume that the order of the subtraction equation will be the same as the order of the word problem. In this case: Let $x =$ a number $\rightarrow x - 3 = 2$.

EX: The sum of twice a number and the number is 36. Find the number.

- In this problem, "sum" tells you that you will need to write an addition equation.
- You may choose x to stand for "the number." You can do this by writing a *let statement*: Let $x =$ the number.
- "is" tells you where to put the equals sign.

The sum of twice a number and the number is 36.

$$2x + x = 36 \quad Check$$
$$2x + x = 36 \quad 2(12) + 12 = 36$$
$$3x = 36 \quad 24 + 12 = 36$$
$$x = 12 \quad 36 = 36 \quad \text{This is your answer.}$$

Formulas

Formulas are special types of equations that express a relationship between variables.

EX: $A = \frac{1}{2}bh$ This the formula for the area of a triangle:

Usually you will be given values for all but one of the variables, and you will need to solve the equation for that variable.

$A =$ area
$b =$ base
$h =$ height

EX: Find the area of triangle with base of 10 and height of 15.

$A = \frac{1}{2}bh$ Use this formula, and substitute 10 for b and 15 for h.

$A = \frac{1}{2}(10)(15)$ Simplify.

$A = 75$ This is your answer.

Inequalities

Earlier we defined an equation as two equal expressions. An inequality *is two unequal expressions.*

EX: $2x < 8$ $y^2 - 9 > 0$ $a^2 + b^2 \leq c^2$ $13x + 4 \geq -75$

"<" is less than   "≤" is less than or equal to
">" is greater than   "≥" is greater than or equal to

The rules for solving inequalities are the same as for solving equations, with one important difference. Your goal and method are still the same: to isolate the variable, and to do the same thing to both sides of the inequality using inverse operations.

EX: $2x < 8$ Divide both sides by 2 to solve for x.
     $x < 4$ This is your answer. All values less than (but not including) 4.
EX: $8a - 7 > 17$ Add 7 to both sides.
     $8a > 24$ Divide both sides by 8.
      $a > 3$ This is your answer.

Here is the crucial new rule that applies only to inequalities: *When multiplying or dividing by a negative number, reverse the inequality sign.*

EX: $-5y + 6 \geq 11$ Subtract 6 from both sides.
    $-5y \geq 5$ Now divide by -5. Here is where this new rule comes in!
       $y \leq -1$ Notice that the sign reversed from ≥ to ≤. Don't forget it!

Exponent Rules

There are certain rules you must follow when working with variables and exponents.

1. When multiplying similar bases, *add the exponents.*

    EX: $j^3 \cdot j^4 = j^{3+4} = j^7$

2. When dividing similar bases, *subtract the exponents.*

    EX: $r^4 \div r^3 = r^{4-3} = r$

3. When raising a power to another power, *multiply the exponents.*

    EX: $\left(s^2\right)^3 = s^{2 \cdot 3} = s^6$

4. When the exponent is negative, *move its base to the denominator and make the exponent positive. Take care to only move the bases with negative exponents.*

EX: $d^{-2} = \dfrac{1}{d^2}$

EX: $mr^{-3} = \dfrac{m}{r^3}$ In this example, leave "m" in the numerator and move "r" to the denominator.

5. *Any base (except zero) to the zero power = 1.*

EX: $k^0 = 1$ and $4^0 = 1$

Factoring

Factoring is the opposite of distributing. Recall that the distributive property involved multiplying factors to find a product. When factoring, then, *start with the product and try to find its factors.*

EX: $4y + 10 - 8x$

To factor this expression, examine each term for a common factor (the factor found in every one of the terms). In this case, there is a "2" in each term. Factor out the "2" (divide each term by 2). $4y + 10 - 8x$ becomes $2(2y + 5 - 2x)$. Note that if you were to distribute the "2," you would arrive at the original expression. This means you've factored correctly!

EX: $24x + 72y + 8$ The common factor is 8.
    $8(3x + 9y + 1)$ This is your answer.

EX: $5x + 2x^2 + x^3$ The common factor is x.
    $x(5 + 2x + x^2)$ This is your answer. Remember, when you divide like bases, you subtract exponents.

GEOMETRY

Geometry is the study of shapes and figures in two dimensions (planar geometry) and in three dimensions (solid geometry). Below is a table of formulas about area, perimeter, and volume.

Area of a circle

$A = \pi r^2$
A = area
π = 3.14
r = radius

Area of a rectangle

$A = lw$
l = length
w = width

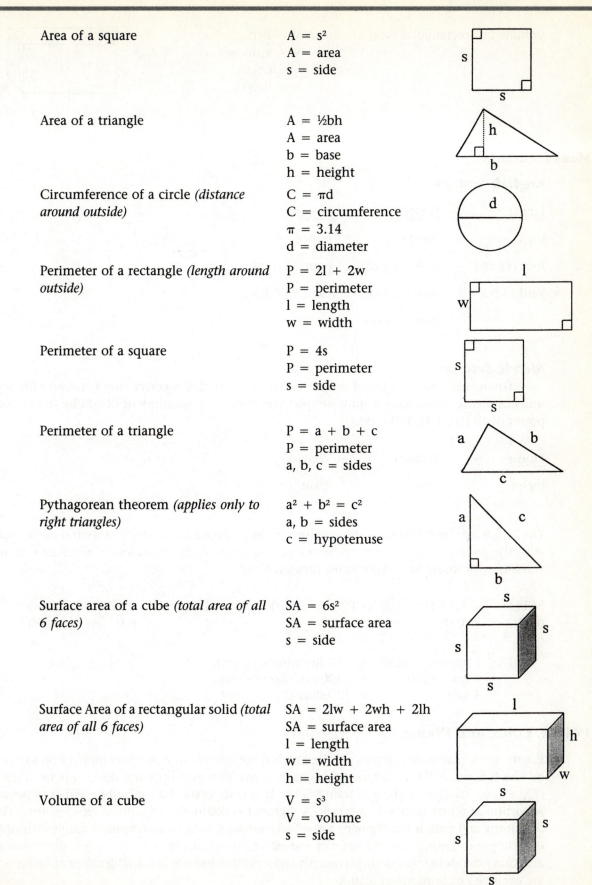

Area of a square

$A = s^2$
A = area
s = side

Area of a triangle

$A = \frac{1}{2}bh$
A = area
b = base
h = height

Circumference of a circle *(distance around outside)*

$C = \pi d$
C = circumference
π = 3.14
d = diameter

Perimeter of a rectangle *(length around outside)*

$P = 2l + 2w$
P = perimeter
l = length
w = width

Perimeter of a square

$P = 4s$
P = perimeter
s = side

Perimeter of a triangle

$P = a + b + c$
P = perimeter
a, b, c = sides

Pythagorean theorem *(applies only to right triangles)*

$a^2 + b^2 = c^2$
a, b = sides
c = hypotenuse

Surface area of a cube *(total area of all 6 faces)*

$SA = 6s^2$
SA = surface area
s = side

Surface Area of a rectangular solid *(total area of all 6 faces)*

$SA = 2lw + 2wh + 2lh$
SA = surface area
l = length
w = width
h = height

Volume of a cube

$V = s^3$
V = volume
s = side

Volume of a rectangular solid

$V = lwh$
V = volume
l = length
h = height

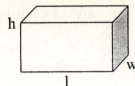

Measurements

English System

Linear	Capacity	Weight
inch	ounce	ounce
foot (12 in.)	pint (16 oz.)	pound (16 oz.)
yard (3 ft.)	quart (2 pts.)	ton (2000 lbs.)
	gallon (4 qts.)	

Metric System

The metric system is based on powers of 10. This makes converting between different units of metric measurement quite simple: you need only multiply or divide by the correct power of 10 (10, 100, 1000, etc.).

Linear	Capacity	Weight
meter	liter	gram

The following chart illustrates the relationship between metric units. You should be familiar with the prefixes. The prefixes always mean the same thing, regardless of whether you are working with linear, square, or cubic measurements.

MILLI	CENTI	DECI	UNIT	DEKA	HECTO	KILO
0.001	0.01	0.1	1	10	100	1000

EX: 1 kilometer (km) = 10 hectometers (hm)
      1 gram (gm) = 1000 milligrams (mg)
      1 liter = 10 deciliters

Points, Lines, and Planes

Points, lines, planes, and angles are the basics of geometry—the building blocks upon which all else follows. A *line* is always a straight line, extending in opposite directions to infinity (EX: a beam of light or straight train tracks). It is composed of an infinite number of *points*. A portion of a line is called a *segment*. A segment is composed of a finite set of points. The beginning and end of the segment are called *endpoints*. A *ray* is a portion of a line with only one endpoint. Thus, it extends only in one direction to infinity. A *plane* is a two-dimensional area that extends in two directions (length and width) to infinity (ex: a tabletop or a blackboard are examples of portions of planes).

In a plane, lines are either:

parallel lines—line that never meet; parallel lines have no points in common

EX: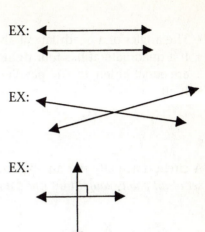

intersecting lines—lines that cross at one point; intersecting lines have one point in common

EX:

perpendicular lines—lines that intersect and form an angle of 90 degrees.

EX:

The small box (□) in the figure to the right indicates a right angle (90 degrees).

Angles

Angles are two rays with a common endpoint. The endpoint is called the *vertex* of the angle, and the rays are called the *sides* of the angle. The size of an angle is measured in degrees.

acute angle	an angle greater than 0 degrees and less than 90 degrees
right angle	an angle that measures exactly 90 degree
obtuse angle	an angle greater than 90 degrees and less than 180 degrees
straight angle	an angle that measures exactly 180 degrees
complementary angles	two or more angles whose degree measures sum 90
supplementary angles	two or more angles whose degree measures sum to 180

Polygons

A *polygon* is a closed, two-dimensional figure with more than two sides. A polygon is composed of segments. Polygons are named by the number of sides they have. If all the sides of a polygon are the same length, it is called a *regular* polygon (ex: equilateral triangle, square).

triangle—a polygon with three sides

- The angles of a triangle always sum to 180 degrees.
- If no two sides of a triangle are the same length, then it is a *scalene* triangle. No two angles of a scalene triangle are equal to each other.
- If two sides of a triangle are the same length, then it is *an isosceles triangle*. An isosceles triangle also has two equal angles.
- If all three sides of a triangle are the same length, then it is an *equilateral triangle*. All three angles of an equilateral triangle measure 60 degrees.
- If a triangle has a right angle, then it is a *right triangle*. The side opposite the right angle is the *hypotenuse*. The *Pythagorean theorem* applies to right triangles.
- If all three angles of a triangle are less than 90 degrees, then it is an *acute* triangle.
- If one angle of the triangle is greater than 90 degrees, then it is an *obtuse* triangle.

quadrilateral   a polygon with four sides

- The angles of a quadrilateral always sum to 360 degrees.
- If a quadrilateral has four right angles, then it is a *rectangle.* In a rectangle, opposite sides are equal in length and parallel.
- If all four sides of a rectangle are the same length, then it is a *square.*

Circles

A circle is actually not a polygon, because it has an infinite number of sides. A circle is *the set of all points equidistant (the same distance) from the center point.* Refer to the diagram.

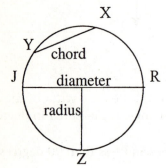

The segment from X to Y is called a *chord.* It has both endpoints on the circle.

The segment from J to R is called a *diameter.* It passes through the center of the circle. All diameters are chords.

The segment from the center to Z is called a *radius.* All radii are equal in length. A radius is always half the length of the diameter.

Every circle contains 360 degrees.

Area

The area of a polygon is the space inside the polygon—the number of square units inside the polygon. Unlike linear, or straight line, measurements (inches, meters), area is measured in square units (square yards, square centimeters). Refer to the chart of formulas for important area formulas. If you need to find the area of a figure for which you have no formula, you may subdivide the figure into polygons you recognize.

EX: To find the area of the following figure, you may introduce one perpendicular line, and find the total area of the resulting two figures: one triangle and one rectangle.

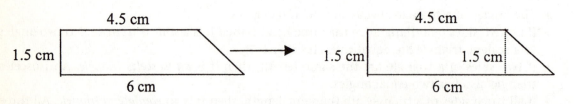

Area of rectangle: $(1.5)(4.5) = 6.75$ sq cm

Area of triangle: $\frac{1}{2}(1.5)(1.5) = 1.125$ sq cm

Area of figure: $6.75 + 1.125 = 7.875$ sq cm

Congruent polygons have the same size and the same shape. Polygons with the same area are not always congruent:

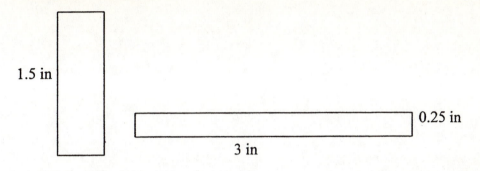

These two rectangles have the same area (0.75 sq in), but they are not congruent.

   Similar polygons have the same shape, but are not always the same size. The corresponding angles of similar polygons are equal to each other. The *ratios* of corresponding sides are equal to each other:

   EX: The following equilateral triangles are similar. The corresponding sides all have the same ratio. The corresponding angles are all equal.

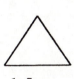 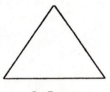

1.5 cm   2.5 cm

I. Mathematics

45 Minutes

Work each problem carefully. Use scrap paper to do your calculations. The correct answers will be found at the end of section B.

Directions

The Mathematics Test section consists of four tests of computations and word problems. You should be able to answer all the questions per test in 45 minutes.

Each test question consists of an incomplete sentence or a question followed by four choices. Read each question carefully, then decide which choice is the correct answer.

Your score will be the total number of correct answers. You may answer a question even if you are not completely sure of the correct response. Do not spend too much time on any one question. If you cannot answer a question, go on to the next question.

1. 6,143 − 387 =
    a. 5,756
    b. 5,766
    c. 5,856
    d. 5,866

2. Bill's heart beats 80 times in 1 minute. How many times will it beat in 15 seconds?
    a. 8
    b. 13
    c. 16
    d. 20

3. 2.06 × 5.08 =
    a. 11.948
    b. 10.5648
    c. 10.4648
    d. 10.0048

4. 6⁵⁄₁₂ − 2⅔ =
    a. 3¼
    b. 3¾
    c. 4¼
    d. 4¾

5. The American Diabetes Association estimates that 1 in 20 people will be diabetic at some time during their lives. In a city of 120,000 people, how many are expected to be diabetic at some time?
    a. 24,000
    b. 6,000
    c. 2,400
    d. 600

6.   0.15 =
      a. $\frac{1}{5}$
      b. $\frac{1}{6}$
      c. $\frac{3}{20}$
      d. $\frac{1}{15}$

7.   Which pair of values of x and y makes both these mathematical statements true: $4x + 3y = 14$ and $6x - 5y = 40$?
      a. $(x = 10, y = 4)$
      b. $(x = 8, y = -6)$
      c. $(x = 5, y = 2)$
      d. $(x = 5, y = -2)$

8.   1 mg = 0.001 gm. How many grams are in 256 mg?
      a. 0.2560
      b. 0.0256
      c. 0.00256
      d. 0.000256

9.   If $\frac{1}{2}$ of x = 64, then $\frac{1}{8}$ of x =
      a. 8
      b. 16
      c. 128
      d. 256

10.   A penicillin solution contains 300,000 units in 1 ml of solution. How many milliliters of solution are needed for a dose of 60,000 units?
      a. $\frac{1}{5}$
      b. $\frac{1}{2}$
      c. $1\frac{1}{5}$
      d. 5

11. $\dfrac{\sqrt{64}}{4} =$
      a. 16
      b. 8
      c. 4
      d. 2

12.   The daily cost of patient care in a certain hospital is $250. If the cost rises by 18%, what will the daily cost be?
      a. $268
      b. $295
      c. $322
      d. $450

13.   0.022 ÷ ? = 0.55
      a. 25
      b. 0.4
      c. 0.04
      d. 0.0121

14. Rectangle A has a perimeter of 36 cm. If the rectangle is 6 cm wide, how many centimeters long is it?
     a. 30
     b. 12
     c. 9
     d. 6

15. The difference between the boiling point and the freezing point of mercury is 396°C. The boiling point is 357°C. What is the freezing point?
     a. −39°C.
     b. −41°C.
     c. 39°C.
     d. 41°C.

16. Which is *NOT* a set of prime numbers?
     a. {5, 13}
     b. {2, 7}
     c. {19, 27}
     d. {3, 23}

17. $\dfrac{3/4}{6} =$
     a. 8
     b. 4½
     c. ⅔
     d. ⅛

18. Assume that the ratio of deaths resulting from heart disease to deaths resulting from cancer is about 5:2. For every 100 deaths resulting from cancer, how many deaths would we expect from heart disease?
     a. 40
     b. 225
     c. 250
     d. 500

19. 3.5% of 1,400 =
     a. 40
     b. 49
     c. 400
     d. 490

20. A baby's temperature dropped an average of 0.15° Fahrenheit per hour over a 12-hour period. If her initial temperature was 104.3°F. at 3 p.m., what was the reading at 3 a.m.?
     a. 102.5°F.
     b. 102.8°F.
     c. 103.5°F.
     d. 104.15°F.

21. In the expression $3a^3b^2c + 12a^4bc^3$ the greatest common factor is
     a. $12a^4b^2c^3$
     b. $3a^3b^2c$
     c. $3a^3bc$
     d. $3abc^2$

22.   A 32-oz. bottle of medicine is on hand. Each person (x) receives 4 oz. Which of these formulas shows the amount of medicine (M) left in the bottle?
   a.   M = $^{32}\!/_{4x}$
   b.   M = $^{28}\!/_x$
   c.   M = $4x - 32$
   d.   M = $32 - 4x$

23.   Labels measuring 2½ × 1½ in. are to be cut from a tape measuring 48¾ × 1½ in. What is the maximum number of labels that can be made?
   a.   17
   b.   19
   c.   24
   d.   39

24.   A circle graph indicates that ⅗ of the hospital budget is spent for staff salaries. How many degrees of the circle represent staff salaries?
   a.   60
   b.   108
   c.   144
   d.   216

25.   Two-fifths of one percent =
   a.   0.004
   b.   0.025
   c.   0.04
   d.   0.4

26.   A child's dose of medicine may be calculated from an adult dose according to the following rule:

$$child's\ dose = \frac{y}{y + 12} \times adult\ dose$$

where y represents the age of the child in years. How many milligrams are to be given to an 8-year-old child when the adult dose is 30 mg?

   a.   10
   b.   12
   c.   20
   d.   22

27.   In which of these problems is the value of ⅔ *changed* by the calculation?
   a.   ⅔ + 0
   b. $\frac{⅔}{1}$
   c.   ⅔ × ⅔
   d.   ⅔ ÷ ⅔

28.   The two shorter sides of a right triangle are 12″ and 9″. How long is the third side?
   a.   10½″
   b.   15″
   c.   18″
   d.   21″

29.   Suppose that 3¾ quarts of blood have been donated for blood transfusions, and 2¾ pints have been used. How many pints are left?
a.   2
b.   4¼
c.   4¾
d.   5¼

30.   If $3^{3x} = 729$, then x =
a.   2
b.   6
c.   27
d.   81

31.   What percent of 180 is 225?
a.   405
b.   145
c.   125
d.   80

32.   In a survey of community needs, 380 of 1,900 respondents said they wanted "purer drinking water." What percent did *NOT* request "purer drinking water"?
a.   20
b.   98
c.   72
d.   80

33.   ¾ of (½ + ¼) =
a.   ⁹⁄₃₂
b.   1
c.   ⁹⁄₁₆
d.   ³⁄₃₂

34.   Two rectangles are similar. One rectangle has a length of 12 cm and a width of 8 cm. The other rectangle has a length of 15 cm. What is its width?
a.   5 cm
b.   10 cm
c.   11 cm
d.   22½ cm

35.   A certain drug constitutes 2% of a solution. If there are 30 ml of the drug available, how many milliliters of solution can be made?
a.   150
b.   294
c.   600
d.   1,500

36.   If $A = \frac{1}{2}h(b_1 + b_2)$, then h =
a. $\dfrac{2A}{b_1 + b_2}$
b. $\frac{1}{2}A(b_1 + b_2)$
c. $\dfrac{A}{2(b_1 + b_2)}$
d. $\dfrac{b_1 + b_2}{2A}$

37. A medication has 3 parts of drug A to 7 parts of drug B. If there are 420 ml of the medication, how many milliliters of drug A are there?
    a. 60
    b. 126
    c. 140
    d. 180

38. $\dfrac{a^2 - ab}{b^2 - ab} =$
    a. $-\dfrac{a}{b}$
    b. $\dfrac{a}{b}$
    c. $\dfrac{a^2}{b^2}$
    d. $\dfrac{a^2}{b^2} - 1$

39. A rectangular room A has an area of 400 sq. ft. What is the area of a similar rectangular room the sides of which are all half as long as those of room A?
    a. 200 sq. ft.
    b. 160 sq. ft.
    c. 100 sq. ft.
    d. 80 sq. ft.

40. 120 ml of alcohol have been combined with 480 ml of water. The percentage of alcohol in the resulting solution is
    a. 20
    b. 25
    c. 33
    d. 40

II. Mathematics

45 Minutes

Work each problem carefully. Use scrap paper to do your calculations. The correct answers will be found at the end of section B.

1. When taking a patient's pulse, one counts 23 beats in 15 seconds. How many times will the patient's heart beat in 1 minute?
   a. 115
   b. 92
   c. 82
   d. 69

2. If $3y = 2x + 8$, and $x = 20$, then $y =$
   a. 48
   b. 18⅔
   c. 16
   d. 9⅓

3. $76.2 \times 1.04 =$
   a. 106.68
   b. 79.248
   c. 78.248
   d. 76.08

4. $3¾ + 1⅖ =$
   a. 4³⁄₂₀
   b. 4³⁄₁₀
   c. 5³⁄₂₀
   d. 5⅝

5. A cube measures 12 cm by 15 cm by 8 cm. What is its volume?
   a. 1440 cu cm
   b. 1360 cu cm
   c. 1584 cu cm
   d. 1225 cu cm

6. Which of the following fractions has the largest value?
   a. $\dfrac{1}{9 \times 3}$
   b. $\dfrac{1}{9 + 3}$
   c. $\dfrac{1}{9 - 3}$
   d. $\dfrac{1}{9 \div 3}$

7. A group of 25 runners recorded a total weight loss of 225 pounds after completing a marathon. What was the average weight loss per runner?
   a. 225 lbs
   b. 25 lbs
   c. 10 lbs
   d. 9 lbs

8. How many seconds are there in 3⅓ minutes?
   a. 200 sec
   b. 188 sec
   c. 180.33 sec
   d. 80 sec

9. Which of the following percentages equals 0.18?
   a. 18%
   b. 1.8%
   c. 0.18%
   d. 0.018%

10. 3.45 ÷ 0.15 =
   a. 0.023
   b. 0.23
   c. 2.3
   d. 23

11. The price of a certain medication is $8.50 per bottle. If the price increases by 7%, how much will a bottle of that medication cost?
   a. $8.57
   b. $9.10
   c. $9.20
   d. $14.45

12. To the nearest 3 decimal places, 367 ÷ 35 =
   a. 1.049
   b. 10.408
   c. 10.486
   d. 14.857

13. In order to allow tape recorders in class, school policy states that ⅔ of the students in that class must request to use a tape recorder. If 15 students out of 48 have requested to use a tape recorder, how many more must do so before tape recorders will be allowed in class?
   a. 16
   b. 17
   c. 32
   d. 33

14. At the start of a diet, Mr. Smith weighed 184 lbs. Eight days later, he weighed 179 lbs. What was his average weight loss per day?
   a. 5 lbs
   b. ¾ lb
   c. ⅝ lb
   d. ½ lb

15. The amount of iron recommended for a typical adult woman is 18 mg daily. One woman's average daily diet contains only 75% of the recommended daily amount. How much more mg of iron should her daily diet contain to supply the recommended daily amount?
    a. 3.5 mg
    b. 4.5 mg
    c. 10.5 mg
    d. 13.5 mg

16. $8a^3 \times 5a^4 =$
    a. $40\ a^7$
    b. $40\ a^{12}$
    c. $13\ a^7$
    d. $13\ a^{12}$

17. Of the children coming into a clinic, 7.5% have a certain condition. For every 150 children that visit the clinic, how many are expected to have this condition?
    a. 112.5
    b. 20
    c. 11.25
    d. 1.125

18. A patient is given three tablets (250 mg each) of a medication daily for 5 days. How many grams of this medication was the patient given?
    a. 0.375
    b. 3.750
    c. 37.50
    d. 375.0

19. Which of the following decimals is most closely equivalent to $5/7$?
    a. .35
    b. .57
    c. .71
    d. .75

20. A recipe requires 1⅓ cups of nonfat milk. A person already has ¾ cup. How much more is needed?
    a. $7/12$ cup
    b. $5/12$ cup
    c. ⅔ cup
    d. ⅚ cup

21. Which of the following values equals 0.35×10^4?
    a. 350,000
    b. 3,500
    c. 0.0035
    d. 0.000035

22. $3⅜ \times 2⅓ =$
    a. 6⅛
    b. $6^{17}/24$
    c. 7¾
    d. 7⅞

23. One tablet of children's aspirin contains 1¼ grains of aspirin, and an adult aspirin contains 5 grains. How many children's aspirin will contain the same amount of medication as two adult aspirin tablets?
    a. 12½
    b. 8
    c. 6¼
    d. 4

24. If your annual salary of $17,200 were increased by 5½%, what would your new annual salary be, to the nearest dollar?
    a. $17,209
    b. $17,295
    c. $18,146
    d. $18,150

Use the following diagram to answer the next question.

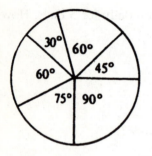

25. The central angle of 45° represents what percent of the circle? (to the nearest whole percent)
    a. 7%
    b. 13%
    c. 15%
    d. 20%

26. The triangles below are similar, with the sides of lengths 3m and 5m corresponding and those of lengths 9m and x corresponding. Find x.

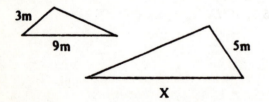

    a. 12m
    b. 15m
    c. 18m
    d. 20m

27. If 10 ml of a blood specimen contain 1.2 g of hemoglobin, how many g of hemoglobin would 15 ml of the same blood contain?
    a. 1.35 g
    b. 1.5 g
    c. 1.8 g
    d. 2 g

28. $6(.83) + .3(100) - 29.09 =$
    a. -23.81
    b. 5.89
    c. 34.37
    d. 64.07

29. The 6% sales tax on textbooks was $3.54. How much did the textbooks themselves cost?
    a. $3.75
    b. $21.24
    c. $55.46
    d. $59.00

30. If 30% of a number is 90, what is that number?
    a. 300
    b. 270
    c. 120
    d. 27

31. On a road map ⅛ inch equals 50 miles. How many inches will equal 125 miles?
    a. ⅔
    b. ⅖
    c. ⅜
    d. ⁵⁄₁₆

32. Which of the following illustrates the distributive property of multiplication?
    a. $3x + 4(a - 2) = 3x + 4a - 8$
    b. $3x + 4(a - 2) = 3x + 4a - 2$
    c. $3x + 4(a - 2) = (3x + 4)(a - 2)$
    d. $3x + 4(a - 2) = 4(a - 2) + 3x$

33. Solve the following system of equations

    $$3x + 2y = 16$$
    $$4x + 2y = 24$$

    a. $x = -4, y = 14$
    b. $x = 4, y = 2$
    c. $x = 8, y = -4$
    d. $x = 8, y = -8$

34. A baby drank an average of 7¼ oz during each of four feedings. If the baby drank 6⅜ oz, 7½ oz, and 7⅜ oz in the first three feedings, how many ounces were taken during the fourth feeding?
    a. 29
    b. 7¾
    c. 7¼
    d. 7¹⁄₁₂

35. If x% of 150 = 12, then x =
    a. 8
    b. 12.5
    c. 18
    d. 80

36. Which of the following values equals $\frac{9}{3/8}$?
    a. ½₄
    b. ⁸⁄₂₇
    c. 3⅜
    d. ²⁴⁄₁

37. Two rectangles have the same ratio of length to width. The first rectangle is 6 cm wide and 9 cm long. If the second rectangle is 12 cm long, how wide is the second rectangle?
    a. 8 cm
    b. 9 cm
    c. 15 cm
    d. 18 cm

38. Two angles of a parallelogram measure 60° each. How large is each of the remaining two angles?
    a. 30°
    b. 60°
    c. 90°
    d. 120°

39. What percent of 75 is 5?
    a. 15
    b. 6.67
    c. 5
    d. 3.75

40. What is the area of a triangle having a base of 10 cm and a height of 5 cm?
    a. 100 sq cm
    b. 50 sq cm
    c. 25 sq cm
    d. 15 sq cm

III. Mathematics

45 Minutes

Work each problem carefully. Use scrap paper to do your calculations. The correct answers will be found at the end of section B.

1. How many $2\frac{1}{4}$ fluid ounce bottles can be filled from a bottle that contains 9 fluid ounces?
   a. 20
   b. 7
   c. 6
   d. 4

2. $1\frac{3}{4} + 2\frac{5}{6} =$
   a. $4\frac{7}{12}$
   b. 4
   c. $3\frac{4}{5}$
   d. $2\frac{7}{24}$

3. 873.65 − 24.344 =
   a. 630.21
   b. 849.306
   c. 849.314
   d. 859.31

4. 50.29 ÷ 0.47 =
   a. 1.07
   b. 1.7
   c. 17
   d. 107

5. $\frac{4}{5} \div 4 =$
   a. $\frac{1}{5}$
   b. $\frac{5}{16}$
   c. $3\frac{1}{5}$
   d. 5

6. A tablet contains 2.5 grains of aspirin. If a patient takes 2 tablets every 4 hours, how many grains of aspirin will be taken in 24 hours?
   a. 60
   b. 30
   c. 20
   d. 15

7. A dieter lost 2.4 lb during the first week, 3.5 lb the second, 2.9 lb the third, and 3.0 the fourth week. What was the dieter's average weekly weight loss?
   a. 2.20 lb
   b. 2.70 lb
   c. 2.95 lb
   d. 11.8 lb

8. $\frac{5}{6} \div \frac{1}{3} =$
   a. $\frac{5}{18}$
   b. $\frac{6}{15}$
   c. $3\frac{3}{5}$
   d. $2\frac{1}{2}$

9. What is the maximum number of 1½ inch strips of tape that can be cut from a 480-inch roll of tape?
   a. 160
   b. 240
   c. 320
   d. 720

10. An income tax system requires that persons having a net income between $10,000 and $16,000 pay a tax of $800 plus 24% of that part of the income in excess of $10,000. How much tax should be paid on an income of $12,500?
    a. $600
    b. $1,400
    c. $3,000
    d. $3,840

11. Which of these decimals is approximately equal to ⅜?
    a. 0.21
    b. 0.37
    c. 0.43
    d. 0.73

12. What is the prime number that lies between 95 and 100?
    a. 96
    b. 97
    c. 98
    d. 99

13. A 3-oz serving of corned beef hash supplies 155 calories. Approximately how many calories will be supplied in a 5-oz serving?
    a. 274
    b. 258
    c. 248
    d. 93

14. A jogger travels x miles each morning. Which of these equations represents the number of days needed to jog 200 miles?
    a. $200x = $ days
    b. $\dfrac{200}{x} = $ days
    c. $\dfrac{x}{200} = $ days
    d. $200 + x = $ days

15. $176 - (-64) =$
    a. 112
    b. 240
    c. 11,264
    d. $-11,264$

16. $3y^2 \times 2y^4 =$
    a. $5y^6$
    b. $6y^6$
    c. $5y^8$
    d. $6y^8$

17. Factor completely: $4a^2 - 49$
    a. $(2a - 7)$
    b. $\sqrt{4a^2 - 49}$
    c. $2a(2a - 7)$
    d. $(2a + 7)(2a - 7)$

18. A man estimates that ⅕ of his salary is spent for taxes, ¼ for rent, and ⅒ for insurance. What fraction of his salary is left for other expenses and savings?
    a. ⁹⁄₂₀
    b. ¹¹⁄₂₀
    c. ³⁄₁₉
    d. ¹⁶⁄₁₉

19. If ⅔ of x = 48, then ½ of x =
    a. 16
    b. 24
    c. 36
    d. 72

20. Which of these values $= -(2^4)$?
    a. 8
    b. 16
    c. -8
    d. -16

21. If 33% of x = 99, x =
    a. 3
    b. 32.67
    c. 33.33
    d. 300

22. What percentage of 200 is 250?
    a. 150
    b. 125
    c. 80
    d. 50

23. If x is an integer, then the solution set of $6 < x \le 7$ is
    a. {6,7}
    b. {7}
    c. {6}
    d. Ø

24. How many degrees are in each unmarked angle of the parallelogram shown below?

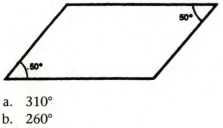

    a. 310°
    b. 260°
    c. 130°
    d. 80°

25. $\sqrt{45} =$
    a. $3\sqrt{5}$
    b. 9×5
    c. 15×3
    d. $5\sqrt{3}$

26. Barry has 4 more cards than Ken. Together, they have 44 cards. If x represents the number of cards Ken has, then which of these equations will represent the total number of cards?
    a. $x + 4 = 44$
    b. $2x - 4 = 44$
    c. $2x + 4 = 44$
    d. $x + 4x = 44$

27. A patient is to receive 3 grams of a medication over 6 days. If he is to receive 2 equal doses of the medication per day, how many milligrams will he receive with each dose?
    a. 1,500 mg
    b. 500 mg
    c. 250 mg
    d. 0.250 mg

28. If 75 ml of solution contain 30 ml of a specific medication, how much of that medication will be needed to provide 120 ml of the same solution?
    a. 18.75 ml
    b. 45 ml
    c. 48 ml
    d. 75 ml

29. How many liters are equivalent to 300 milliliters?
    a. 10
    b. 3⅓
    c. 3
    d. ³⁄₁₀

30. Four squares have been placed side by side to form the rectangle shown below. If the perimeter of the rectangle is 120 cm, what is the area of one square?
    a. 96 cm²
    b. 144 cm²
    c. 225 cm²
    d. 576 cm²

31. Which of these numbers has the smallest value?
    a. ¹⁄₁₁
    b. 0.45
    c. 0.7%
    d. ³⁄₂₀

32. Of 60 patients treated with a certain medication, 24 showed no improvement. What percentage of patients improved?
    a. 60%
    b. 40%
    c. 36%
    d. 24%

33. A temperature of $-15°$ Celsius (C) is equal to how many degrees on the Fahrenheit (F) scale? ($F = \frac{9}{5}C + 32$)
    a. 5°F
    b. 17°F
    c. 59°F
    d. −27°F

34. A state's sales tax is 7%. If a student paid $37.45 for a uniform, what was the price of the uniform without the tax?
    a. $30.45
    b. $34.83
    c. $35.00
    d. $40.07

35. If $\frac{3}{7} = \frac{5}{x}$ then x =
    a. $\frac{35}{3}$
    b. $\frac{15}{7}$
    c. $\frac{5}{21}$
    d. $\frac{7}{15}$

36. What percent of 80 is 15?
    a. 18.75
    b. 15
    c. 12
    d. 5.33

37. If the monthly expenses for a family are represented by a circle graph, how many degrees of the circle will be needed to show that 20% of the expenses are used for clothes?
    a. 20°
    b. 36°
    c. 54°
    d. 72°

38. How many 8-inch-by-8-inch tiles will be needed to cover a 12-foot-by-12-foot floor?
    a. 64
    b. 144
    c. 192
    d. 324

39. Which of these fractions is equal to 0.04%?
    a. $\frac{1}{2500}$
    b. $\frac{1}{25}$
    c. $\frac{1}{4}$
    d. $\frac{2}{5}$

40. The decimal that equals $\frac{1}{8}$% is
    a. 0.00125
    b. 0.125
    c. 1.25
    d. 12.5

IV. Mathematics

45 Minutes

Work each problem carefully. Use scrap paper to do your calculations. The correct answers will be found at the end of section B.

1. What is the arithmetic average of 7, 9, 21, 1, and 2?
   a. 5
   b. 8
   c. 21
   d. 40

2. On a certain day, 85% of a school's student body is in attendance. Which of the following statements can be made with certainty?
   a. 85% of each class is present.
   b. 15% of the student body is absent.
   c. 85% attendance rate is normal for the student body.
   d. 15% of most classes is absent.

3. $5a = 10b + 15$. If $b = 2$, then $a =$
   a. 3
   b. 5
   c. 7
   d. 35

4. A solution contains 9 mg of salt per 1,000 ml. How much salt would be needed to make 250 ml of that solution?
   a. 0.036 mg
   b. 2.25 mg
   c. 36 mg
   d. 2,250 mg

5. If $x = 6$, then $x^3 =$
   a. 18
   b. 36
   c. 216
   d. 1,296

6. How many liters are in 2,750 milliliters?
   a. 275,000
   b. 2,750
   c. 2.75
   d. 0.00275

7. Round off 6,845.0793 to the nearest hundredth.
   a. 6,845.079
   b. 6,800.079
   c. 6,845.08
   d. 6,845.07

8. The daily cost of a bed in a certain hospital is $225. If the cost rises 12%, what will the daily cost be?
   a. $237
   b. $252

    c. $260
    d. $270

9. $\dfrac{\sqrt{81}}{3} =$

    a. 27
    b. 13.5
    c. 9
    d. 3

10.   Withdrawal from a savings account left ⅔ of the original amount. Which of these decimals is approximately equal to ⅔?
    a. 0.92
    b. 0.86
    c. 0.67
    d. 0.42

11.   Ms. Smith went into labor at 10:35 p.m. Her labor lasted 11 hours 45 minutes. At what time was her baby born?
    a. 9:55 a.m.
    b. 10:10 a.m.
    c. 10:20 a.m.
    d. 11:15 a.m.

12.   If the replacement set for x is a set of positive integers, then the solution set for $x + 3 \leq 5$ is
    a. {1, 2, 3, 4, 5}
    b. {1, 2, 3}
    c. {1, 2}
    d. {1}

13.   Which of the following is a set of prime numbers?
    a. {7, 11}
    b. {0, 5}
    c. {−1, 7}
    d. {19, 39}

14.   Which of the following pairs of values are equivalent?
    a. 0.053 and $^{53}/_{100}$
    b. 0.499 and ⅘
    c. 0.0756 and $^{756}/_{10,000}$
    d. 0.6 and $^{6}/_{100}$

15.   From a bottle holding 1½ liters of solution, ⅝ liter was used. How much solution remains in the bottle?
    a. ⅞ liter
    b. 1⅛ liter
    c. ¾ liter
    d. $^{15}/_{16}$ liter

16.   Simplify: $6 - 2(x - 2y) =$
    a. $6 - 2x - 4y$
    b. $6 - 2x + 4y$
    c. $6 - 2x + 2y$
    d. $6 - 2x - 2y$

17. 39 is 30% of what number?
    a. 1,170
    b. 130
    c. 69
    d. 11.7

18. ½ of (⅓ + ⅙) =
    a. ¼
    b. 1
    c. ⁴⁄₉
    d. ⅑

19. On a scale drawing of a room, 1 inch represents 3 feet. How many feet are represented by 5¾ inches?
    a. 15¾
    b. 18
    c. 17¼
    d. 19

20. A survey shows 0.45 students in a class have brown hair. Which of these fractions indicates the proportion of students with brown hair?
    a. ¹⁄₄₅
    b. ⁹⁄₂₀
    c. ⅘
    d. ⁵⁄₉

21. In a health club, the ratio of joggers to swimmers is 7:2. For every 40 swimmers, how many joggers would we expect to find in this club?
    a. 280
    b. 140
    c. 129
    d. 11

22. One and a quarter cups of powdered concentrate are used to make 25 8-ounce bottles of infant's formula. How many cups of powdered concentrate are needed to make 80 8-ounce bottles of formula?
    a. 2.56
    b. 3.2
    c. 4
    d. 6.4

23. 4.6% of 150 =
    a. 690
    b. 32.6
    c. 6.9
    d. 3.26

24. What is the perimeter of a rectangle that is 15 cm long and 6 cm high?
    a. 21 cm
    b. 42 cm
    c. 90 cm
    d. 180 cm

25.   A cough syrup provides 15 mg of medication per 5 ml dose. How many milliliters are needed to provide 50 mg of that medication?
    a.   16⅔ ml
    b.   15 ml
    c.   10 ml
    d.   3⅓ ml

26.   The difference between the boiling point and the melting point of a specific substance is 80 degrees Celsius. The boiling point is 56°C. What is the melting point?
    a.   24°C
    b.   −24°C
    c.   36°C
    d.   −36°C

27.   If ⅔ cup coleslaw provides 60 calories, how many calories are provided by ½ cup coleslaw?
    a.   20
    b.   30
    c.   40
    d.   45

28.   A jogger averages ⅘ mile in 9 minutes. If this speed is maintained, how many miles can the jogger run per hour?
    a.   5⅓
    b.   7⅕
    c.   8⅕
    d.   8⅓

29.   A salesperson earns a salary of $250 for a five-day week plus a percentage of the total sales for each day. If the percentages of sales is earnings during one week were $83, $116, $49, $94, and $67, what was the salesperson's total income that week?
    a. $750
    b. $659
    c. $409
    d. $250

30.   What is the maximum number of ¾ lb bags of nuts that can be made from 48 lb?
    a.   16
    b.   36
    c.   60
    d.   64

31.   If a patient receives 300 mg of a certain medication four times per day, how many grams of that medication will that patient take each day?
    a.   1,200
    b.   300
    c.   1.2
    d.   0.3

32.   Before starting a diet, a person consumed an average of 3,000 calories per day. While dieting, that person consumed an average of 1,800 calories per day. By what percentage did the calories consumed decrease?
    a.   16.6%
    b.   40%
    c.   60%
    d.   66%

33. A shopper bought 6.3 lb of potatoes for $4.41 and 4.9 lb of tomatoes for $3.92. Which vegetable costs less per pound, and by how much?
    a. Potatoes cost 18 cents per pound less.
    b. Tomatoes cost 10 cents per pound less.
    c. Tomatoes cost 18 cents per pound less.
    d. Potatoes cost 10 cents per pound less.

34. A circle graph shows that 30% of a hospital's direct patient costs are for nursing care. How many degrees in this circle represent direct patient care?
    a. 108°
    b. 81°
    c. 54°
    d. 27°

35. Which of these fractions is exactly halfway between ½ and ¾?
    a. ⅝
    b. ⅔
    c. ⁹⁄₁₆
    d. ⅞

36. A multivitamin that contains 0.5 mg of vitamin B_6 supplies 23% of the U.S. Recommended Daily Allowance (USRDA) of that vitamin for adults. Find, to the nearest tenth of a milligram, the USRDA of vitamin B_6 for adults.
    a. 2.2 mg
    b. 2.0 mg
    c. 0.2 mg
    d. 0.5 mg

37. $(x-5)^2 =$
    a. $x^2 - 25$
    b. $x^2 + 25$
    c. $x^2 - 5x + 25$
    d. $x^2 - 10x + 25$

38. The expression 5.15x may be used to indicate the increase in the price of a daily newspaper over its price 30 years ago. Which of these percentages also expresses this increase?
    a. 515% of x
    b. 51.5% of x
    c. 5.15% of x
    d. 0.0515% of x

39. When packed in water, fruit cocktail provides 35 calories per ½ cup; and in heavy syrup, 80 calories per ½ cup. Water packing provides what percentage fewer calories than heavy syrup?
    a. 56.25
    b. 43.75
    c. 28
    d. 14

40. The area of a triangle with a base of 15 inches and an altitude of 6 inches is
    a. 21 in²
    b. 30 in²
    c. 45 in²
    d. 90 in²

Answers

I. Mathematics

1. **The answer is a.** This problem requires you to borrow twice.

$$
\begin{array}{r}
6143 \\
-\ 387 \\
\hline
5756
\end{array}
$$

2. **The answer is d.** You may set up a proportion to solve this problem. You will need to convert 1 minute to 60 seconds. Be sure to align the units correctly: beats across from beats, and seconds across from seconds.

   $\dfrac{80\ beats}{60\ sec} = \dfrac{x}{15\ sec}$ Cross multiply.

   $60x = 1200$ Divide both sides by 60 to solve for x.

   $x = \dfrac{1200}{60} = \dfrac{120}{6} = 20$ This is your answer.

3. **The answer is c.** Remember to line up the decimal points:

$$
\begin{array}{r}
2.06 \quad \text{2 decimal places} \\
\times\ 5.08 \quad \text{2 decimal places} \\
\hline
1648 \\
0000 \\
+\ 103000 \\
\hline
10.4648 \quad \text{4 decimal places}
\end{array}
$$

4. **The answer is b.** You will need to find the lowest common denominator before you add the mixed numbers. The LCD is 12, because 3 and 12 are both factors of 12.

$$
6\frac{5}{12} = 6\frac{5}{12} = 5\frac{17}{12}
$$

$$
-\ 2\frac{2}{3} = 2\frac{8}{12} = 2\frac{8}{12}
$$

$$
\rule{6cm}{0.4pt}
$$

$$
3\frac{9}{12} = 3\frac{3}{4}
$$

5. **The answer is b.** You may set up a proportion to solve this problem. Remember to align the units correctly: diabetics across from diabetics, and total across from total.

   $\dfrac{1\ diabetic}{20\ total} = \dfrac{x}{120{,}000}$ Cross multiply.

   $20x\ total = 120{,}000$ Divide both sides by 20 to solve for x.

   $x = \dfrac{120{,}000}{20} = \dfrac{12{,}000}{2} = 6{,}000$ This is your answer.

6.   **The answer is c.** Because 0.15 ends in the hundredths place, you may change it to a fraction by placing 15 over 100, and reducing the fraction.

$$\frac{15}{100} = \frac{15 \div 5}{100 \div 5} = \frac{3}{20}$$

7.   **The answer is d.** You can solve this "system of equations" by adding them together, in order to eliminate either the x-terms or the y-terms. However, to eliminate the x-terms or y-terms, they need to have the same coefficient but be opposite in sign (ex: 3y and −3y). To accomplish this, multiply the equations by the appropriate number. Make sure to multiply *each term* in the equation by the number you choose.

Multiply the first equation by 5, and the second equation by 3:

$5(4x + 3y) = 5(14) \rightarrow 20x + 15y = 70$ Now the equations can be added together.
$3(6x - 5y)\ 3(40) \rightarrow 18x - 15y = 120$ This will eliminate the y-terms.

Add the equations together:
$$\begin{array}{r} 20x + 15y = 70 \\ +\ 18x - 15y = 120 \\ \hline 38x = 190 \\ x = 5 \end{array}$$
Divide both sides by 38 to solve for x.

Now substitute 5 for x in either of the original equations to solve for y:

$4x + 3y = 14$ One of the original equations.
$4(5) + 3y = 14$ Substitute 5 for x, and simplify.
$20 + 3y = 14$ Subtract 20 from both sides.
$3y = -6$ Divide both sides by 3 to solve for y.
$y = -2$
$(x = 5, y = -2)$ This pair of values makes both equations true.

8.   **The answer is a.** You may set up a proportion to solve this problem. As usual, make sure you align the units correctly: mg across from mg, and gm across from gm.

$$\frac{1\ mg}{0.001\ gm} = \frac{256\ mg}{x}$$ Cross multiply to solve for x.
$x = 0.2560$ This is your answer.

9.   **The answer is b.**

Solve the first equation: $\frac{1}{2}$ of x = 64   "of" means multiply

$\frac{1}{2}x = 64$ Multiply both sides by 2 to solve for x.

$x = 128$ Plug this value in to the second equation.

Second equation: $\frac{1}{8}$ of x = ?

$\frac{1}{8} \cdot 128 = \frac{1}{8} \cdot \frac{128}{1} = \frac{128}{8} = 16$ This is your answer.

10. **The answer is a.** You may set up a proportion to solve this problem. As usual, make sure you align the units correctly: units across from units, and ml across from ml.

$$\frac{300,000\ units}{1\ ml} = \frac{60,000\ units}{x}$$ 　Cross multiply.

$300,000x = 60,000$ 　Divide both sides by 300,000 to solve for x.

$x = \dfrac{60,000}{300,000} = \dfrac{6}{30} = \dfrac{1}{5}$ 　This is your answer.

11. **The answer is d.**

$$\frac{\sqrt{64}}{4} = \frac{8}{4} = 2$$

12. **The answer is b.** Solve this problem in 3 steps:

First, change 18% to a decimal by dividing by 100:　18% ÷ 100 = 0.18

Second, calculate 18% of $250 by multiplying:

250	0 decimal places
× 0.18	2 decimal places
2000	
+ 2500	
45.00	2 decimal places

Third, add $45 (the 18% increase) to $250 (the original cost) to find the new cost:

$250 + $45 = $295

13. **The answer is c.** Rewrite this problem as a proportion in order to solve it:

$0.022 \div x = 0.55$ 　The problem again.

$\dfrac{0.022}{x} = \dfrac{0.55}{1}$ 　Cross multiply.

$0.55x = 0.022$ 　Divide both sides by 0.55 to solve for x.

$x = \dfrac{0.022}{0.55} = \dfrac{22}{550} = \dfrac{1}{25} = 0.04$ 　This is your answer.

14. **The answer is b.** Use the formula for perimeter of a rectangle to solve this problem:

$2L + 2W = P$
$2L + 2(6) = 36$ 　Substitute 36 for P and 6 for W.
$2L + 12 = 36$ 　Subtract 12 from both sides.
$2L = 24$ 　Divide both sides by 2 to solve for L.
$L = 12$ 　This is your answer:

15. **The answer is a.** The freezing point of mercury is certainly below its boiling point of 357° C. In fact, it is 396° C below that temperature. To find this value, subtract 396 *from* 357.

$357 - 396 = -39$ 　This is your answer.

16. **The answer is c.** 27 is not prime. Its factors are 1,3,9, and 27. The other choices are all comprised of 2 prime numbers.

17. **The answer is d.** Rewrite the complex fraction as a division problem, and then divide.

$$\frac{3/4}{6} = \frac{3}{4} \div 6 = \frac{3}{4} \cdot \frac{1}{6} = \frac{3}{24} = \frac{1}{8}$$

18. **The answer is c.** Set up a proportion to solve this problem. As always, remember to align the units correctly: heart disease across from heart disease, and cancer across from cancer.

$\frac{5}{2} = \frac{x}{100}$ Cross multiply.
$2x = 500$ Divide both sides by 2 to solve for x.
$x = 250$ This is your answer.

19. **The answer is b.** Change 3.5% to a decimal by dividing by 100: 3.5% ÷ 100 = 0.035

Next, multiply 0.035 by 1400:

```
   1400    0 decimal places
× 0.035    3 decimal places
   7000
+ 42000
 49.000    3 decimal places
```

20. **The answer is a.** Over 12 hours, the baby's temperature dropped 0.15° F each hour. To find the total drop in temperature, multiply 0.15 by 12:

```
    12     0 decimal places
× 0.15     2 decimal places
    60
+ 120
  1.80     2 decimal places
```

Subtract 1.8 from the original temperature to find the new temperature:

```
104.3
−  1.8
102.5   This is your answer.
```

21. **The answer is c.** The greatest common factor of the expression $3a^3 b^2 c + 12a^4bc^3$ is a factor that divides evenly into both terms. Only $3a^3bc$ has factors found in both terms of the original expression.

22. **The answer is d.** If each person (x) receives 4 oz., then 4x represents the total amount of medicine doled out:

EX: if it were 1 person, then 4 · 1 = 4 oz.
if it were 2 people, then, 4 · 2 = 8 oz.
if it were x people, then 4 · x = 4x oz.

Subtract 4x from the original amount to find how much remains: M = 32 − 4x.

23. **The answer is b.** First, find the area of each label you wish to make:

$$2\frac{1}{2} \cdot 1\frac{1}{2} = \frac{5}{2} \cdot \frac{3}{2} = \frac{15}{4}$$

Second, find the total area of the tape:

$$48\frac{1}{2} \cdot 1\frac{1}{2} = \frac{97}{2} \cdot \frac{3}{2} = \frac{291}{4}$$

Finally, divide $\frac{291}{4}$ by $\frac{15}{4}$ to find the maximum number of labels:

$$\frac{291}{4} \div \frac{15}{4} = \qquad \text{Invert the divisor and multiply.}$$

$$\frac{291}{4} \cdot \frac{4}{15} = \qquad \text{(cross cancel the 4's)}$$

$$\frac{97}{1} \cdot \frac{1}{5} = \qquad \text{Multiply.}$$

$$\frac{97}{5} = 19.4 = \qquad \text{19 maximum labels}$$

24. **The answer is d.** To find ⅗ of 360° (the total number of degrees in a circle), multiply ⅗ by 360:

$$\frac{3}{5} \cdot \frac{360}{1} =$$

$$\frac{3}{1} \cdot \frac{72}{1} = 216° \qquad \text{This is your answer.}$$

25. **The answer is a.**

Change two-fifths to a decimal: $\frac{2}{5} = 0.4$

Change 1% to a decimal: $1\% \div 100 = 0.01.$

To find $\frac{2}{5}$ of 1%, multiply 0.4 by 0.01:

$$
\begin{array}{rl}
0.01 & \text{2 decimal places} \\
\times\ 0.4 & \text{1 decimal places} \\
\hline
0.004 & \text{3 decimal places}
\end{array}
$$

26. **The answer is b.**

$$\frac{y}{y + 12} \cdot \text{adult dose} \quad \text{Substitute 8 for y, and 30 for ``adult dose''}$$

$$\frac{8}{8 + 12} \cdot 30 \quad \text{Simplify.}$$

$$\frac{8}{20} \cdot \frac{30}{1} \quad \text{Cross cancel.}$$

$$\frac{8}{2} \cdot \frac{3}{1} \quad \text{Multiply.}$$

$$\frac{24}{2} = 12 \quad \text{This is your answer.}$$

27. **The answer is d.** Adding zero, dividing by 1, and multiplying by $1 \left(\frac{3}{3} = 1 \right)$ do not change the value of a number. Only choice D alters the value of $\frac{2}{3} : \left(\frac{2}{3} \div \frac{2}{3} = 1 \right)$.

28. **The answer is b.** Use the *Pythagorean theorem* to solve this problem: $a^2 + b^2 = c^2$
The two shorter sides of the triangle (a and b) are 9 and 12. Plug them into the equation and solve for c:

$9^2 + 12^2 = c^2$ Simplify
$81 + 144 = c^2$ Combine like terms.
$225 = c^2$ Take the square root of both sides.
$15 = c$ This is your answer.

29. **The answer is c.** Change $3\frac{3}{4}$ quarts to pints by multiplying by 2 (there are 2 pints in every quart):

$$3\frac{3}{4} \cdot 2 = \frac{15}{4} \cdot \frac{2}{1} = \frac{30}{4} = 7\frac{2}{4} = 7\frac{1}{2} \text{ (pints)}$$

Subtract $2\frac{3}{4}$ *from* $7\frac{1}{2}$ to find out how many pints of blood are left:

$$7\frac{1}{2} = 7\frac{2}{4} = 6\frac{6}{4}$$
$$- 2\frac{3}{4} = 2\frac{3}{4} = 2\frac{3}{4}$$
$$\overline{}$$
$$4\frac{3}{4} \quad \text{This is your answer.}$$

30. **The answer is a.**

$3^{3x} = 729$ The question is asking: 3 to the what power = 729?
3 to the 6th power is 729. To make the exponent "3x" equal 6, x must equal 2.

31. **The answer is c.** This is one of three common types of percent problems. Turn it into an equation to solve it.

What percent of 180 is 225? Turn the problem into an equation.
$x\% \cdot 180 = 225$ Deal with the x percent at the end.
$x(180) = 225$
$180x = 225$ Divide both sides by 180 to solve for x.
$x = \frac{225}{180} = \frac{225 \div 45}{180 \div 45} = \frac{5}{4}$ Change $\frac{5}{4}$ to a decimal.
$\frac{5}{4} = 1.25$ Finally, multiply by 100 to get a percent.
$1.25 \cdot 100 = 125\%$ This is your answer.

32. **The answer is d.** If 380 of 1900 respondents want purer drinking water, then the remainder $(1900 - 380 = 1520)$ did NOT request purer drinking water.
To find what percent of the total this is, divide 1900 by 1520:

$$\frac{1520}{1900} = \frac{1520 + 19}{1900 + 19} = \frac{8}{10} = 80\%$$

33. **The answer is c.** Add the fractions within the parentheses first, and then multiply their sum by $\frac{3}{4}$.

$$\frac{3}{4} \cdot \left(\frac{1}{2} + \frac{1}{4} \right) =$$

$$\frac{3}{4} \cdot \left(\frac{2}{4} + \frac{1}{4} \right) =$$

$$\frac{3}{4} \cdot \left(\frac{3}{4} \right) = \frac{9}{16}$$

34. **The answer is b.** Because the two rectangles are similar, their sides are in proportion to one another:

$$\frac{12\ l}{8\ w} = \frac{15\ l}{x} \quad \text{Cross multiply.}$$

$12x = 120$ Divide both sides by 12 to solve for x.

$x = 10$ This is your answer.

35. **The answer is d.** You may set up a proportion to solve this problem. As always, make sure to align the units correctly: amount of drug across from amount of drug, and amount of solution across from amount of solution.

$$\frac{2}{100} = \frac{30}{x} \quad \text{Cross multiply.}$$

$2x = 3000$ Divide both sides by 2 to solve for x.

$x = 1500$ This is your answer.

36. **The answer is a.**

$A = \frac{1}{2}h(b_1 + b_2)$ Multiply both sides by 2 to clear the fraction.

$2A = h(b_1 + b_2)$ Divide both sides by $(b_1 + b_2)$ to solve for h.

$\dfrac{2\ A}{(b_1 + b_2)} = h$ This is your answer.

37. **The answer is b.** The two drugs are in the ratio 3:7. Because we know the total number of milliliters of the drug (420), we can write an equation, using the ratio that's been provided.

$3x + 7x = 420$ Combine like terms.

$10x = 420$ Divide both sides by 10 to solve for x.

$x = 42$ Now plug 42 back into our original equation to find out how much of each drug there is.

$3(42) = 126$ ml of Drug A

$7(42) = 294$ ml of Drug B $126 + 294 = 420$

38. **The answer is a.** First, simplify the numerator and denominator by factoring out common factors:

$$\frac{a^2 - ab}{b^2 - ab} = \frac{a(a - b)}{b(b - a)}$$

Now, factor out $a - 1$ in the denominator. This will make the expressions within the parentheses identical.

$$\frac{a(a - b)}{b(b - a)} = \frac{a(a - b)}{b(-1)(-b + a)} = \frac{a(a - b)}{-b(a - b)}$$

Now you can cancel the factor "$(a-b)$" in both the numerator and the denominator:

$$\frac{a}{-b} = -\frac{a}{b} \quad \text{This is your answer.}$$

39.   **The answer is c.** If the scale factor of two similar figures is a:b, then the ratio of their areas is $a^2 : b^2$.
The sides of the original rectangle are twice as long as the sides of the smaller triangle. This is a scale factor of 2:1.

Thus, the scale factor of the areas is 4:1. This means the area of the smaller rectangle is ¼ that of the larger rectangle.

¼ of 400 = 100 sq. ft.   This is your answer.

40.   **The answer is a.**
120 ml alcohol + 480 ml of water = 600 ml of solution.
120 ml of 600 ml = alcohol. To calculate this percent, divide 120 by 600:

$$\frac{120}{600} = \frac{120 \div 60}{600 \div 60} = \frac{2}{10} = 20\%$$

II. Mathematics

1. **The answer is b.** You may set up a proportion to solve this problem. As always, make sure to align your units correctly: beats across from beats, and seconds across from seconds. You will need to change 1 minute to 60 seconds.

    $$\frac{23\ beats}{15\ seconds} = \frac{x}{60\ seconds}$$ Cross multiply.

    $15x = 1380$ Divide both sides by 15 to solve for x.
    $x = 92$ This is your answer.

    Another way to solve this proportion is to note that $15 \cdot 4 = 60$. Therefore, multiplying 23 by 4 will give you 92, the answer to our problem!

2. **The answer is c.**

    $3y = 2x + 8$ Substitute 20 for x.
    $3y = 2(20) + 8$ Simplify.
    $3y = 40 + 8$ Combine like terms.
    $3y = 48$ Divide both sides by 3 to solve for x.
    $y = 16$ This is your answer.

3. **The answer is c.**

    $$\begin{array}{rl} 76.2 & \text{1 decimal place} \\ \times\ 1.04 & \text{2 decimal places} \\ \hline 3048 & \\ +\ 76200 & \\ \hline 79.248 & \text{3 decimal places} \end{array}$$

4. **The answer is c.**
    Find the lowest common denominator (LCD) before adding. The LCD is 20, because 4 and 5 are both factors of 20.

    $$3\frac{3}{4} = 3\frac{15}{20}$$
    $$+\ 1\frac{2}{5} = 1\frac{8}{20}$$
    $$4\frac{23}{20} = 5\frac{3}{20}$$

5. **The answer is a.**

    Use this formula to find the volume of a rectangular prism: $V = LWH$
    $V = 12 \cdot 15 \cdot 8$
    $V = 1440$

6. **The answer is d.** Because all of the numerators are the same, the fraction with the *smallest* denominator will have the largest value.

7. **The answer is d.** To find the average weight loss per runner, divide the total number of pounds lost by the number of runners.

$$25)\overline{225} \;\; \frac{9}{}$$

8. **The answer is a.** If each minute contains 60 seconds, then $3\frac{1}{3}$ minutes must contain $60 \cdot 3\frac{1}{3}$ seconds.

    $$\frac{60}{1} \cdot 3\frac{1}{3} = \qquad \text{Change } 3\frac{1}{3} \text{ to an improper fraction.}$$

    $$\frac{60}{1} \cdot \frac{10}{3} = \frac{600}{3} = 200 \quad \text{This is your answer.}$$

9. **The answer is a.** To change a decimal to a percent, multiply the decimal by 100, and tack on the percent sign:

    $$0.18 \cdot 100 = 18\%$$

10. **The answer is d.**

    $$0.15)\overline{3.45} = \qquad \text{Change the divisor into a whole number by multiplying by 100.}$$
    $$15)\overline{345} = \qquad \text{You must also multiply the dividend by 100.}$$
    $$15)\overline{345} \;\; \frac{23}{} \qquad \text{Divide to find your answer.}$$

11. **The answer is b.**

    First, change 7% to a decimal by dividing by 100: $7 \div 100 = 0.07$

    Next, find 7% of 8.50 by multiplying:

8.5	1 decimal place
x .07	2 decimal places
0.595	3 decimal places

    Add this product to $8.50:

    $$
    \begin{array}{r}
    8.500 \\
    + \; 0.595 \\
    \hline
    9.095
    \end{array}
    $$

    Finally, because we are working with money, round your answer to the nearest penny (or hundredths place): $9.095 \approx \$9.10$

12. **The answer is c.** When the problem asks for the answer to the "nearest 3 decimal places," this means you must round to this place (the thousandths place). To round this place, you must carry out your division to one place more than this: the 4th decimal place, or to the ten-thousandths place.

    $$35)\overline{367.00000} \;\; \frac{10.4857 \ldots}{} \qquad 10.4857 \approx 10.486$$

    Recall the rounding rules: if the number is 5 or bigger, round up. Because "7" is in the 4th decimal place, you must round the "5" up 1 in value.

13.   **The answer is b.** First find out what $\frac{2}{3}$ of 48 is: $\frac{2}{3} \cdot \frac{48}{1} = \frac{96}{3} = 32$

There need to be 32 students who request tape recorders. Since there are already 15 who have requested them, then 32 − 15, or 17 more students, need to request tape recorders.

14.   **The answer is c.** Solve this problem in two steps.
First: Subtract 179 from 184 to find the total weight loss. 184 − 179 = 5

Second: Divide the 5 pounds by the 8 days it took to lose this weight: $\frac{5}{8}$

15.   **The answer is b.** First, find out what 75% of 18 mg is by multiplying.

$$
\begin{array}{r}
0.75 \\
\times\ 18 \\
\hline
13.5
\end{array}
$$

Next, subtract 13.5 *from* 18 to find out how many more mg of iron are needed.

$$
\begin{array}{r}
18.0 \\
-13.5 \\
\hline
4.5
\end{array}
$$
   (It's ok to tack on a zero to the right of the decimal place.)

4.5   This is your answer.

16.   **The answer is a.** When you multiply powers with like bases, **add** the exponents.

$8a^3 \cdot 5a^4 = 40a^7$

17.   **The answer is c.** Change 7.5% to a decimal by dividing by 100:

$7.5\% \div 100 = 0.075$

Multiply 0.075 by 150 to find your answer:

$$
\begin{array}{r}
0.075 \\
\times\ 150 \\
\hline
11.250
\end{array}
$$
   This is your answer.

18.   **The answer is b.** First, calculate how many mg the patient is given each day:

250 mg · 3 = 750 mg each day

Next, calculate how many mg the patient is given over 5 days:

750 · 5 = 3750

Finally, the tricky part! These calculations give the answer in mg, but the question asks for the answer in grams! Change mg to grams by dividing by 1000, because there are 1000 mg in every gram.

3750 ÷ 1000 = 3.75

19. **The answer is c.** To change $\frac{5}{7}$ to a decimal, divide 5 by 7:

$$\begin{array}{r} .714 \\ \hline 7\overline{)5.000} \end{array}$$

$0.714 \approx 0.71$ Round the quotient to the nearest hundredth.

20. **The answer is a.** First, change $1\frac{1}{3}$ into $\frac{4}{3}$.

Next, find a common denominator for 3 and 4. The LCD is 12, because 3 and 4 are both factors of 12.

$$\begin{array}{r} \frac{4}{3} = \frac{16}{12} \\ -\frac{3}{4} = \frac{9}{12} \\ \hline \frac{7}{12} \end{array}$$ This is your answer.

21. **The answer is b.**

$10^4 = 10,000$

$$\begin{array}{r} 10,000 \\ \times\ 0.35 \\ \hline 3500 \end{array}$$

The shortcut for multiplying decimals by a power of 10 is to move the decimal to the **right** the same number of places as there are zeros in the power of 10. Following this rule, 0.35 becomes 3500!

22. **The answer is d.** Change each mixed number into an improper fraction and then multiply them.

$2\frac{1}{3} = \frac{7}{3}$ and $3\frac{3}{8} = \frac{27}{8}$

$\frac{7}{3} \cdot \frac{27}{8} = \frac{189}{24} = 7\frac{21}{24} = 7\frac{7}{8}$

23. **The answer is d.** Two adult tablets contain 10 grains of aspirin, so the question is really: How many children's tablets, each with $\frac{11}{4}$ (or 2.75) grains, will yield 10 grains?

$2.75 \cdot 3 = 8.25$ This is not enough.
$2.75 \cdot 4 = 11$ This is enough. The answer is 4.

24. **The answer is c.** This problem involves percent increase. Solve this problem in three steps:

    First, turn 5½%, or 5.5% into a decimal by dividing by 100:   5.5% = 0.055

    Second, calculate 5.5% of $17,200 by multiplying:

    $$\begin{array}{rl} 17{,}200 & \text{no decimal places} \\ \times\ 0.055 & \text{3 decimal places} \\ \hline 946.000 & \text{3 decimal places} \end{array}$$

    Third, add this amount to the
    original price to find your new annual salary: $17,200 + $946 = $18,146

25. **The answer is b.** Recall that all circles contain 360 degrees. (If you had forgotten this, you could have added up all of the angles.) Write a fraction of the information:

    $\dfrac{45}{360} = \dfrac{1}{8}$ Change the fraction into a decimal.

    $\dfrac{1}{8} = 0.125$ Change the decimal into a percent.

    $0.125 = 12.5\%$ Finally, round to the nearest whole percent.
    $12.5\% \approx 13\%$

26. **The answer is b.** Similar polygons have their sides in proportion. This means the ratio of corresponding sides is constant. Set up a proportion according to the relationship in the problem.
    The first ratio is → 3 cm side of first triangle: 5 cm side of second triangle
    The second ratio is → 9 cm side of first triangle: x cm side of second triangle

    Here is the proportion: $\dfrac{3}{5} = \dfrac{9}{x}$ Cross multiply.

    $3x = 45$ Divide both sides by 3 to solve for x.
    $x = 15$ This is your answer.

27. **This answer is c.** You may set up a proportion to solve this problem. As always, make sure you align the units correctly: ml across from ml, and g across from g.

    $\dfrac{10\ ml}{1.2\ g} = \dfrac{15\ ml}{x}$ Cross multiply.

    $10x = 18$ Divide both sides by 10 to solve for x.
    $x = 1.8$ This is your answer.

28. **The answer is b.** Multiply first, and then work the problem from left to right.

    $6(.83) + .3(100) - 29.09 =$

    $4.98 + 30 - 29.09 =$

    $34.98 - 29.09 = 5.89$

29. **The answer is d.** To solve this problem, turn it into an equation.

    6% of *the original cost* = 3.54
    0.06 of x = 3.54
    0.06x = 3.54   Divide both sides by 0.06 to solve for x
    x = 59.00   This is your answer.

30.   **The answer is a.** To solve this problem, turn it into an equation.

30% of a number is 90   The problem again.
30% · x = 90
0.3x = 90   Divide both sides by 0.3 to solve for x:
x = 300   This is your answer.

31.   **The answer is d.** You may set up a proportion to solve this problem. As always, make sure to align the units correctly: inches across from inches, and miles across from miles.

$$\frac{\frac{1}{8}\ in}{50\ miles} = \frac{x}{125\ miles}$$ Cross multiply.

$$50\,x = \frac{125}{8}$$ Multiply both sides by $\frac{1}{50}$ to solve for x.

$$x = \frac{125}{8} \cdot \frac{1}{50}$$ Multiply.

$$x = \frac{125}{400} = \frac{125 \div 25}{400 \div 25} = \frac{5}{16}$$ This is your answer.

32.   **The answer is a.** The distributive property of multiplication allows you to distribute across a sum or difference. This is easier shown then explained:

EX: 3 · (4 + 5)   The 3 is distributed across (4 + 5).
    3 · 4 + 3 · 5 Each addend in the parentheses is multiplied by 3.
    12 + 15
    27

In the problem, the only answer that illustrates this property is choice A:

3x + 4(a − 2) = 3x + 4a − 8   In this answer, "4" is distributed across "a" and "−2"

33.   **The answer is c.** You can solve this "system of equations" by adding the equations together in order to eliminate either the x-terms or the y-terms. However, to eliminate the x-terms or y-terms, they need to have the same co-efficient, but be opposite in sign (EX: 3y and −3y). To accomplish this, multiply the equations by the appropriate number. Make sure to multiply *each term* in the equation by the number you choose.

Multiply either the first or second equation by −1. For this problem, we'll multiply the first equation by −1.

−1 (3x + 2y) = −1 (16) →   −3x − 2y = −16   Now the equations can be added
              4x + 2y = 24 →   4x + 2y = 24   together to eliminate the y-terms.

Add the equations together:
$$\begin{array}{r} -3x - 2y = -16 \\ +\ 4x + 2y = 24 \\ \hline x = 8 \end{array}$$

Now plug in 8 for x into either of the original equations to solve for y:

```
4x + 2y = 24        One of the original equations.
4(8) + 2y = 24      Simplify.
32 + 2y = 24        Subtract 32 from both sides.
2y = −8             Divide both sides by 2 to solve for y.
y = −4
(x = 8, y = −4)     This pair of values makes both equations true.
```

34. **The answer is b.** Solve this problem in two steps:

First, multiply the average feeding by the total number of days: $7\frac{1}{4} \cdot 4 = 29$

Then, subtract each of the 3 feedings from this total. $29 = 27\frac{16}{8}$

You will need to find a common denominator.

$$6\frac{3}{8} = 6\frac{3}{8}$$
$$7\frac{1}{2} = 7\frac{4}{8}$$
$$-7\frac{3}{8} = 7\frac{3}{8}$$
$$\overline{\quad\quad\quad}$$
$$7\frac{6}{8} = 7\frac{3}{4}$$

35. **The answer is a.**

```
x% of 150 = 12      Deal with "x" being a percent at the end of the problem.
150x = 12           Divide both sides by 150 to solve for x.
x = 0.08            Now, turn 0.08 into a percent by multiplying by 100.
8% is your answer.
```

36. **The answer is d.**

$\frac{9}{3/8}$ is a complex fraction, but do not be alarmed. Remember that fractions mean division.

Just turn this complex fraction into a division problem.

$$\frac{9}{3/8} = 9 \div \frac{3}{8}$$

$$9 \div \frac{3}{8} = \frac{9}{1} \cdot \frac{8}{3}$$ To divide fractions, multiply by the reciprocal of the divisor.

$$\frac{9}{1} \cdot \frac{8}{3} = \frac{72}{3} = \frac{24}{1}$$ This is your answer.

37. **The answer is a.** You may set up a proportion to solve this problem. It is especially important to align the units correctly here, as the problem tries to be tricky, and lists the dimensions out of order! Make sure you put length across from length, and width across from width!

$$\frac{9\ length}{6\ width} = \frac{12\ length}{x}$$ Cross multiply.

```
9x = 72             Divide both sides by 9 to solve for x.
x = 8               This is your answer.
```

38.   **The answer is d.** You must recall a few geometry facts to solve this problem.
All quadrilaterals (a parallelogram is a quadrilateral—4 sides) have a total of 360 °.
Opposite angles in a parallelogram are congruent (same size, same shape).
Once you recall these facts, you're all set!
First, determine how many degrees are left in the 2 remaining angles:

$$360 - 2(60) =$$

$$360 - 120 = 240$$

Second, since each angle must be the same, divide 240 by 2 to find the measure of each:

$$240 \div 2 = 120°$$ This is your answer.

39.   **The answer is b.** Turn this problem into an equation:
What percent of 75 is 5?

x% of 75 = 5	We'll worry about the x% at the end.
x(75) = 5	Divide both sides by 75.
$x = \dfrac{5}{75} = \dfrac{1}{15}$	Change $\dfrac{1}{15}$ to a decimal.
$x = 15\overline{)1.00000}^{.06666}$	Multiply by 100 to find the percent.
$x = 0.06666 \cdot 100 = 6.666\ldots$	Round to find the answer.
$x = 6.666 \approx 6.67$	This is your answer.

40.   **The answer is c.**

Use this formula to find the area of a triangle:	$A = \dfrac{1}{2}bh$
Plug in the values from the problem:	$A = \dfrac{1}{2}(10)(5)$
Simplify:	$A = \dfrac{1}{2} \cdot 50$
This is your answer:	$A = 25$

III. Mathematics

1. **The answer is d.** This question is really asking: "How many 2¼'s are there in 9?" This is division!

    $$9 \div 2\frac{1}{4} = \qquad \text{Change } 2\frac{1}{4} \text{ to an improper fraction.}$$

    $$9 \div \frac{9}{4} = \qquad \text{Invert the divisor and multiply.}$$

    $$\frac{9}{1} \cdot \frac{4}{9} = \frac{36}{9} = 4 \quad \text{This is your answer.}$$

2. **The answer is a.** Find the lowest common denominator (LCD) before adding. The LCD is 12, because both 4 and 6 are factors of 12.

    $$1\frac{3}{4} = 1\frac{9}{12}$$
    $$+\ 2\frac{5}{6} = 2\frac{10}{12}$$
    $$\overline{}$$
    $$3\frac{19}{12} = 4\frac{7}{12} \quad \text{Remember to simplify your answer.}$$

3. **The answer is b.** Make sure you line up the decimal places before subtracting.

    873.650   It's ok to add this extra zero at the end of the number.
    − 24.344
    849.306   This is your answer.

4. **The answer is d.**

    $0.47\overline{)50.29} = \qquad$ Change both the divisor and dividend to whole numbers.

    $\phantom{47\overline{)}}107$
    $47\overline{)5029} \qquad$ 107 is your answer.

    Another way to solve this problem is by inspection. Once you've multiplied both the divisor and dividend by 100, inspect your answer choices. Of the four answers given, only "107" makes sense for this problem; all the others are too small. It is possible to answer this problem without dividing at all!

5. **The answer is a.**

    $$\frac{4}{5} \div 4 = \qquad \text{Change 4 to an improper fraction.}$$

    $$\frac{4}{5} \div \frac{4}{1} = \qquad \text{Invert the divisor and multiply.}$$

    $$\frac{4}{5} \cdot \frac{1}{4} = \frac{4}{20} = \frac{1}{5} \quad \text{Remember to reduce your answer.}$$

6. **The answer is b.** The patient takes 2 tablets every 4 hours. Because each tablet contains 2.5 grains of aspirin:

    2 tablets = 2 · 2.5 = 5 grains of aspirin every 4 hours

If the patient takes 5 grains of aspirin every 4 hours, then in 24 hours the patient takes aspirin a total of 6 times ($24 \div 4 = 6$).

6 doses $\cdot$ 5 grains each = 30 grains of aspirin.

7. **The answer is c.** Solve this problem in 2 steps:

Total the weight loss over 4 weeks: $2.4 + 3.5 + 2.9 + 3.0 = 11.8$

Divide the total weight loss by the number of weeks (4):

$$\begin{array}{r} 2.95 \\ 4\overline{)11.80} \end{array}$$

8. **The answer is d.**

$$\frac{5}{6} \div \frac{1}{3} = \qquad \text{Invert the divisor and multiply.}$$

$$\frac{5}{6} \cdot \frac{3}{1} = \frac{15}{6} = \frac{5}{2} = 2\frac{1}{2} \quad \text{Remember to simplify your answer.}$$

9. **The answer is c.** The question is really asking: "How many $1\frac{1}{2}$'s are there in 480?" This is division!

$$480 \div 1\frac{1}{2} = \qquad \text{Change } 1\frac{1}{2} \text{ to an improper fraction.}$$

$$480 \div \frac{3}{2} = \qquad \text{Invert the divisor and multiply.}$$

$$\frac{480}{1} \cdot \frac{2}{3} = \frac{960}{3} = 320 \quad \text{This is your answer.}$$

10. **The answer is b.** The tax to be paid will be $800 plus 24% of $2,500 (the income in excess of $10,000).

Calculate 24% of $2,500: $0.24 \cdot \$2500 = \$600$
Add $600 to $800 to obtain total taxes: $1,400.

11. **The answer is c.**

To change $\frac{3}{7}$ to a decimal, divide 7 into 3: $7\overline{)3.000}^{\,.428} \approx 0.43$

12. **The answer is c.** Recall that a prime number has exactly two factors: 1 and the number itself. The only prime number between 95 and 100 is 97: 96 and 98 are both even, and 99 is divisible by 3, 9, and 11.

13. **The answer is b.** You may set up a proportion to solve this problem. As always, be sure to align your units correctly: ounces across from ounces, and calories across from calories.

$$\frac{3\ oz}{155\ cal} = \frac{5\ oz}{x} \qquad \text{Cross multiply.}$$

$3x = 775$ Divide both sides by 3 to solve for x.
$x = 258.\overline{3}$ Round this to the nearest whole number.
$x = 258$ This is your answer.

14. **The answer is b.** The rate of the jogger is x miles each morning, or x miles each day. To help you figure out the problem, let's pretend that x stands for 10 miles each day (I just made up that number). Plug that in to the equations and see if it makes any sense:

    a. $200 \cdot 10 = 2000$ days. 2000 days, at 20 miles each day? If this were right, the jogger would travel a total of 40,000 miles! *Try another choice.*

    b. $\frac{200}{10} = 20$ days. 20 days, at 10 miles each day, would allow the jogger to travel 200 miles. *This is our answer!*

15. **The answer is b.** Recall the rules for subtracting negative numbers: *Subtracting a negative is like adding a positive.* Therefore,

$$176 - (-64) = 176 + 64 = 240$$

16. **The answer is b.** Recall the rules for multiplying powers with similar bases: ADD the exponents. Therefore,

$$3y^2 \cdot 2y^4 = 6y^{2+4} = 6y^6$$

17. **The answer is d.** The product $4a^2 - 49$ is known as a difference of two squares, because both the first and last terms are perfect squares, and one is being subtracted from the other. When this is the case, there is a short cut for factoring such a product. Knowing that your answer will be two binomials, you may assume the first term of each will be the square root of $4a^2$, and that the second term will be the square root of 49, and that the second terms will be opposite in sign. The signs must be opposite so that when multiplied together, their terms will cancel each other out.
    Thus, $4a^2 - 49 = (2a + 7)(2a - 7)$

18. **The answer is b.** Find the lowest common denominator (LCD) for all three fractions, and then change each of the fractions to an equivalent fraction with the new denominator. 4, 5, and 10 are all factors of 20, so 20 is the LCD. Then add them together.

$$\frac{1}{4} = \frac{5}{20}$$
$$\frac{1}{5} = \frac{4}{20}$$
$$+ \frac{1}{10} = \frac{2}{20}$$
$$\overline{\qquad\qquad}$$
$$\frac{9}{20}$$

If $\frac{9}{20}$ of the man's salary is spent already, then $\frac{11}{20}$ must remain.

19. **The answer is c.** Solve the first equation for x by multiplying both sides by $\frac{3}{2}$.

$$\frac{2}{3}x = 48$$

$$x = 72$$

Now substitute 72 for x in the second equation:

$$\frac{1}{2} \cdot 72 = \qquad \text{Change 72 to an improper fraction and multiply.}$$

$$\frac{1}{2} \cdot \frac{72}{1} = \frac{72}{2} = 36 \quad \text{This is your answer.}$$

20. **The answer is d.** Following the order of operations, first simplify the expression *inside* of the parentheses: $2^4 = 16$. Then, apply the negative sign: -16.

21. **The answer is d.** This is one of three types of common percent problems: finding the base when you know the percent and the percentage.

   33% of x is 99? Turn the problem into an equation.
   $33\% \cdot x = 99$
   $0.33x = 99$ Divide both sides by 0.33 to solve for x.
   $x = 300$ This is your answer.

22. **The answer is b.** This is another of three types of common percent problems: finding the percent when you know the base and the percentage.

   What percent of 200 is 250? Turn the problem into an equation.
   $x\% \cdot 200 = 250$ Deal with "x" being a percent at the end.
   $200x = 250$ Divide both sides by 200 to solve for x.
   $x = 1.25$ Change 1.25 to a percent by multiplying by 100.
   125% is your answer.

23. **The answer is b.** The problem calls for x to be greater than 6 (and therefore not equal to 6), and, *at the same time,* less then or equal to 7. Furthermore, because, x is restricted to being an integer (nor fractions or decimals), the only choice for x is 7.

24. **The answer is c.** You must know two things about parallelograms to solve this problem.

   1. There are 360 degrees in a parallelogram.
   2. Opposite angles in a parallelogram are equal.

   Once you recall these facts, the rest is simple:
   Subtract 100 (50 + 50) from 360 to calculate how many degrees the two unmarked angles have in total.
   Divide this amount (260) in half, because the two angles are equal. $260 \div 2 = 130$.

25. **The answer is a.**

   $\sqrt{45} = \qquad$ Split 45 into factors.
   $\sqrt{9 \cdot 5} = \qquad$ Assign each factor its own radical sign.
   $\sqrt{9} \cdot \sqrt{5} = \qquad$ Simplify.
   $3 \cdot \sqrt{5} = 3\sqrt{5}$

26. **The answer is c.**
   x = Ken's cards
   If Ben has four more cards than Ken, then Ben has x + 4 cards.
   If their total number of cards is 44, then $x + x + 4 = 44$
   $2x = 44$

27. **The answer is d.** The trick to this problem is not to forget to change grams to milligrams. The original amount of medication is given in grams, *yet the answer needs to be in milligrams.* Before starting any other work, multiply 3 grams by 1000 (1000 milligrams in each gram) to get 3000 milligrams.

    The patient receives 3000 milligrams of medicine over 6 days. Dividing 6 into 3000 yields the amount of medication each day:

    $$3000 \div 6 = 500 \text{ grams of medication each day}$$

    The patient receives 2 equal doses of medication each day, so divide 500 by 2:

    $$500 \div 2 = 250$$

28. **The answer is c.** You may set up a proportion to solve this problem. As always, be sure to align the units correctly: ml of solution across from ml of solution, and ml of medication across from ml of medication.

    $\dfrac{75}{30} = \dfrac{120}{x}$ Cross multiply.

    $75\,x = 3600$ Divide both sides by 75 to solve for x.

    $x = 48$ This is your answer.

29. **The answer is d.** There are 1000 milliliters in every liter. Therefore, 300 milliliters is less than a full liter. To calculate how many liters (or what part of a liter) 300 milliliters represents, divide:

    $$300 \div 1000 = 0.3, \text{ or } \frac{3}{10} \text{ of a liter.}$$

30. **The answer is b.** The rectangle is made up of four squares, each with the same length. The rectangle's perimeter is made up of 10 of these equal segments. Therefore, divide the perimeter by 10 to find the length of one of these segments.

    $120 \div 10 = 12.$ The length of a side of each square is 12 cm.

    To find the area of one of the squares, use the following formula: $A = s^2$
    $A = 12^2$
    $A = 144 \ cm^2$

31. **The answer is c.** To compare the four numbers, change them all to decimals.

    $\dfrac{1}{11} = 0.\overline{09}$ In this form, it is clear that 0.07 has the smallest value.

    $0.45 = 0.45$

    $0.7\% = 0.07$

    $\dfrac{3}{20} = 0.15$

32.   **The answer is a.** If 24 of 60 patients showed no improvement, then $60 - 24$, or 36 patients, showed improvement. To calculate what percent 36 is of 60, write a fraction, and change that fraction to a percent. You may reduce the fraction first to make your work easier.

$$\frac{36}{60} = \frac{3}{5}$$ Divide 5 into 3: $3 \div 5 = 0.6$

Change 0.6 to a percent: $0.6 \cdot 100 = 60\%$

You could also recall that $\frac{3}{5} = 60\%$. This is why it is helpful to know the common fraction-to-decimal-to-percent equivalents.

33.   **The answer is a.**

$F = \frac{9}{5}C + 32$ Substitute -15 for C in the equation provided.

$F = \frac{9}{5} \cdot \left(\frac{-15}{1}\right) + 32$ Change -15 to an improper fraction and multiply.

$F = \frac{-135}{5} + 32$ Simplify the fraction.

$F = -27 + 32$ Combine like terms.

$F = 5$ This is your answer.

34.   **The answer is c.** To find the original cost of the uniform (cost without tax), use algebra.

Let x = original cost of the uniform
Let 0.07x = the sales tax (7% of the original cost)

Therefore, $x + 0.07x = \$37.45$ Combine like terms.
$1.07x = \$37.45$ Divide both sides by 1.07 to solve for x.
$x = \$35.00$ This is your answer.

35.   **The answer is a.** By now, you are no doubt comforted by the familiar set up of a proportion!

$\frac{3}{7} = \frac{5}{x}$ Cross multiply.

$3x = 35$ Divide both sides by 3 to solve for x.

$x = \frac{35}{3}$ This is your answer.

36.   **The answer is a.** This one of three types of common percent problems: finding the percent when you know the base and the percentage.

What percent of 80 is 15?   Turn the problem into and equation.
$x\% \cdot 80 = 15$ Deal with "x" being a percent at the end.
$80x = 15$ Divide both sides by 80 to solve for x.
$x = 0.1875$ Change 0.1875 to a percent.
18.75% is your answer.

37.   **The answer is d.** Recall that there are 360 degrees in a circle. Once you know this, calculate 20% of 360:

$0.2 \cdot 360 = 72.$ 72 degrees represents 20% of the whole.

38.   **The answer is d.** *The trick to this problem is not to forget to make the units the same.* The tiles are measured in inches, but the floor is measured in feet. Convert the 8 inch by 8 inch tiles to feet.

To change inches to feet, divide by 12 (12 inches for every foot): $8 \div 12 = \frac{2}{3}$ ft.

Thus, the 8 inch x 8 inch squares are really $\frac{2}{3}$ ft. by $\frac{2}{3}$ ft. squares.

Each square measures $\frac{2}{3} \cdot \frac{2}{3} = \frac{4}{9}$ square feet.

The 12 foot by 12 foot floor measures $12 \cdot 12 = 144$ square feet.

To find out how many $\frac{4}{9}$ square feet there are in 144 square feet, divide.

$\frac{144}{1} \div \frac{4}{9} =$ Invert the divisor and multiply.

$\frac{144}{1} \cdot \frac{9}{4} =$ Multiply.

$\frac{1296}{4} =$ Simplify.

324 This is the number of tiles that will be needed.

39.   **The answer is b.** *Beware of this tricky problem!* You must realize that 0.04% is still in percent form, even though there is a decimal present. Change the percent to a decimal by dividing by 100.

$0.04\% = 0.0004$

Now, change the decimal to a fraction.

$0.0004 = \frac{4}{10,000}$ Reduce the fraction to find your answer.

$\frac{4}{10,000} = \frac{1}{2500}$ This is your answer.

40.   **The answer is a.** *This problem is tricky, too!* Basically, you must realize that the number given is still in percent form, even though you see a fraction.
Convert the fraction to a decimal, but remember that the decimal is still really a percent:

$\frac{1}{8}\% = 0.125\%$ Now change the percent to a decimal by dividing by 100.

$0.125\% = 0.00125$ This is your answer.

IV. Mathematics

1.   **The answer is b.** To find the average of a set of numbers, add up the numbers, and divide by the number of numbers added together.

   $$7 + 9 + 21 + 1 + 2 = 40$$

   $40 \div 5 = 8$ This is your answer.

2.   **The answer is b.** If 85% of the student body is present, then 15% of the same group—the student body—must be absent, because the two percentages must total 100% (the entire student body).

3.   **The answer is c.**

   $5a = 10b + 15$ The problem again.
   $5a = 10(2) + 15$ Substitute 2 for b.
   $5a = 20 + 15$ Combine like terms.
   $5a = 35$ Divide both sides by 5 to solve for a.
   $a = 7$ This is your answer.

4.   **The answer is b.** You may set up a proportion to solve this problem. As always, make sure you align the units correctly: mg across from mg, and ml across from ml.

   $\dfrac{9\ mg}{1000\ ml} = \dfrac{x}{250\ ml}$ Cross multiply.
   $1000\ x = 2250$ Divide both sides by 1000 to solve for x.
   $x = 2.25$ This is your answer.

5.   **The answer is c.** The equation $x = 6$ means that x and 6 are equivalent. Wherever you see x, you may substitute 6. Therefore, when you see x^3, substitute 6 for x.

   $$x^3 = 6^3 = 6 \cdot 6 \cdot 6 = 216.$$

6.   **The answer is c.** There are 1000 milliliters in every liter. Therefore, to change milliliters to liters, divide by 1000.
   If there are 2750 ml, then there are $2750 \div 1000 = 2.75$ liters.

7.   **The answer is c.** To round off the nearest hundredth, examine the digit in the *thousandths* place:
   If it is 5 or bigger, round the hundredths digit up 1.
   If it is less than 5, the hundredths digit remains the same.
   Here is the number again: 6,845.0793
   In this example, the digit in the thousandths place is larger than 5. Therefore, you round the digit in the hundredths place up one, from 7 to 8.

   6,845.0793 rounds up to 6,845.08

8. **The answer is b.** This problem involves percent increase. Solve this problem in three steps:

First, turn 12% into a decimal by dividing by 100:   12% = 0.12

Second, calculate 12% of $225 by multiplying:

$$\begin{array}{r} 225 \\ \times\ 0.12 \\ \hline 450 \\ +\ 2250 \\ \hline 27.00 \end{array}$$

Third, add this amount to the
original price to find the new price: $225 + $27 = $252

9. **The answer is d.**

$$\frac{\sqrt{81}}{3} = \frac{9}{3} = 3$$

10. **The answer is b.**

To change $\frac{6}{7}$ to a decimal, divide 7 into 6: $7\overline{)6.000}$ → .857 . . .

Round the quotient to the nearest hundredth to match one of the choices:

0.857 . . . ≈ 0.86   This is your answer.

11. **The answer is c.** If Ms. Smith's labor had lasted a full 12 hours, her baby would have been delivered at 10:35 a.m. However, her labor was 15 minutes shy of 12 hours, so subtract 15 minutes from 10:35 a.m. to arrive at her delivery time of 10:20 a.m.

12. **The answer is c.**

First, let's solve the inequality: $x + 3 \le 5$ Subtract 3 from both sides to solve for x.
     $x \le 2$ The first solution.

The problem states, in a rather fancy way, that only positive integers can be substituted for x. Our solution says these values must be less than or equal to 2. Therefore, the only possible values that are positive integers less than or equal to 2 are 1 and 2!

13. **The answer is a.** Only set A contains two prime numbers (numbers with exactly 2 factors, 1 and the number itself). The other sets are disqualified because 0 and 1 (and −1) are neither prime nor composite (have more than 2 factors), and 39 has factors other than 1 and itself (namely, 3 and 13).

14. **The answer is c.** You need to know the names of the decimal places to solve this problem. In choices A and D, the denominators of 100 do not match the decimal place names, while in choice B, 4/9 = 0.444 . . . , not 0.499. Only choice C displays the correct match: 0.0756 extends to the ten-thousandths place, and there is a 10,000 in the denominator of the accompanying fraction.

15.   **The answer is a.**

This problem calls for subtraction:

$$1\frac{1}{2} = \frac{3}{2} = \frac{12}{8}$$
$$-\frac{5}{8} = \frac{5}{8} = \frac{5}{8}$$
$$\overline{}$$
$$\frac{7}{8} \quad \text{This is your answer.}$$

16.   **The answer is b.** This problem uses the distributive property. The -2 outside of the parentheses is distributed (multiplied together with) each term inside of the parentheses. If you do not recognize the 2 as negative, consider changing the subtraction to addition:

$6 - 2(x - 2y)$ becomes $6 + -2(x - 2y)$
$\phantom{6 - 2(x - 2y) \text{ becomes } } 6 + -2x + 4y$ which is the same as $6 - 2x + 4y$

17.   **The answer is b.**

39 is 30% of what number?   Change this problem to an equation.
$39 = 0.3 \cdot x$
$39 = 0.3x$ Divide both sides by 0.3 to solve for x.
$130 = x$ This is your answer.

18.   **The answer is a.** Add the fractions within the parentheses first, and then multiply their sum by $\frac{1}{2}$. Remember to reduce the final answer.

$$\frac{1}{2}\left(\frac{1}{3} + \frac{1}{6}\right) =$$
$$\frac{1}{2}\left(\frac{2}{6} + \frac{1}{6}\right) =$$
$$\frac{1}{2} \cdot \frac{3}{6} =$$
$$\frac{3}{12} = \frac{1}{4}$$

19.   **The answer is c.** You may set up a proportion to solve this problem. As always, make sure you align the units correctly: inches across from inches, and feet across from feet.

$$\frac{1\ inch}{3\ feet} = \frac{5\frac{3}{4}}{x} \qquad \text{Cross multiply to solve for x.}$$

$$x = 5\frac{3}{4} \cdot 3 \qquad \text{Convert } 5\frac{3}{4} \text{ into an improper fraction.}$$

$$x = \frac{23}{4} \cdot \frac{3}{1} = \frac{69}{4} = 17\frac{1}{4} \qquad \text{Remember to simplify your answer.}$$

20.   **The answer is b.** You need to know the names of the decimal places to solve this problem. Because 0.45 ends in the hundredths, change 0.45 to a fraction with a denominator of 100, and reduce.

$$0.45 = \frac{45}{100} = \frac{9}{20}$$

21.   **The answer is b.** You may set up a proportion to solve this problem. As always, make sure you align the units correctly: joggers across from joggers, and swimmer across from swimmers.

$$\frac{7 \text{ joggers}}{2 \text{ swimmers}} = \frac{x}{40 \text{ swimmers}}$$ Cross multiply.

$2x = 280$ Divide both sides by 2 to solve for x.

$x = 140$ This is your answer.

22.   **The answer is c.** You may set up a proportion to solve this problem. As always, be sure to align the units correctly: cups across from cups, and 8-ounce bottles across from 8-ounce bottles.

$$\frac{1\frac{1}{4} \text{ cups}}{25} = \frac{x}{80}$$ Cross multiply.

$25\,x = 80 \cdot 1\frac{1}{4}$ Simplify.

$25\,x = 100$ Divide both sides by 25 to solve for x.

$x = 4$ This is your answer, in cups.

23.   **The answer is c.** First, change 4.6% to a decimal by dividing by 100: $4.6\% = 0.046$

Next, multiply 0.046 by 150:

$$\begin{array}{r} 0.046 \\ \times\ 150 \\ \hline 2300 \\ +\ 4600 \\ \hline 6.900 \end{array}$$ This is your answer.

24.   **The answer is b.** Use this formula to find the perimeter of a rectangle: 2W + 2L = perimeter

Substitute 15 for length and 6 for width: $2(15) + 2(6) =$
$30 + 12 = 42$

25.   **The answer is a.** You may set up a proportion to solve this problem. As always, be sure to align the units correctly: mg across from mg, and ml across from ml.

$$\frac{15 \text{ mg}}{5 \text{ ml}} = \frac{50 \text{ mg}}{x}$$ Cross multiply.

$15x = 250$ Divide both sides by 15 to solve for x.

$x = 16\frac{10}{15} = 16\frac{2}{3}$ Remember to reduce your answer.

26.   **The answer is b.** The difference between the boiling point and melting point is 80 degrees Celsius. This means that there 80 units (degrees) between the two points. If one of those points is 56, then you may find the other by subtracting: $56 - 80 = -24$.

27.   **The answer is d.** You may set up a proportion to solve this problem. As usual, make sure you align the units correctly: cups across from cups, and calories across from calories.

$$\frac{\frac{2}{3}\ cup}{60\ calories} = \frac{\frac{1}{2}\ cup}{x} \qquad \text{Cross multiply.}$$

$$\frac{2}{3}x = 60 \cdot \frac{1}{2} \qquad \text{Simplify.}$$

$$\frac{2}{3}x = 30$$

$$\frac{3}{2} \cdot \frac{2}{3}x = 30 \cdot \frac{3}{2} \qquad \text{Multiply both sides by } \frac{3}{2}$$

$$x = \frac{90}{2} = 45 \qquad \text{This is your answer.}$$

28.   **The answer is a.** You may set up a proportion to solve this problem. As always, make sure you align the units properly: miles across from miles, and minutes across from minutes:

$$\frac{\frac{4}{5}\ miles}{9\ minutes} = \frac{x}{60\ minutes} \qquad \text{Cross multiply.}$$

$$9x = 60 \cdot \frac{4}{5} \qquad \text{Simplify.}$$

$$9x = \frac{240}{5} \qquad \text{Simplify.}$$

$$9x = 48 \qquad \text{Divide both sides by 9 to solve for x.}$$

$$x = \frac{48}{9} = 5\frac{3}{9} = 5\frac{1}{3} \qquad \text{This is your answer.}$$

29.   **The answer is b.** Total the five sums (the percentages of sales for each day), and add this sum to the salesperson's base salary of $250.

First: 83 + 116 + 49 + 94 + 67 = 409
Second: 409 + 250
Answer: $659

30.   **The answer is d.** This question is really asking how many groups of ¾ there are in 48. Division!

$$48 \div \frac{3}{4} = \qquad \text{Invert the divisor and multiply.}$$

$$48 \cdot \frac{4}{3} =$$

$$\frac{48}{1} \cdot \frac{4}{3} = \frac{192}{3} = 64 \qquad \text{This is your answer.}$$

31.   **The answer is c.** *Don't be fooled by this problem!* It gives you information in milligrams, and asks for the answer in grams! To avoid being tricked, change mg to grams right away!

300 mg = 0.3g   (divide by 1000, because there are 1000 mg in every g)

If the patient receives 0.3 g of medication four times daily, this amounts to 0.3 · 4, or 1.2 grams of medication each day.

32. **The answer is b.** This problem involves percent decrease. Solve this problem in 2 steps:

First, calculate the drop in average daily calorie consumption:
$$\begin{array}{r} 3000 \\ -1800 \\ \hline 1200 \end{array}$$

Second, calculate what percentage 1200 (the drop) is of 3000 (the original total):

$$\frac{1200}{3000} = \frac{12}{30} = \frac{2}{5}$$

Convert $\frac{2}{5}$ into a decimal $(2 \div 5) \rightarrow 0.4$

Multiply 0.4 by 100 to find the percentage: $0.4 \times 100 = 40\%$

33. **The answer is d.** To find out how much each pound of potatoes cost, divide the total cost by the total number of pounds. Do the same for the tomatoes. Then compare the costs.

$$\frac{\$\,4.41}{6.3\ lbs} = \$0.70 \quad \$0.70/\text{lb. for potatoes} \qquad \frac{\$\,3.92}{4.9\ lbs} = \$0.80 \quad \$0.80/\text{lbs for tomatoes}$$

The potatoes cost $0.10 per pound less.

34. **The answer is a.** Recall that there are 360 degrees in a circle. To solve this problem, calculate 30% of 360 by multiplying:

30% of 360 =

$0.3 \cdot 360 = 108$

35. **The answer is a.** This problem asks for the average of two numbers. To find the average, add up the numbers, and divide by how many there are (in this case, divide by two):

$$\frac{1}{2} + \frac{3}{4} = \qquad \text{Now, divide } \frac{5}{4} \text{ by 2:}$$

$$\frac{2}{4} + \frac{3}{4} = \frac{5}{4} \quad \frac{5}{4} \div \frac{2}{1} =$$

$$\frac{5}{4} \cdot \frac{1}{2} = \frac{5}{8} \qquad \text{This is your answer.}$$

36. **The answer is a.** The problem states 0.5 mg is equal to 23% of the USDRA of vitamin B_6 for adults. Restating this as an equation, we have:

$$0.5 = 23\% \text{ of } x,$$
$$\text{or}$$

$0.5 = 0.23x$ Divide both sides by 0.23 to solve for x.

$2.1739\ldots \approx x$ The problem asks for the answer to nearest tenth. Round to the nearest tenth by examining the digit in the hundredths place. Because the digit in the hundredths place is 5 or bigger, you round the tenths digit up one.

$2.2 = x$ This is your answer.

37. **The answer is d.** Recall how to multiply binomials (expressions with two terms). This process is often called F.O.I.L., because it tells you what order to multiply the binomials together.

$(x - 5)^2 = (x - 5)(x - 5)$ In this problem, F.O.I.L. tells us to multiply:
the two First terms together: $x \cdot x = x^2$
the two Outside terms together: $x \cdot {}^-5 = {}^-5x$
the two Inside terms together: ${}^-5 \cdot x = {}^-5x$
the two Last terms together: ${}^-5 \cdot {}^-5 = 25$

When you add these products together, you get:

$x^2 - 5x - 5x + 25$ Combine like terms.
$x^2 - 10x + 25$ This is your answer.

38. **The answer is a.** 5.15x represents an increase in price. To find its percent equivalent, change the decimal to a percent by multiplying by 100:

$$5.15x \cdot 100 = 515\% \text{ of } x$$

39. **The answer is a.** First, determine how many fewer calories packing in water provides: $80 - 35 = 45$. Next, determine what percent 45 is of 80:

$$\frac{45}{80} = \frac{9}{16}$$ Change $\frac{9}{16}$ to a decimal.

$$16\overline{)9.0000} \xrightarrow{.5625} \to 56.25\%$$

40. **The answer is c.** The area of a triangle can be found using this formula: $A = \frac{1}{2}(bh)$

From the figure, substitute the appropriate dimensions: $A = \frac{1}{2}(15)(6)$

$$A = \frac{1}{2}(90)$$

$$A = 45$$

Bibliography

Dolciani, Swanson, & Graham, *Algebra 1*, Houghton Mifflin, 1992
Jurgensen, Brown, & Jurgensen, *Geometry*, Houghton Mifflin, 1988
Lowry, Ockenga, & Rucker, *Pre-Algebra*, D.C. Heath and Co., 1986
Moise & Downs, *Geometry*, Addison-Wesley, 1991
Smith, Charles, Keedy, Bittinger, & Orfan, *Algebra*, Addison-Wesley, 1988

SECTION B
MATHEMATICS ANSWERS

Science Content Review

General Biology

Cell Structure and Function

Cells are the smallest living units in all living things. Living cells are approximately 60% water and vary in size and shape. For example, a red blood cell is disk-shaped while nerve cells can be very long and have extensions on their main body. Cells also vary in terms of the role they play in the body. Despite these differences, there are features and functions common to many cells. The following description is that of a general animal cell.

The **nucleus** contains the genetic information, or **DNA** (deoxyribonucleic acid), and controls the activities of the cell. The **plasma membrane** is a semi-permeable membrane, that separates the contents of the cell from the surrounding fluid, the interstitial fluid. The **interstitial fluid** contains substances such as amino acids, sugars, fatty acids, hormones, neurotransmitters, and salts. The term **semi-permeable** refers to the selective nature of the plasma membrane. It contains pores and channels which only allow particles of the right size or chemical nature to pass through. Additionally, the plasma membrane contains receptors that bind specific substances. This allows for special entry or serves to signal the cell to perform a certain activity.

The cytoplasm is the fluid matrix found between the plasma membrane and the nucleus that acts as a scaffolding for the organelles. **Organelles**, which means "little organs", are specialized units in the cell that perform specific functions. The **mitochondria** is the location of cellular respiration, which is a process that converts foods to energy at the cellular level. Thus, the mitochondria is in charge of energy production, and it is where most of the ATP required by the cell is formed. **Ribosomes** are the sites of protein synthesis in the cell and, some ribosomes float freely while others are attached to the **endoplasmic reticulum (ER)**. The ER serves as a means for transport within the cell and is made up of many channels.

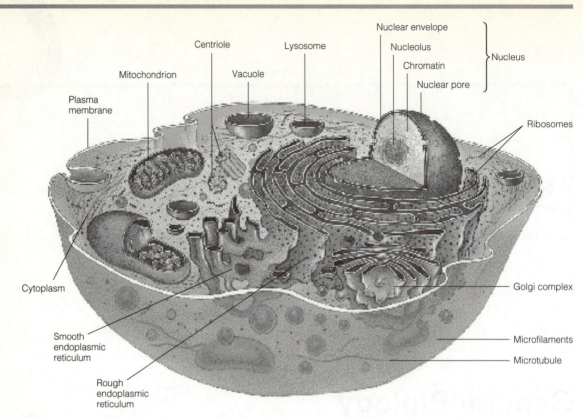

Figure 1.   Structure of a Cell

Rough ER, named for the fact that it has ribosomes on its surface, serves to store and deliver the proteins made by the attached ribosomes. Smooth ER is free of ribosomes and found mostly in liver cells. It is thought to be involved in detoxification of chemicals and the metabolism of fats. The **golgi apparatus** modifies and packages proteins destined for export of the cell. **Lysosomes** are sacs that contain strong digestive enzymes. They are responsible for digesting cell structures that are no longer living or malfunctioning and for digesting waste.

Plant cells can be distinguished by the fact that they are surrounded by a cell wall and that they contain chloroplasts. The cell wall is essential for protection of the cell, maintenance of the shape, and water balance. Chloroplasts contain chlorophyll, which is necessary for photosynthesis.

Cells divide for a number of reasons: growth, repair, and production of gametes. The most important aspect of cell division is that the genetic material, DNA, is transmitted to the offspring. DNA is a nucleic acid and is made up of nucleotides. Nucleotides are made up of a nitrogenous base, a phosphate group, and a 5-carbon sugar. There are two groups of nitrogenous bases: the **pyrimidines** and the **purines.** The pyrimidines are **cytosine** and **thymine** (C and T) while the purines are **adenosine** and **guanine** (A and G). Cytosines attach by covalent bonds to guanines while adenines attach in the same manner to thymines. In **RNA**, the thymines are replaced by the base, **uracil** (U), another nucleic acid important in protein synthesis, DNA is found in the nucleus in the form of chromatin and chromosomes. When a cell is not dividing, DNA is found in the form of loosely structured **chromatin**, while when a cell is dividing the DNA is seen in condensed rod-shaped bodies called **chromosomes.**

When cells divide, the appropriate amount of genetic material must be passed on to the new, or "daughter," cells. In the case of somatic cells, the new cells are identical copies of the parent cells. This is achieved by a doubling of the chromosomes prior to the division.

This type of cell division is referred to as **mitosis** and is useful in growth and repair in our bodies. Another type of division takes place in the production of gametes, or sperm and eggs. These cells contain half of the normal complement of chromosomes so that the **zygote**, created by the union of a sperm and egg, contains a full set of chromosomes, half from each parent. This type of division, or **meiosis**, consists of a doubling of chromosomes and two subsequent divisions. Thus, the products are four daughter cells with half the normal number of chromosomes.

Levels of Organization

Cells with common structure and function make up **tissues.** Tissues can be classified in four main categories: **muscle tissue** (skeletal, cardiac, and smooth), **epithilial tissue** (skin, lining of organs), **nervous tissue** (neurons) and **connective tissue** (cartilage, blood, fat, bone). Various tissues are combined into an organ that performs a specialized function in the body. For instance, the stomach is involved in digestion and is made up of three types of tissue. The next level of organization is the **organ system**, which is made up of a number of organs working together to carry out a major function. For example, the circulatory system includes many organs such as the heart, blood vessels, spleen, tonsils, and lymph nodes. These organs work together to circulate and deliver necessary products throughout the body. The highest level of organization is the **organism** itself.

Evolution: Evidence and Theories

In 1859 Charles Darwin published "On the Origin of Species by Means of Natural Selection" which presented evidence for evolution. Evolution is a theory regarding the processes that have produced the biological diversity that we see today. Darwin's two main arguments were that present species have evolved from ancestral ones and that evolution occurs via a mechanism called **natural selection.** Natural selection refers to the process by which those traits that promote or enhance an organism's ability to survive and reproduce are passed on to following generations. Evidence for the theory of evolution does exist. For instance, the **fossil record** supports the idea of evolution. Fossils that have been dated show a timeline of the appearance of different organisms in the order: fish, then amphibians, then reptiles, and finally mammals and birds. This finding supports Darwin's first evolutionary argument and contradicts the theory that all species were created at the same time. Many other types of evidence have been found through studies of biogeography, comparative anatomy, and molecular biology.

Evolution: Classification of Organisms

Due to the great degree of biological diversity on our planet, it has been necessary to establish a means of organizing the different species into groups. **Taxonomists** place separate species into groups according to their similarities and differences, and there are many different levels of classification, each more specific than the level above it. The broadest units of classification are the **kingdoms,** of which there are five: animal, plant, bacteria, protist, and fungi. The next six classifications become increasingly specific: **phylum, class, order, family, genus, and species.** The scientific name of an organism is always the genus and the species of the organism.

Diffusion and Osmosis

The processes through which the plasma membrane controls entry and exit can be either passive or active. **Active transport** involves the use of energy in the form of ATP to move substances across the membrane. **Passive transport** does not require energy and includes diffusion and filtration. **Diffusion** is the process by which particles moving in a random matter spread evenly throughout an available space, moving from regions of high concentration to low concentration. For instance, perfume or smoke pervade an entire room due to this process. A specific type of diffusion is the diffusion of water, **osmosis.** Water moves from an area of low particle concentration to high particle concentration (or, high water concentration to low water concentration). Red blood cells provide a good example of osmosis. When these cells are in a solution of the same concentration, or an **isotonic** solution, the amount of water that leaves and enters is equal. In the case in which the solution is more concentrated, or **hypertonic**, water leaves the cell due to osmosis. Thus, the cell shrinks. If the concentration outside the cell is less than that inside the cell, or **hypotonic**, water flows into the cell and the cell bursts.

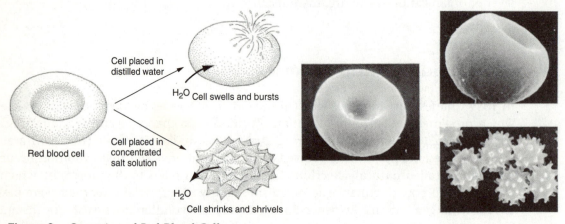

Figure 2.   Osmosis and Red Blood Cell

Filtration involves the movement of water and solutes through the membrane by fluid pressure, or hydrostatic pressure.

Ecology: Interrelationships

Autotrophs produce their own food from inorganic substances. Plants are autotrophs and are discussed in greater detail below. **Heterotrophs,** on the other hand, obtain their food by consuming plants or other animals. They are also referred to as ''**consumers.**'' **Primary consumers** are herbivores while **secondary consumers** are carnivores that eat herbivores. **Tertiary consumers** are carnivores that eat other carnivores. These divisions, that are made on the basis of how the organism meets its nutritional needs make up the **trophic levels** of an **ecosystem.** The autotrophs are the most important trophic level in the ecosystem, and the next levels are made up of the different types of consumers mentioned earlier. The pathway along which food is transferred between these levels is called a **food chain**, and the relationship between many food chains is called a **food web.** An important part of an ecosystem is the **decomposers**, such as bacteria and fungi, which consume non-living organic material and release inorganic material. Thus, material is recycled through the ecosystem and inorganic material is made available to the plants.

On a larger scale, a **biosphere** is the entire portion of our planet that is inhabited by living things in a variety of ecosytems and communities. Within the biosphere are groups of organisms that are common to a type of geographical area. These are called **biomes.** Many of the terrestrial biomes are based upon differences in climate. Some of the most familiar terrestrial biomes are **deserts, tropical forests, deciduous forests, coniferous forests,** and **tundras.** Tropical forests typically have a constant temperature and daylight length throughout the year with variable amounts of precipitation. Deserts on the other hand have little precipitation and are more arid than all of the other biomes. Temperate deciduous forests are usually found in midlatitude regions where the air contains enough moisture to support the growth of large trees. Deciduous trees, such as oaks and maples, are ones that drop their leaves during dry months. The temperatures in this biome are not constant and can range from season to season. Coniferous forests (taigas) are found at high and cool elevations and the seasons consist of short summers and long and chilly winters. Conifers, such as pine and firs, are found in these areas. Finally, tundras are biomes that are characterized by very cold temperatures and high altitude. Here the conditions allow for the growth of shrubs and bushes, but no trees.

Aquatic biomes are abundant as well. Some familiar ones include swamps, wetlands, rivers and streams, coral reefs, and estuaries.

Plants and Photosynthesis

All organisms obtain the organic substances they need via **autotrophic** or **heterotrophic** means. Autotrophs make their own organic molecules from inorganic molecules in the environment. Autotrophs for this reason are also referred to as "**producers.**" The method by which they accomplish this is called **photosynthesis**, in which light energy is absorbed by the pigment chlorophyll which is located in the chloroplasts of plant cells. This energy drives the synthesis of food molecules:

$$6CO_2 + 6H_2O + \text{light energy} \rightarrow C_6H_{12}O_6 + 6O_2$$

Plants have acquired some unique characteristics to help them survive in a terrestrial environment. Most plants have a **cuticle** covering their stems and leaves, which is a waxy layer that aids in the prevention of water loss via evaporation. Additionally, the leaves have **stomata**, which are pores in the surface so that carbon dioxide can enter and oxygen can be released during photosynthesis. The flower in flowering plants, or **angiosperms**, is responsible for reproduction of an angiosperm. The **sepals** encase the flower before it blooms, and the **petals** are useful in attracting pollinators. In the center of the petals are the **stamen** and **carpels.** The stamen consists of the **filament**, which supports the **anther** where pollen is produced. At the base of the carpel is a **style**, which leads to the **ovary.** After fertilization, the ovules within the ovary develop into **seeds.** After fertilization the walls of the ovary thicken to protect the seed, and this thick fleshy protective layer is what we know and love as **fruit!**

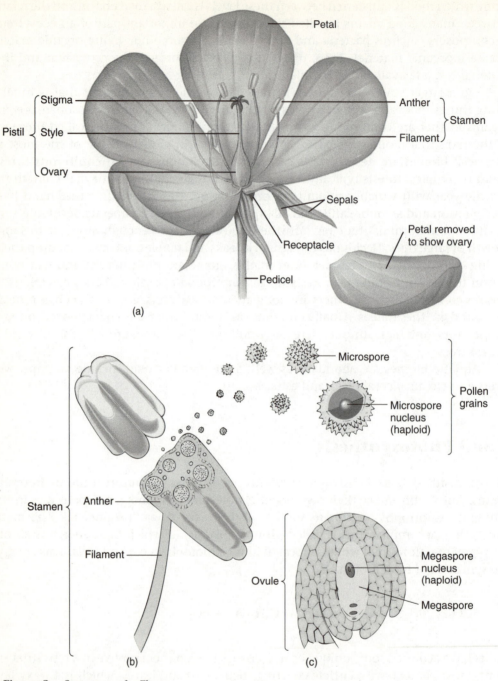

Figure 3.   Structure of a Flower

Genetics

In 1857, **Gregor Mendel** began breeding garden peas in the abbey garden of the monastery in which he resided. Heredity was not a new question, but it had not been researched in an organized manner through the collection of data and use of controls. It is thought that Mendel chose to work with peas because they have many distinguishable characteristics such as color or shape. Mendel followed many generations of pea plants in a very controlled and meticulous manner and discovered two fundamental principles of heredity.

The first principle is that alternate versions of genes account for the variation in characters that are inherited. These alternate versions are now called **alleles.** For instance, the green seed allele and the yellow seed allele are two DNA variations possible at the seed-color location, or locus, on one of the pea plant's chromosomes.

Additionally, Mendel found that for every character, an organism inherits two alleles, one from each parent. The two alleles can be different, for instance, one may be the dominant allele which is fully expressed, while one may be the recessive allele which has no affect on the appearance of the organism. For example, if the character under study is eye color, it is known that brown eyes are dominant over blue eyes. If B represents the **dominant** allele, and b represents the **recessive** allele then there are three possibilities due to different combinations of the two alleles. An individual who is BB has brown eyes and is termed **homozygous** dominant due to the presence of two dominant alleles. A person who is Bb is **heterozygous** and is brown-eyed due to the presence of the one dominant allele. Finally, a person who is bb for this character will be blue-eyed and is termed **homozygous recessive.** When gametes are made during meiosis, each contain one of the alleles for each character from each parent. Thus, the progeny's genetic make-up have contributions from both parents.

Unfortunately all of genetics is not a simple as yellow versus green seeds and blue versus brown eyes! For instance, some characters are sex-linked, meaning that they are located on the sex chromosomes and thus are transmitted to the progeny in a different way. Or, for example, not all characters are controlled by one allele as some are contributed to by many. However, Gregor Mendel's work supplied the basis for modern genetics and his contributions have been indispensible in the study of heredity.

Research Procedures

Microscopes greatly affected the progress of science, allowing scientists to see cells, when they were introduced in the seventeenth century. In a **light microscope**, light is first passed through a specimen and then through a glass lens, which bends light in such a manner that the image of the specimen under observation is magnified. Many internal structures of the cell are too small to be seen through the light microscope and thus the invention of the electron microscope in the 1950s greatly enhanced the study of cell biology. The **electron microscope** sends a beam of electrons through a specimen and can be used to see structures that are too small to be seen through the light microscope. The light microscope can be used for objects between 1 and 100 μm while an electron microscope can be used to see objects from 0.2 to 100 nm.

Human Anatomy and Physiology

Digestion

Humans, as opposed to more simple animals such as jellyfish, have a digestive system that is composed of a tube that extends between two openings, the mouth and the anus. This tube, or the **alimentary canal**, is organized into specialized regions that carry out specific portions of the digestive process. Food enters through the mouth where it is chewed, increasing the surface area, which makes it easier to both swallow and digest. The presence of food also stimulates the salivary glands to release saliva which contains the enzyme amylase. **Amylase** breaks down starch into smaller polysaccharides and disaccharides. As the food is swallowed it is pushed by the tongue into the **pharynx** (throat) which leads to both the windpipe and the **esophogus.** During swallowing, the top of the windpipe is covered by the **glottis** to prevent food from entering the respiratory system. From the esophogus, the food is passed

Figure 4. Digestive System

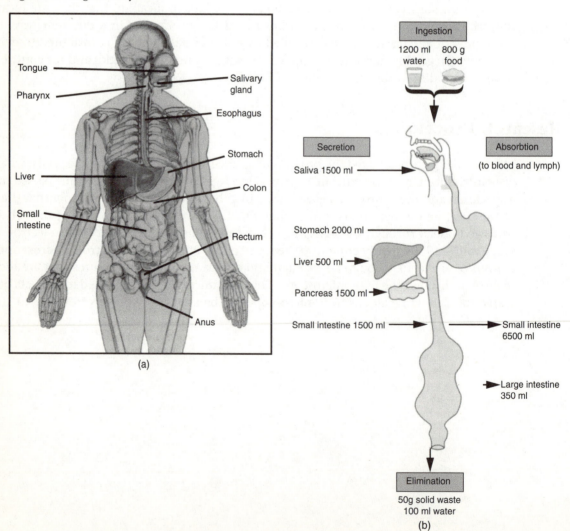

(a)

(b)

to the **stomach.** The lining of the stomach releases **gastric juice** which mixes with the food. It contains a great deal of hydrochloric acid, which has a very acidic pH (around 2). This helps to break down proteins and activates other enzymes. Fortunately, cells in the stomach lining secrete mucus, which protects the stomach wall from the action of the very acidic gastric juice. The smooth muscles of the stomach mix the partially digested food, and the result is a liquid called **chyme.** Small portions of this chyme are released to the **small intestine** through the **pyloric sphincter**, and it is here that most of the digestion of the food takes place. The small intestine can be up to 6 meters long in humans and is not only the major site of digestion but also the major site for absorption of nutrients into the blood stream. Contributing to the digestion taking place here are the liver, the **pancreas**, and the **gallbladder.** The liver produces **bile**, a substance stored in the gall bladder, which helps in the break down of fats. The pancreas supplies a number of enzymes needed for digestion. Next, the food travels to the **large intestine**, or **colon**, which is responsible for reabsorbing water that has entered the alimentary canal. Thus the waste, or feces, that moves along the colon by **peristalsis** (contractions of the tube) becomes increasingly solidified and is ultimately stored in the rectum until excretion. Diarrhea is a result of peristalsis moving feces through the colon too quickly so that water is not reabsorbed, whereas constipation results from too little persitalsis and thus too much reabsorption of water.

Circulation: Cardiovascular and Lymphatic Systems

Circulation refers to the internal transport of fluid throughout the body, which allows for the exchange of gases, absorption of nutrients, and the disposal of waste. The circulatory system is thus made up of the cardiovascular system and the lymphatic system, which function together to achieve these goals.

The cardiovascular system in humans is made up of the heart, blood vessels, and blood. The heart contains two **atria** (receive blood) and two **ventricles** (pump blood). The pathway of blood through the heart, beginning arbitrarily at the lungs, is as follows: blood leaves the

Figure 5.   Human Heart

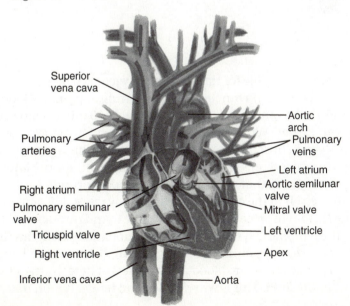

lungs via the **pulmonary veins**, where it picks up oxygen and unloads carbon dioxide and is thus oxygenated. The pulmonary veins take the blood to the left atrium where it fills this chamber until the pressure is great enough to force open the **atrioventricular valve.** Blood then enters the left ventricle and when the pressure is great enough, the atrioventricular valve closes, and the blood is expelled through the **aortic valve** into the **aorta**, which supplies the body's tissues with oxygen and picks up carbon dioxide. As the blood leaves the tissues by way of the **systemic veins**, or inferior and superior vena cavae, it is deoxygenated or without oxygen. This deoxygenated blood enters the right atrium and passes to the right ventricle through another atrioventricular valve. From here it is pumped through the semilunar valve into the **pulmonary artery**, which carries the blood to the lungs where the cycle begins again.

Interestingly, **blood** is considered a type of connective tissue that is made up of a variety of cells suspended in a liquid called plasma. Red blood cells, white blood cells, and platelets make up 45% of whole blood while **plasma**, which contains proteins, ions, hormones, and gases, makes up the other 55%.

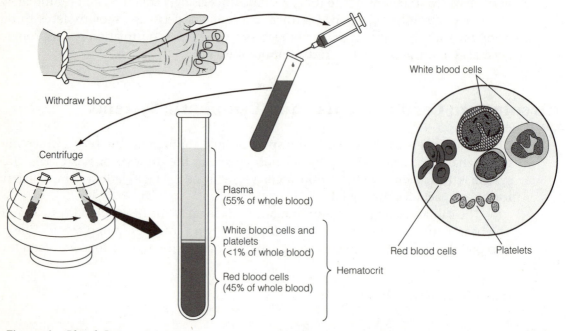

Figure 6. Blood Composition

Red blood cells, or erythrocytes, are responsible for transporting oxygen. Red blood cells do not have nuclei or mitochondria. To suit their main function of transporting oxygen, red blood cells are small and thin (to allow for diffusion) and contain approximately 250 million molecules of **hemoglobin**, which is an oxygen carrier. White blood cells, or leukocytes, are less abundant than red blood cells and are involved in host immune defense. Not surprisingly, an infection is indicated when the number of white blood cells exceed the normal concentration. **Platelets** are also found in plasma and are pieces of cells that are important in blood clotting.

As blood passes through the vessels of the circulatory system, leakage of fluid and proteins can occur. This lost fluid diffuses into **lymph capillaries**, which are found throughout the cardiovascular system, and enters the lymphatic system. Inside the lymphatic system, this fluid, or **lymph**, returns to the circulatory system. **Lymph nodes** are special pockets in the lymphatic system where filtering of the lymph occurs. White blood cells are present here to attack bacteria and viruses that may be present in the fluid. This is why swollen and tender lymph nodes are a sign of an infection!

Figure 7. Lymphatic System

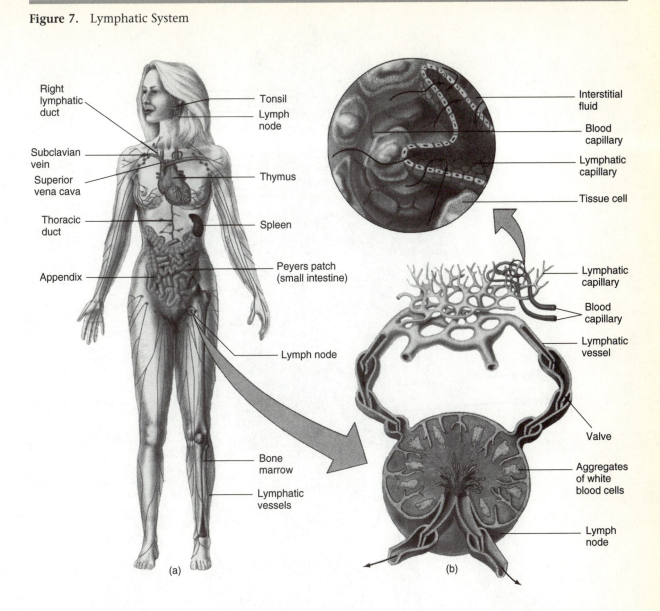

Respiration

Air enters the respiratory system through the nasal cavities, which lead to the **pharynx.** Here, the glottis remains open, and the air travels to the **larynx,** or the voicebox. From the larynx, the air travels to the trachea, or windpipe, which branches into **two bronchi,** which lead to each lung. Inside each lung, the branching continues, creating thinner and thinner tubes. Finally, at the end of the bronchioles, there are a cluster of air sacs called **alveoli.** These thin and permeable air sacs are the functional units of the lung. The deoxygenated blood arrives at the lung via the pulmonary arteries from the right ventricle. The arteries branch into smaller and smaller vessels and finally become capillaries. These capillaries surround the alveoli, and it is here that simple exchange occurs across the alveolar membrane via diffusion: the blood picks up oxygen and releases carbon dioxide, which will be exhaled.

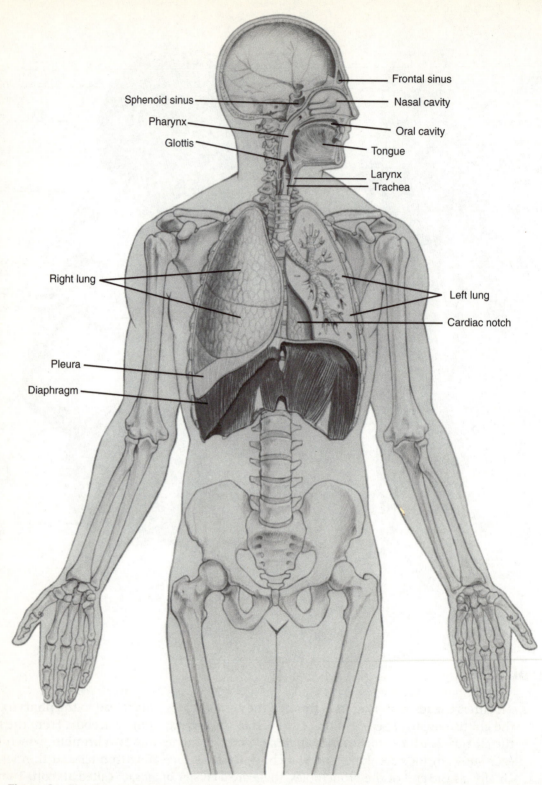

Figure 8. Respiratory System

Inhalation is an active process in which the diaphragm, a sheet of muscle lining the bottom of the thoracic cavity, and the rib muscles contract. This increases the volume in the thoracic cavity and lungs and thus the pressure in them drops (Boyle's Law: volume and pressure are inversely related) causing outside air to rush in to equalize the pressure. When these muscles relax, the volume decreases and thus the pressure increases causing air to be pushed out and exhaled.

Figure 9.   Inhalation and Exhalation

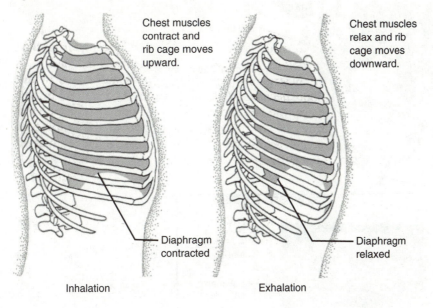

Inhalation

Exhalation

Cellular Respiration

Cellular respiration can be anaerobic or aerobic and is the process by which we get energy from the food that we eat. **Aerobic respiration** occurs when oxygen is present and is the opposite process to that of photosynthesis. During photosynthesis, a plant uses energy to convert water and carbon dioxide to glucose. Aerobic respiration is the way in which we use glucose, at a cellular level, to obtain energy. Its formula is:

$$C_6H_{12}O6 + 6O_2 \rightarrow 6CO_2 + 6H_2O$$

Aerobic respiration, a very efficient process, begins in the cytoplasm of the cell and ends in the mitochondria where the energy from glucose is made in the form of ATP. If oxygen is not present, **anaerobic respiration** ensues, which is less efficient, producing a lower amount of ATP. **Lactic acid** is produced during aerobic respiration and is a cause of sore muscles after strenuous exercise. Anaerobic respiration is also called fermentation because yeast undergoing anaeorbic respiration produce ethanol rather than lactic acid.

Excretion

The kidneys are made up of microscopic tubules called **nephrons** and collecting ducts. The nephron is the functional unit of the kidney. The nephron is made up of the **glomerulus**, **Bowman's capsule**, the **proximal tubule**, the **loop of Henle**, and the **distal tubule**.

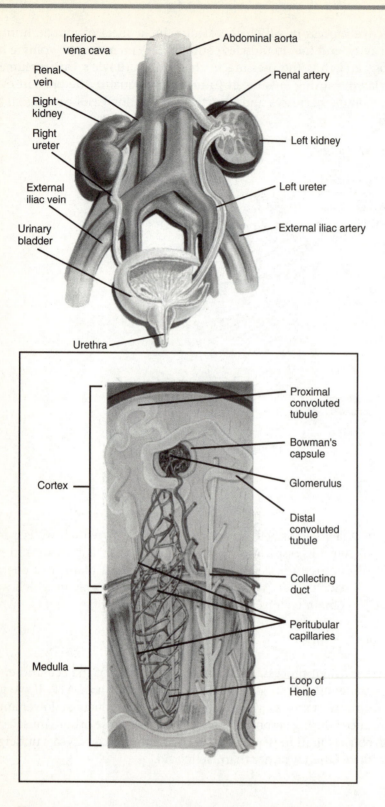

Figure 10. Urinary System and Cross Section of Kidney

Approximately 20% of the volume of blood that is pumped with each heartbeat is brought to the kidney to be filtered. Blood that has entered the ball of capillaries, the glomerulus, is forced into Bowman's capsule which, due to the size of the pores, only allows water and small particles through. This filtrate composed of the water and small particles passes through the nephron where particles and water are either secreted into the filtrate from surrounding plasma or reabsorbed into the plasma to be returned to the body. In this way, urine is formed at an appropriate concentration to meet the needs of the individual. After passing through the nephron, the filtrate travels to the collecting duct to the ureters which are tubes connected to the urinary bladder. Finally, the urine leaves the bladder through the urethra, which is near the vagina in females or through the penis in males.

Regulation: Endocrine System

The function of this system is to maintain **homeostasis**, which is the body's way of maintaining a stable internal environment. One example of a homeostatic process is perspiration. When we get hot, our pores secrete a substance that is mostly water, which coats our skin and quickly evaporates, leaving us cooler. Thus, our body temperature is maintained. Another way in which our bodies maintain a stable internal environment is through endocrine glands, which secrete **hormones.** Hormones are chemicals, that act as messengers and help control the important processes of growth, metabolism, reproduction, osmotic balance, and development. Most work by binding to a specific type of cell via a receptor and influencing the activity of the cell. Most often hormones are activated in response to some type of stimulus. One example is the hormone insulin. When we ingest a meal, it is broken down by our digestive system, and glucose is released from starches into our bloodstream. The presence of glucose triggers the release of insulin from the pancreas, and insulin binds to cells causing them to uptake glucose present in the bloodstream. Thus cells are able to use this glucose for energy. When the glucose levels in the bloodstream start to decline, the stimulus for the release of insulin declines as well. This sort of regulation of hormone release is called a negative-feedback mechanism, and prevents over-secretion of hormones.

Reproduction

Sexual reproduction involves the fusion of two **gametes** (sperm and egg) to form a **zygote** (union of sperm and egg). Each gamete is **haploid**, meaning it contains half the normal complement of chromosomes. Thus, since the zygote is created from the union of a sperm and an egg, it contains the full complement of chromosomes and is thus called **diploid.**

In the male, the genitalia, or the external reproductive organs, are the **penis** and the **scrotum.** Internal reproductive organs consist of the **testes**, the primary male reproductive organs, which contain **seminiferous tubules** where sperm form and **interstitial cells** which produce male sex hormones such as **testosterone.** When sperm is produced in the seminiferous tubules, it then travels into the **epididymis**, which is made of coiled tubes that store sperm while they mature. The sperm are sent through the epididymis during ejaculation into the **vas deferens** to the **ejaculatory duct** to the **urethra.** The urethra, which runs the length of the penis and opens to the external environment, is common to both the reproductive and urinary systems.

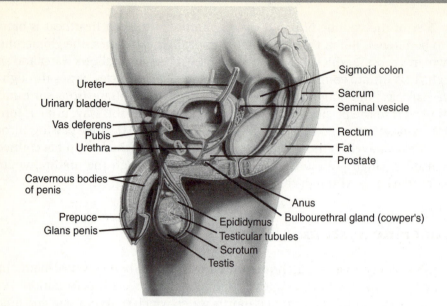

Figure 11. Male Reproductive System

In the female, the primary reproductive organs are the **ovaries,** which produce both eggs and the hormones **progesterone** and **estrogen.** Inside the ovaries are ovarian follicles, each of which contains an immature egg called an **oocyte.** As the egg develops, the follicle matures as well and enlarges. Finally, when fully matured, the follicle releases the egg in the stage called **ovulation,** which occurs approximately every 28 days. The egg then travels through the **fallopian tubes** where it can be fertilized. If this occurs, the fertilized egg travels to the **uterus** where it implants in the lining of the uterus, the **endometrium,** and remains here for the rest of its development. If a woman is not pregnant, the endometrial lining sheds and then thickens again in preparation for the possibility of implantation in the next cycle. The shedding is a process known as **menstruation.**

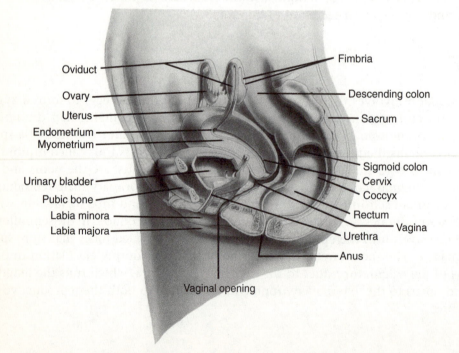

Figure 12. Female Reproductive System

Senses

Eye

At the front of the eyeball, the transparent **cornea** allows light to enter the eye and serves as a lens. Behind the cornea is the **iris**, which not only gives our eyes color but also changes size, regulating how much light will be allowed to enter the **pupil**, which is found in the middle of the iris. The **retina** is the innermost layer of the eyeball and contains two types of photoreceptor cells. **Rod cells** are sensitive to light and distinguish between black and white and allow us to see at night. **Cone cells** allow us to distinguish between colors in the day. When they are stimulated by light, the photoreceptor cells transmit the information via the **optic nerve** to the brain.

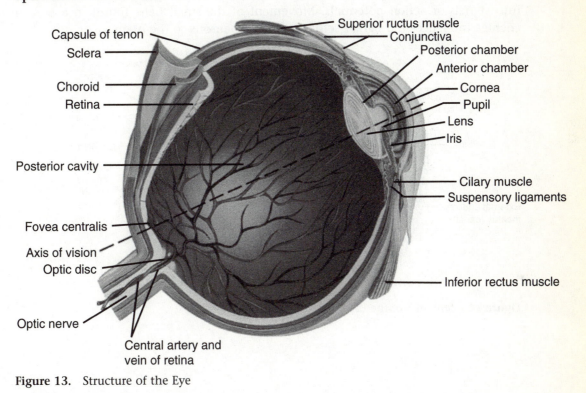

Figure 13. Structure of the Eye

Ear

The ear is not only responsible for hearing but balance as well. Its anatomy can be divided into 3 regions: the **outer ear**, the **middle ear**, and the **inner ear.** The outer ear collects sounds and transmits them to the **tympanic membrane**, which separates the outer ear from the middle ear. In the middle ear, the vibrations produced by sound are transmitted through 3 small bones (ossicles)—the **malleus, incus,** and **stapes.** As they pass through the oval window, the vibrations enter the inner air. The middle ear also is connected to the **eustachian tube,** which opens into the pharynx. This equalizes the pressure between the middle ear and the atmosphere—this is "popping" your ears. The inner ear has many channels that contain fluid that moves in response to your movement or to sound. Sound coming into the inner ear moves the fluid that causes the **cochlea**, a part of the inner ear, to transduce this movement into signals or action potentials. Movement of the small hairs found in a portion of the cochlea influences the signals sent via sensory neurons to the brain.

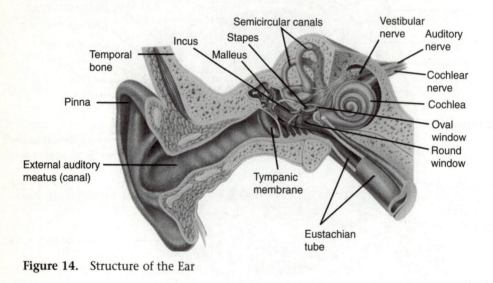

Figure 14. Structure of the Ear

Basic Chemistry

Atomic Structure, Isotopes, Ions, and the Periodic Table

Non-living substances are made up of atoms, the smallest unit of an object that still retain the properties of that object. Atoms contain three types of subatomic particles: **protons**, **neutrons**, and **electrons**. Protons carry a positive charge and are found in the nucleus of an atom. Neutrons are neutral and found in the nucleus as well. Electrons carry a negative charge and are found outside the nucleus and arranged according to their energy level. An **element** is made up of atoms of the same type and is defined by the number of protons. For example, let us look at the element carbon. The **atomic number**, or number of protons, of carbon is 6. We can infer from this that the number of electrons is also 6 since carbon carries no charge, or is neutral. The **atomic mass** of carbon, or the sum of the number of protons and neutrons, is 12. Thus, the number of neutrons in carbon is 6. However, some types of carbon can be found with a different atomic mass and this is due to a varying number of neutrons, never protons. Atoms of the same element that contain the same number of protons but a different number of neutrons are called **isotopes.** A different number of protons means a different element. Thus, nitrogen always has 5 protons and carbon always has 6 protons. The number of electrons can change as well. When the number of electrons does not equal the number of protons, the atom carries a charge. Charged atoms are called **ions.** For instance, neutral sodium has 23 protons and 23 electrons. However, it often tends to lose an electron and thus carries a charge of +1. (Remember, losing an electron means losing one unit of negative charge.) An ion with a positive charge is called a **cation**, while an ion with a negative charge is called an **anion.**

Elements are arranged on the periodic table in rows in order of increasing atomic number. The columns represent similar configurations of electrons, which confer their chemical characteristics.

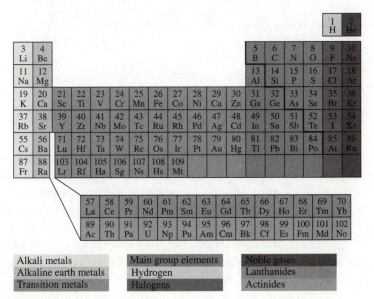

Figure 15. Periodic Table

Elements, Compounds, and States of Matter

Elements can be found in different phases: **gases**, **liquids**, and **solids.** In the gas form the attractions between the atoms or molecules are weak and the atoms move around in a random and erratic manner. If placed in a container, a gas will spread to fill the volume of that container. A liquid has more attractions between its particles and will also take the shape of the container it is in. A solid will not take the shape of the container it is in, does not flow, and its particles have very little movement. The process that takes a solid to a liquid is **melting** and liquid to a gas is **evaporation.** In reverse, a gas to a liquid is called **condensation** and a liquid turns into a solid by **freezing.** During a phase change, the amount of heat that is input or extracted from the substance changes while the temperature remains the same. This is due to the fact that all of the heat is being used to change the phase of the substance, not the temperature. Thus, the evaporating and condensing points of water are both 100 degrees Celsius.

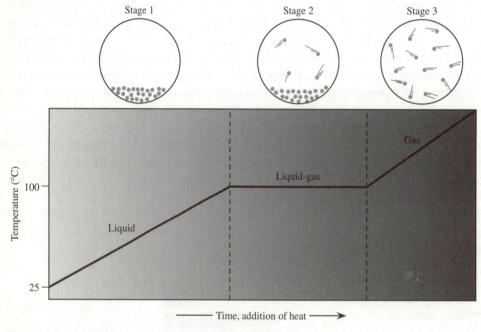

Figure 16. Liquid/Gas

Mixtures, Solutions, Tinctures, and Emulsions

Soil, air, and sea water are examples of **mixtures** since their composition varies. For instance, the air in a city is not identical to that found in a nearby suburb. A **homogeneous** mixture is one in which the composition does not vary from place to place and is referred to as a **solution.** An example of a solution is a tablespoon of sugar thoroughly dissolved in a hot cup of water. In this situation, each teaspoon of the water should contain an equal amount of sugar dissolved in it. In a solution, the substance that does the dissolving is called the **solvent** while the substance that is being dissolved is called the **solute.** A **tincture** refers to a solution in which the solvent is alcohol. For instance, a tincture of iodine contains iodine dissolved in alcohol. Finally, an **emulsion** refers to a liquid dispersed in another liquid in which it is not **soluble** (or, it cannot be dissolved). Take for instance oil and vinegar. Oil remains suspended as droplets in vinegar, in which it is not soluble. The addition of certain substances, called emulsifiers, will stabilize emulsions. For instance, adding an egg to oil and vinegar makes mayonnaise, which is uniform throughout.

Chemical versus Physical Changes

Iron left exposed to the environment will react with oxygen in the air. The result is a new compound, iron oxide, otherwise known as rust. This type of change where a substance changes into a new and different substance is a **chemical change.** Now, take for instance the melting of a cup of ice cubes. The result is a glass of water. A change has occurred but the substance has not been changed into a new substance. A **physical change** refers to a change where the same type of matter of the substance remains the same. Ice and the results of melting are both water.

Types of Chemical Change

There are many types of chemical changes, or chemical **reactions.** The substances that are react with each other, and are written on the left side of the equation, are called the **reactants.** The substances that are the end result of the reaction and written on the right side of the equation, are called the **products.** Remember the law of conservation of mass, too! The same number of atoms of each element must be present on each side of an equation, and this is accomplished by coefficients, the numbers placed in front of the each substance. In this section we will review four main categories under which reactions fall.

Synthesis or Combination Reactions

These reactions involve 2 or more reactants that combine to create 1 ultimate product.

$$2H_2 + O_2 \rightarrow 2H_2O$$

In this reaction, 2 molecules of hydrogen react with 1 molecule of oxygen to produce 2 molecules of water. As you can see there are 4 atoms of hydrogen and 2 atoms of oxygen on each side. Thus, this is a balanced equation for a synthesis reaction.

Single Replacement Reactions

These reactions involve an element reacting with a compound. During this reaction, an atom of the single element replaces an element in the compound.

$$3Al + 3NaCl \rightarrow 3Na + AlCl_3$$

Double-Displacement Reactions

These reactions involve 2 ionic compounds. The positive ions, or metal, in each compound switch positions. A common type of double-dispacement reaction is an **acid-base reaction.** The products, as you will see in the example below, are always a salt and water. Since the products are neutral, these specific types of displacement reactions are called **neutralization reactions.**

$$NaOH + HCl \rightarrow NaCl + H_2O$$

A reminder: an acid is classified as a substance that donates hydrogen ions (H+) while a base is one that donates hydroxide ions (OH−). The **pH scale** was created to identify the strength of an acid or a base based upon the concentration of either hyrogen or hydroxide ions. The scale runs from 0 to 14 where 7 is neutral. A pH of 0 indicates an extremely strong acid, while a pH of 6 indicates that the acid is fairly weak. A pH of 14 on the other hand indicates a very strong base, and a pH of 8 means the base is fairly weak.

Decomposition Reactions

These reactions involve one reactant that is broken down into two or more products. Most often, it is heat that is used to drive this type of reaction.

$$H_2CO_3 \rightarrow H_2O + CO_2$$

Gas Laws

The gas laws relate temperature, volume, and pressure. **Boyle's Law** states that at a constant temperature pressure is inversely related to volume. Thus, as pressure increases, volume decreases and vice versa. **Charles's Law** states that at constant pressure, temperature and volume are directly related. Thus, as temperature increases, volume increases. Finally, **Gay-Lussac's Law** states that at constant volume, as temperature increases, pressure increases.

Reaction Rates and Catalysis

The occurrence of a reaction depends on two things. First, the two substances must come into contact in order to react, and second, there must be enough energy available for the reaction to occur. If the appropriate amount of energy, the **activation energy**, is available, then the reaction is able to proceed. Reaction rates are thus influenced by any factors that affect these two steps. For instance, reaction rate is increased by raising the temperature since this elevation of temperature causes particles to move around in a quicker and more erratic manner. This increased movement increases the probability that two particles will come into contact. Increasing the surface area of a substance also increases reaction rate. Take for instance a cube of sugar versus a crushed cube of sugar. The crushed one will dissolve faster because water will be brought into contact with more surfaces of the sugar. Finally, a very important influence on rate is that of **catalysts**. These are substances that increase the rate of a reaction by lowering the activation energy. It is important to remember that catalysts only affect rate and are not used up in the reaction.

Organic Chemistry

Organic chemistry refers to compounds that contain carbon. Examples of organic compounds include carbohydrates, lipids, and proteins. Carbohydrates contain carbon, hydrogen, and oxygen, and it is usually found that the ratio of hydrogen to oxygen is 2:1. Carbohydrates can be found in different sizes and are classified based on their size. **Monosaccharides** are the "simple sugars," while **disaccharides** are made from two monosaccharides and include table sugar, or sucrose. **Polysaccharides** are chains of monosaccharides and are known as starch and glycogen. **Starch** is formed in plants, while **glycogen** is found in animals.

Lipids refer to fats and steroids. Fats are made of **fatty acids** and **glycerol.** Each fat molecule is made up of one glycerol molecule attached to three fatty acids. In saturated fats the bonds between the carbons are single, while in unsaturated fats, the bonds tend to be double or triple bonds.

Proteins are made up of amino acids of which there are about 20 types. These amino acids are linked in chains, and the sequence determines the properties of the protein. Examples of proteins include enzymes, collagen (cartilage, tendons, bones), and keratin (hair and nails).

Physics

The study of physics focuses on obtaining an understanding of the physical laws and principles that influence every aspect of daily life. Physicists examine the behavior and interaction of energy and matter in the universe to increase understanding of phenomena that occur in everyday life. An understanding of the principles of physics will provide you with an appreciation of your physical world. This physics review will provide you with an overview of the principles of physics.

Mechanics

Terms to be Defined

Displacement	Newton	Work
Motion	Joule	Power
Speed	Friction	Simple Machine
Velocity	Gravity	Inclined plane
Acceleration	Weight	Wedge
Deceleration	Force	Screw
Momentum	Lever-arm	Lever
Conservation of momentum	Torque	Pulley
Newton's first law	Centripetal force	Wheel and axle
Inertia	Energy	Compound machine
Mass	Kinetic energy	Efficiency
Newton's second law	Potential energy	

The ***displacement*** of an object is defined as the distance that the object is from some starting point, and it is measured in units of length. When an object is in ***motion,*** its displacement is constantly changing. Motion is described by displacement, velocity (speed), and acceleration. ***Speed*** is the distance traveled by an object per unit of time.

$$\text{Speed} = \frac{\text{distance travelled}}{\text{time}}$$

Velocity is speed in a given direction. Velocity tells us two things about a moving object: its speed and direction. Sometimes velocity, as well as displacement, can change with time. The rate of change in velocity is called ***acceleration.*** Acceleration refers to any change of velocity. ***Deceleration*** is a decrease in velocity (negative acceleration) and can cause a change in direction.

$$\text{Acceleration} = \frac{\text{final velocity} - \text{original velocity}}{\text{time}}$$

An object traveling at a specific velocity has a quantity called ***momentum.*** All moving objects have momentum. Momentum is equal to the mass of an object multiplied by its velocity. The mass of an object is the amount of matter in an object.

Momentum = mass × velocity

One of the main laws of classical physics is the ***conservation of momentum.*** The total momentum of an isolated system is always constant. During a collision between two bodies the momentum of each body will change; however, the total momentum is conserved. None of the momentum is lost. One object may lose momentum, but the momentum lost by this object is gained by the other. When a moving object hits a stable object, such as a bullet hitting a wall, the bullet delivers an ***impulse*** to the wall. The impulse is defined to be the change in the object's momentum.

Newton's Laws

Classical mechanics is based on the application of Newton's laws. His ***first law*** is the law of ***inertia,*** which states that objects in motion tend to stay in motion, and objects at rest tend to stay at rest. Inertia is the property of matter that resists any change in motion. Newton's ***second law*** describes the relationship between force, mass, and acceleration. It states that the force applied on an object equals the mass of the object times the acceleration of the object.

F = ma
(Force = mass × acceleration)

Newton's second law explains why a small car has better gas mileage than a big car. According to this law, the force required to accelerate the big car with the greater mass is greater than the force required to accelerate the small car. Therefore, the big car will have to burn more gas in its engine to produce the additional force. The ***newton*** (N) is the unit that represents a force that accelerates a mass of 1 kilogram 1 meter per second.

You might think something is wrong with Newton's analysis because in the real world when you slide a box along the floor, giving it a velocity, it does not continue on at that speed forever but stops. This is due to the ***friction*** between the box and the floor. Whenever a force is exerted on an object along a surface, or an object has a velocity along the surface, and the two surfaces touch, such as a box being pushed along the floor, there is a force called friction, which opposes the motion or the force being applied. Note that the force of friction is always in the direction to stop the object from moving.

An example of a ***force*** with which we are all familiar is gravitational force. ***Gravity*** is the force of attraction between all objects in the universe. The greater the mass of an object, the greater its gravitational force. The earth's gravitational force is great because the earth has a large mass. If you drop an object, it falls to the earth. The object falls because earth exerts a gravitational force on it. The force due to gravity is not the same on every object, it depends on the mass of the object. However, the acceleration towards earth is the same for all objects independent of their mass. The pull of gravity on an object determines its ***weight.*** A change in the force of gravity results in a change in the weight of the object but not in its mass. The earth has more mass than the moon. Therefore, the earth exerts a greater gravitational force than the moon. On the moon you would weigh about ⅙th of what you weigh on earth because the gravitational pull of the moon is about ⅙th of the gravitational pull of the earth. Yet, your body mass would stay exactly the same as it is on earth. In addition, the force of gravity between two objects decreases as the distance between the two objects increases. For example, the earth's gravitational pull on a rocket decreases as the rocket moves away from the earth.

The ability of a force that is applied perpendicularly to rotate an object around an axis, such as a ball on a string, is measured by a quantity called ***torque.*** The distance from the axis of rotation to the point where the force is exerted is called the ***lever arm.*** Torque is defined as perpendicular force times lever-arm. The further the force is from the axis of rotation, the easier it is to rotate the object and the more torque is produced. In order to keep the ball at the end of a string moving in a circle, you must continually exert a force pulling the ball toward the center of the circle. This force is called the ***centripetal force,*** and in the case of the ball on a string, the string provides the force.

In mechanics, objects are defined as having energy. ***Energy*** is defined as the ability to do work. There are two types of energy. The first type of energy is called ***kinetic energy.*** Kinetic energy is energy associated with motion. Any moving body has kinetic energy because it is able to do work by moving other bodies. Kinetic energy is defined as one half of the product of mass and velocity squared:

$$KE = \frac{1}{2}mv^2$$

The kinetic energy of a body tells us how much work that body can do by moving other bodies until it is brought to rest.

The other type of energy is ***potential energy.*** Potential energy is the stored energy that a body has because of its position. When you lift an object up you provide it with potential energy. An object has more potential energy at the top of a building than when it is on the first floor.

When a person does work on an object, you change the energy of the object by giving it some of your energy. Work is defined as the product of the force applied to a object and the distance through which the force is applied. A ***joule*** is the unit of energy equal to the work done by a force of one Newton acting over a distance of one meter.

Work = force × distance

Power is the rate at which work is done. The power of a machine is the total work done divided by the time taken. Since work equals force times distance, the formula for power is:

$$\text{Power} = \frac{F \times d}{t} = \frac{\text{Work}}{t}$$

A ***machine*** is a device that makes work easier by changing the force or direction of an applied force. The ***efficiency*** of a machine is the work done divided by the energy used to power the machine or the comparison of work input to work output. Because of friction, no machine can be 100% effective.

There are ***six simple machines:***

inclined plane, a slanted surface used to raise an object
wedge, a moving inclined plane
screw, an inclined plane wrapped around a cylinder
lever, a simple machine that is free to move around a fulcrum when an effort force is applied
pulley, a chain or rope wrapped around a wheel
wheel and axle, a lever that rotates in a circle

A ***compound machine*** is a combination of two or more simple machines.

Thermodynamics

Terms to be Defined

Atoms	Boyle's Law	Celsius
Kinetic theory of energy	Charles's Law	Fahrenheit
Molecules	Temperature	Kelvin
Solid	Heat	Ice point
Liquid	Phase change	Steam point
Gas	Latent heat	Triple point
Pressure		Absolute zero

All matter is made up of *atoms,* which are the smallest particles of an element that retain all the chemical properties of the element. According to the *kinetic theory of energy,* the atoms in matter are in a constant state of motion. The motion and spacing of these atoms determine the state of simple matter. The three ordinary states of matter are solid, liquid, and gas. In the gas and liquid states of matter *molecules,* which are *groups of atoms,* are free to move around. Gases and liquids do not have definite shapes of their own. When a liquid or gas is placed in a container the atoms or molecules move around freely in the container and take the shape of the container. These molecules move in all possible directions and keep colliding with the walls of the container. Each time a molecule collides with the wall of the container it delivers an *impulse* to the wall. The greater the quantity of gas or liquid in a container, the more frequent the collisions will be. *Pressure* is the result of the impulses that result from the collision of molecules with the walls of their containers.

There are two important laws in thermodynamics.

Boyle's Law states that the volume of a fixed amount of gas varies inversely with the pressure of the gas. If the volume of the gas is decreased, the number of particle collisions will increase and the pressure of the gas will increase. If the volume of the gas is increased, the pressure of the gas will decrease.

Charles's Law defines the relationship between temperature and volume of a gas. According to Charles's Law the volume of a fixed amount of gas varies directly with the temperature of the gas. If the temperature of a gas increases, the volume increases.

Temperature is a very familiar concept, but what exactly is temperature? Temperature is a measure of the average kinetic energy of the particles in a substance. It tells how warm or cold a substance is with respect to other substances. Temperature determines whether a substance will gain or give up heat when put into contact with other bodies. A substance with a high temperature is said to be hot, or contain heat. *Heat* is a form of energy that causes the particles of matter to move faster and farther apart. When a substance is heated, its temperature will increase. The *specific heat* of a substance is defined as the heat needed to raise the temperature of one gram by one degree.

When the temperature of a substance changes, the specific phase that the matter is in may change. *Phase change* refers to the physical change of a substance from one state to another. For example, when ice is heated it will eventually melt. The *latent heat* is the heat energy needed per unit mass to change the phase of a substance.

Temperature is measured with a thermometer using different scales. In science the most commonly used temperature scale is the *Celsius* scale. Two other scales are the *Fahrenheit* scale and the *Kelvin,* or absolute temperature scale. The *ice point* is the temperature at which ice melts or water freezes. On the Fahrenheit scale the ice point is 32°; on the Celsius scale the ice point is 0°. The *steam point* is the point at which water at standard pressure boils.

On the Celsius scale the steam point is 100°. On the Fahrenheit scale the steam point is 212°. The *triple point* (273.16 K) on the Kelvin scale is the temperature at which water exists simultaneously as a gas, liquid, and solid. On the Kelvin scale the lowest possible temperature is known as *absolute zero,* or zero Kelvin (0 K).

The relationship of the Celsius scale to the Kelvin scale is:

$$T \text{ (Kelvin)} = T(\text{Celsius}) + 273$$

The relationship of the Celsius scale to the Fahrenheit scale is:

$$T(\text{Fahrenheit}) = \left(\tfrac{9}{5} T(\text{Celsius})\right) + 32$$

Therefore:

$$\text{Change of temperature in Fahrenheit} = \tfrac{9}{5} \text{ change in Celsius degrees}$$

Waves

Terms to be Defined

Motion	Crest	Pitch
Wave	Trough	Loudness
Transverse wave	Wavelength	Doppler effect
Longitudinal wave	Wave speed	Reflection
Periodic motion	Diffraction	Refraction
Periodic wave	Interference	Dispersion
Period	Resonance	Lens
Frequency	Electromagnetic waves	Convex lens
Hertz	Electromagnetic spectrum	Concave lens
Amplitude	Visible light	Focal point

Motion is defined as a change in position relative to a frame of reference. Wave motion is a means of transferring energy. A *wave* is a rhythmic disturbance that travels through matter or space. The two basic waves are the longitudinal and transverse waves. A *transverse wave* is a wave in which matter vibrates at right angles to the direction in which the wave travels. Water waves approximate a transverse wave. Light and heat appear to be transmitted by transverse waves. A *longitudinal wave* is a wave in which matter vibrates back and forth along the path that the wave travels. Sounds are transmitted by longitudinal waves.

Periodic motion is motion that repeats itself over and over again. The motion of a pendulum represents periodic motion. A *periodic wave* can be described as motion that repeats itself at regular intervals and transfers energy but not mass. The time it takes for motion to repeat itself is measured in seconds and is called the *period.* A *cycle* is equal to one complete repetition of a periodic event. The *frequency (f)* of a wave tells us how often a cycle repeats itself in a specific time unit. Frequency is often measured in *hertz (Hz),* which is equivalent to cycles per second.

Amplitude refers to the maximum distance a wave rises or falls as it travels and is related to the energy that the wave carries. Amplitude relates to brightness with light waves and loudness with sound waves. The louder the sound, the higher the amplitude. The *crest* of a transverse wave is the maximum upward displacement while the *trough* is the maximum downward displacement. The *wavelength* of a transverse wave is the distance between two successive wave crests. *Wave speed* is the frequency of the wave times the wavelength.

The phenomena of *diffraction* refers to the bending of waves around an obstacle. When two waves meet each other they combine to make a new wave. The way in which the waves interact with each other when they go through the same portion of a medium at the same time is called *interference. Resonance* between two systems results when the vibration of one system results in the vibration of the other system at the same frequency.

Light waves are made up of streams of *photons,* or tiny packets of energy. The amount of energy in the photons determines the kind of light wave produced. Light waves are called *electromagnetic waves* because the moving photons generate electric and magnetic fields. The complete spectrum of light arranged in order of their wavelengths is called the *electromagnetic spectrum. Visible light* is only a small part of the electromagnetic spectrum; it is the portion of the spectrum that is visible to the human eye. The electromagnetic spectrum consists of

Radio waves
Infrared waves
Visible light
Ultraviolet light
X-rays
Gamma rays

The photons of visible light contain a moderate amount of energy, while x-rays are made up of high-energy photons and radio waves contain low-energy photons. Gamma rays have the highest energy photons and the shortest wavelengths of all the electromagnetic waves.

Sound waves are longitudinal waves; they vibrate in the direction of motion. The *pitch* of a sound wave has to do with the frequency. High frequency sound waves have a high pitch and low frequency waves have a low pitch. The *loudness* of a sound wave is determined by the amplitude of the wave. The *Doppler effect* occurs whenever there is relative motion between the source of waves and the observer. The pitch of a siren will be higher as an ambulance approaches you and lower as it drives away. The siren has not changed its frequency but the motion of the ambulance towards you increases the frequency of the sound waves you hear. As the siren moves away the frequency you hear is less than the source frequency and the pitch is lower.

When a light wave bounces off of a surface that does not absorb its energy it is *reflected.* The type of surface that light strikes determines the kind of reflection. Because a mirror has a smooth, flat surface, the reflected rays are not scattered and the image reflected is clearly defined. *Refraction* refers to the bending of light rays as they pass from one medium to another. Light moves at different speeds through different mediums. As it passes from one medium to another, it either speeds up or slows down. A prism is a piece of glass that separates light into its component colors. This phenomenon is called *dispersion.*

A *lens* is any transparent material that refracts light. When parallel rays of light pass through a lens they are refracted so that they either come together or spread out. A lens that is thicker in the center than it is at the edges is a *convex lens.* When parallel rays of light pass through a convex lens they *converge;* they are bent toward the center. The *focal point* is the point at which the light rays meet. A *concave lens* is thicker at the edges than it is in the middle. When light rays pass through a concave lens, they **diverge** because they are bent toward the edges, or the thickest part, of the lens. Images of an object produced by concave lenses are smaller than the object.

Electricity and Magnetism

Terms to be Defined

Neutron	Generator	Current
Proton	Electrical potential energy	Watts
Electron	Potential difference	Resistor
Coulomb's Law	Transformer	Series circuit
Magnetism	Voltage	Parallel circuit
Magnetic fields	Amperes	Ammeter
Torque	Voltmeter	

Two types of electric charge exist in our universe; positive and negative. Some particles have no charge (*neutron*), some have positive charge (*proton*), and some have negative charge (*electron*). Like charges repel each other and unlike charges attract each other. *Coulomb's law* applies to this force of attraction and repulsion. Coulomb found that the electric force between two charges is proportional to the product of the two charges. Therefore, if one charge is doubled, the electric force is doubled. If both charges are doubled, the electric force increases four times. Coulomb also found that the electric force varied inversely as the square of the distance between the charges. Thus, when the distance between two forces doubles the force between them decreases to ¼ of the original force. When the two forces are brought closer together, the force between them increases.

Electricity is closely related to *magnetism*. All magnets have a north and a south pole that attract their opposite and repel their similar pole. *Magnetic fields* exist whenever electric charges are moving. When the moving charges are in a wire that loops a *torque* result. This is the basis for electric motors. A *generator* is a device that converts mechanical energy, such as water coming down a waterfall, into electric energy. *Electrical potential energy* can be compared to the gravitational force associated with an object's position; there is potential energy associated with this force. Electrical potential energy is associated with the potential interaction of two objects' charges. *Potential difference* refers to the change in electrical potential energy. The device that changes potential difference of electricity is called a *transformer*. *Voltage* is a measure of the electrical energy available; it is another term for potential difference. A *voltmeter* is a device that measures the potential difference between two points in an electric circuit.

Electricity moving through a circuit is called a *current*. An *ampere* is the unit used to measure electrical current. The way by which the ability to flow through a circuit is limited is a *resistor*. The two different types of circuits are called series and parallel. A *series circuit* has all its resistors in a row so that all current must travel through all resistors. A *parallel circuit* has all resistors at the same voltage. An *ammeter* is a device that measures the current going trough any specific point on the circuit. Electrical power is expressed as *watts*.

Power = Voltage × Current

Watts = Voltage × Amperes

Modern Physics

Terms to be Defined

Mass defect	Nuclear reaction	Photoelectric effect
Radioactivity	Fusion	Ionization
Radioactive decay	Fission	Theory of relativity
Transmutation	Quantum mechanics	

In the early twentieth century scientists began to understand the structure of the atom. They discovered that the atom is made up of a nucleus of positively charged protons and uncharged neutrons, surrounded by negatively charged electrons. The mass of a nucleus is heavier then all the protons and neutrons that make it up. This mass difference is known as the *mass defect.* The mass defect represents the energy in the bonds holding the nucleus together. It was also discovered that an atom's nucleus could spontaneously disintegrate while giving off energy in the form of alpha and beta particles and gamma rays. This phenomenon is known as *radioactivity.* The spontaneous change in the nucleus of an atom is known as *radioactive decay.* The conversion of one element into another element is referred to as *transmutation.* When a radioactive nucleus goes through a transmutation it is called a *nuclear reaction.* There are two main processes of nuclear reactions.

Fusion is the process in which the nuclei of several light atoms combine to form a single heavy nucleus with a release of energy.

Fission is the process in which a heavy nucleus splits into two main pieces and with the release of a huge amount of energy.

Another discovery attributable to modern physics is the nature of light. For years scientists have been arguing over whether light consists of particles or acts like waves. As it turns out the only theory that can accurately explain the behavior of light is *quantum mechanics.* The behavior of light is actually an interesting combination of particles and waves. An example which illustrates this wave-particle duality is the *photoelectric effect.* When a light wave strikes certain metallic surfaces electrons are emitted. This process is called *ionization,* and it means that an atom loses an electron (or several electrons) and becomes an ion.

Albert Einstein's *theory of relativity,* devised in 1905, was one of the greatest accomplishments of modern physics. The main consequence of this theory is the identification of the existence of an upper limit on velocity. This upper limit, c, also known as the speed of light, is the fastest that any particle can travel. According to this theory, the speed of light is absolute and material particles can never reach the speed of light.

Science Bibliography

Avila, Vernon. *Investigating Life on Earth*. Bookmark Publishers: Jamul, CA. 1995

Cambell, Neil A. *Biology*. Benjamin/Cummings Publishing Company Inc.: Menlo Park, CA. 1996.

Marieb, Elaine. *Essentials of Anatomy and Physiology*. Benjamin/Cummings Publishing Company Inc.: Redwood City, CA. 1991.

Olmsead and Williams. *Chemistry: The Molecular Science*. William C. Brown Publishers: Dubuque, Iowa, 1997.

Serway, R. & Jerry Faughn. *Physics*. Holt, Rinehart and Winston: New York, 1999.

I. Science

Read each question carefully, and then select the best answer. The correct answers will be found at the end of section C.

Directions

The Science Tests consist of questions on biology, chemistry, physics, human anatomy and physiology. You should be able to answer all the questions in the test in 60 minutes.

Each test question consists of an incomplete sentence or a question followed by four choices. Read each question carefully, then decide which choice is the correct answer.

If you finish the Science Test before the 60 minutes are up, go back and check your work.

Your score will be the total number of correct answers. You may answer a question even if you are not completely sure of the correct response. Do not spend too much time on any one question. If you cannot answer a question, go on to the next question.

1. An organism with chloroplasts in its cells probably looks
    a. white.
    b. green.
    c. red.
    d. yellow.

2. What is the property of water that allows someone to fill a glass slightly above the rim without the water flowing over?
    a. its specific gravity
    b. its capillarity
    c. its opacity
    d. its surface tension

3. Synapses are spaces
    a. between neurons.
    b. between chromosomes.
    c. in mitochondria.
    d. in nephrons.

4. Which of these groups of chemicals is *NOT* normally found in most living things?
    a. carbohydrates
    b. proteins
    c. silicates
    d. nucleic acids

5. The alimentary canal is another name for the
    a. spinal cord.
    b. digestive system.
    c. urinary tract.
    d. birth canal.

6. The numerous villi in the small intestine serve to
   a. secrete enzymes for digestion.
   b. absorb water from dissolved foods.
   c. secrete hydrochloric acid to dissolve food.
   d. provide greater surface for absorption.

7. As light passes obliquely from air to water, it is bent. This bending is called
   a. diffraction.
   b. reflection.
   c. refraction.
   d. dispersion.

8. Which of the following structures is *NOT* part of the cytoplasm of a cell?
   a. ribosome
   b. mitochondrion
   c. endoplasmic reticulum
   d. nucleus

Questions 9 to 11 refer to the graph below, which shows the amounts of different gases in automobile exhaust at different air-fuel ratios.

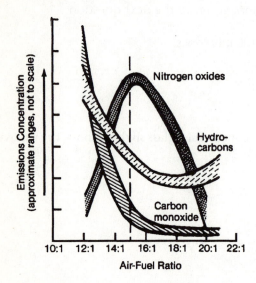

9. The exhaust from the engine contains the most nitrogen oxides when the air-fuel ratio is approximately
   a. 12:1
   b. 16:1
   c. 18:1
   d. 20:1

10. This graph provides an explanation of
    a. engine knock.
    b. lead content of gasoline.
    c. diesel engine operation.
    d. air pollution.

11. The emission of carbon dioxide is probably not included in the graph because carbon dioxide is
    a. included in the hydrocarbons.
    b. not affected by the air-fuel ratio.
    c. a natural part of the atmosphere.
    d. part of the carbon monoxide.

12. To be used by cells, carbohydrates must be changed to
    a. glucose.
    b. sucrose.
    c. glycogen.
    d. glycerol.

13. A neuron that transmits impulses from the spinal cord to a muscle is called
    a. a motor neuron.
    b. an associative neuron.
    c. an interneuron.
    d. a sensory neuron.

14. A ball rolls down an incline, passing through the four positions shown in the diagram.

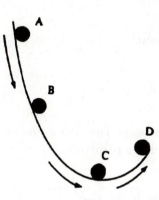

    In which of these positions does the rolling ball have the maximum kinetic energy?
    a. A
    b. B
    c. C
    d. D

15. Which of these organisms help prevent the accumulation of organic wastes in nature?
    a. rabbits
    b. mosses
    c. bacteria
    d. ferns

16. As the eardrum is made to vibrate more rapidly, the sound will be perceived as
    a. louder in intensity.
    b. softer in intensity.
    c. higher in pitch.
    d. lower in pitch.

Questions 17 and 18 refer to the graph below, which shows the heat required as 1 gm of ice at $-40°C$ is changed to steam at 200°C.

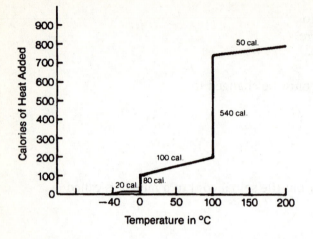

17.   The number of calories needed to change the liquid to steam is
       a.   540.
       b.   590.
       c.   640.
       d.   750.

18.   If the temperature were raised to 300°C, the substance would
       a.   change back to liquid.
       b.   remain a gas.
       c.   ionize.
       d.   break into its constituent elements.

19.   In a field of pure white asters, a grower noticed a single blue aster. How could the grower test whether this change affected the gamete-producing cells of the plant?
       a.   Self-pollinate the flower, and plant the resulting seeds.
       b.   Examine the blue petals under an electron microscope.
       c.   Perform a chemical analysis to find the nature of the blue pigment.
       d.   Perform vegetative propagation on a cutting of the plant.

20.   A human egg will develop into a female if it is fertilized by a sperm containing
       a.   an X chromosome.
       b.   a Y chromosome.
       c.   an XY chromosome.
       d.   an XXY chromosome.

21.   In a food chain involving grass, grasshoppers, birds, and mammals, the original source of energy is
       a.   glucose.
       b.   sunlight.
       c.   chlorophyll.
       d.   ATP.

22.   The action of baking soda is expressed in which of these formulas?
       a. $H^+ + NaHCO_3 \rightarrow CO_2 + NA^+ + H_2O$
       b. $CaCO_3 + 4C \rightarrow 3CO + CaC_2$
       c. $4NH_3 + 5O_2 \rightarrow 6H_2O + 4NO$
       d. $H_2CO_3 + Ca(OH)_2 \rightarrow 2H_2O + CaCO_3$

Questions 23 to 25 are based on the experiment below.

A chemical test for the presence of dissolved vitamin C is that the vitamin C bleaches a dark blue solution of indophenol. A student placed 1 ml of indophenol in each of six different test tubes. Then the student added a different liquid drop by drop to each test tube until the blue color of the indophenol disappeared. As indicated below, each liquid took a different number of drops to bleach out the blue color of the indophenol.

Liquid	Drops required
Lemon juice	5 drops
Fresh orange juice	20 drops
Cooked orange juice	30 drops
Pineapple juice	30 drops
Apple juice	45 drops
Water	100 drops did not bleach it

23. Which liquid had the highest concentration of vitamin C?
    a. fresh orange juice
    b. water
    c. lemon juice
    d. apple juice

24. According to these results, when orange juice is heated, its concentration of vitamin C is
    a. increased.
    b. reduced.
    c. destroyed.
    d. maintained at the same level.

25. Which of the following substances contained *NO* vitamin C when the study began?
    a. the indophenol solution
    b. the cooked orange juice
    c. the lemon juice
    d. none of these

Question 26 refers to the experiment below.

The midday shadow of a flagpole was measured once a month (on the same date) for a year. This bar graph presents that data, in order, beginning with month A.

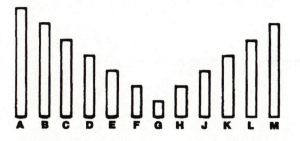

26. In which month does the longest shadow occur?
    a. A
    b. G
    c. K
    d. M

27. Which of these foods is a good source of protein?
   a. nuts
   b. cooked oatmeal
   c. honey
   d. raisins

28. When oxygen goes from air in the lungs into the blood, it does so by
   a. catalysis.
   b. diffusion.
   c. active transport.
   d. osmosis.

Questions 29 to 31 refer to the diagram below of the human endocrine system.

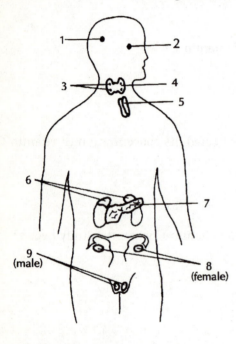

29. The function common to the organs of this system is
   a. reproduction.
   b. secretion.
   c. respiration.
   d. excretion.

30. Which of these organs controls the amount of calcium in the blood?
   a. 1
   b. 2
   c. 3
   d. 6

31. Which of these organs has the added function of producing digestive enzymes?
   a. 2
   b. 5
   c. 6
   d. 7

32. A reading on the Celsius scale is 5°. On the Fahrenheit scale, the reading would be closest to
   a. −25°.
   b. 30°.
   c. 40°.
   d. 95°.

33. Which of these formulas represents an alcohol?
   a. $C_2H_5OC_2H_5$
   b. C_3H_8
   c. CH_3COOH
   d. C_2H_5OH

34. If a car's rate of change of velocity is negative, the car is
   a. speeding up.
   b. maintaining a constant speed.
   c. slowing down.
   d. stopped.

35. Consider the *unbalanced* equation

   $$\_\_N_2 + \_\_H_2 \rightarrow \_\_NH_3.$$
   What is the coefficient of ammonia in the balanced equation that has the smallest whole-number coefficient?
   a. 1
   b. 2
   c. 3
   d. 4

Questions 36 to 38 refer to the graph below of changes in population over a period of time. The graph represents the relationship of the actual population to the capacity of the environment to support it.

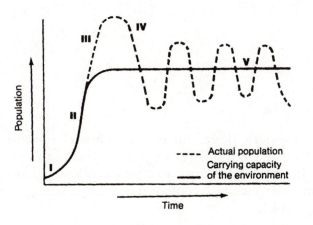

36. At which point is the population growth most rapid?
   a. I
   b. II
   c. III
   d. IV

37. At which point is there a decrease in population due to competition for a dwindling food supply?
    a. I
    b. II
    c. III
    d. IV

38. For which type of organism is this graph believed to be typical?
    a. bacteria only
    b. plants only
    c. all animals except humans
    d. all organisms, including humans

39. Which of these compounds contain 5-carbon sugars and nitrogen bases?
    a. nucleic acids
    b. carbohydrates
    c. proteins
    d. fats

40. A substance with a pH of 8 is a
    a. strong acid.
    b. weak acid.
    c. strong base.
    d. weak base.

41. Paramecia may reproduce by binary fission and by conjugation. This shows that some one-celled organisms are capable of
    a. asexual reproduction only.
    b. sexual reproduction only.
    c. spontaneous generation and sexual reproduction.
    d. sexual and asexual reproduction.

42. Which of these substances will form an alkaline solution in water?
    a. $Mg(OH)_2$
    b. H_2SO_4
    c. $MgSO_4$
    d. NaCl

Questions 43 and 44 are based on the study below.

A student was testing the colored materials in spinach. He ground up some spinach leaves in acetone. He then filtered the mixture and obtained a dark green filtrate. He placed a spot of this filtrate on spot X on a strip of filter paper. Then he hung the dried paper in a tube containing a mixture of petroleum ether and acetone at the bottom. After a while, he observed moisture creeping up on the paper and several bands of yellow and green color.

43. This experiment uses the technique of
    a. fluorescence.
    b. photosynthesis.
    c. centrifugation.
    d. chromatography.

44. The student should conclude that
    a. spinach contains two kinds of chlorophyll—green and yellow.
    b. spinach contains more than one kind of pigment.
    c. all organic pigments are soluble in acetone and petroleum ether.
    d. all organic pigments migrate on filter paper at the same rate.

45. Which diagram represents a nonpolar covalent bond?

    a. $:\ddot{C}l:\ddot{C}l:$

    b. $H:\ddot{B}r:$

    c. $(Li^+)(:\ddot{C}l:)$

    d. $H:\ddot{N}:H$
       $\quad H$

46. Certain seaweeds accumulate iodine in a concentration as much as a million times greater than that of the surrounding ocean. How must this intake be accomplished?
    a. osmosis
    b. diffusion
    c. active transport
    d. passive transport

47. Hydrogen can be prepared in the laboratory by combining Zn and HCl. In the resulting reaction, the metallic zinc (Zn)
    a. is changed to another element.
    b. reacts with the water in the acid.
    c. replaces the combined hydrogen in the acid.
    d. serves as a catalyst.

48. Which of the following organisms has a nutritive process most similar to that of animals?
    a. seaweed
    b. oak tree
    c. grass
    d. bread mold

49. As moist air rises, it becomes
    a. warmer.
    b. lighter.
    c. saturated.
    d. capable of holding more water.

Questions 50 and 51 are based on the diagram below, which shows the state of water at equilibrium at different pressure and temperature conditions.

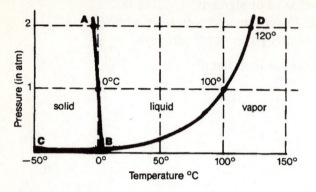

50.   Which of these substances has the lowest boiling point?
        a.   ether
        b.   ethanol
        c.   water
        d.   glycerol

51.   If the pressure on water is increased from 1 atm. to 2 atm., how, if at all, is its boiling point affected?
        a.   The boiling point decreases by 20°C.
        b.   The boiling point is not affected.
        c.   The boiling point increases by 20°C.
        d.   The boiling point increases by 120°C.

52.   In humans, if the diaphragm were pushed upward, there would be a decrease in chest volume. This decrease would be followed by
        a.   an increase in pressure in the chest cavity, and inhalation.
        b.   an increase in pressure in the chest cavity, and exhalation.
        c.   a decrease in pressure in the chest cavity, and inhalation.
        d.   a decrease in pressure in the chest cavity, and exhalation.

53.   Which of these biological processes includes the other three?
        a.   cell respiration
        b.   krebs cycle
        c.   electron transport chain
        d.   anaerobic splitting of glucose

54.   A 5-year-old and her father each lifted identical chairs from the floor to a table top. Which person did the most work?
        a.   the father
        b.   the 5-year-old
        c.   They both did the same amount.
        d.   Not enough information is given.

55.   An excess of which of these ions tends to make a solution acidic?
        a.   chloride
        b.   hydroxyl
        c.   hydronium
        d.   Sodium

56. In the classification of two organisms, which of the following is the best evidence of a close relationship?
    a. similar number and arrangement of bones
    b. similar sequence of amino acids in their proteins
    c. similar methods of sexual reproduction
    d. similar methods of cell respiration

57. In Einstein's equation, $E = mc^2$, which does "c" represent?
    a. the quantum numbers of the atoms involved
    b. the number of coulombs
    c. the number of calories of heat
    d. the speed of light

58. The change from solid dry ice to gaseous carbon dioxide is an example of
    a. sublimation.
    b. evaporation.
    c. precipitation.
    d. condensation.

59. On top of a mountain, the boiling point of water will be
    a. lower than at sea level, because the atmospheric pressure is higher on the mountain.
    b. lower than at sea level, because the atmospheric pressure is lower on the mountain.
    c. the same as at sea level, because the atmospheric pressure is the same in both locations.
    d. higher than at sea level, because the atmospheric pressure is lower on the mountain.

60. Suppose cube A is 10 cm along each edge and cube B is 5 cm along each edge. What is the relationship of the volume of cube A to that of cube B?
    a. Cube A has two times the volume of cube B.
    b. Cube A has four times the volume of cube B.
    c. Cube A has six times the volume of cube B.
    d. Cube A has eight times the volume of cube B.

II. Science

60 Minutes

Read each question carefully, and then select the best answer. The correct answers will be found at the end of section C.

1.   The tissue in the human female that develops to nourish the embryo is called the
     a. amnion.
     b. oviduct.
     c. Fallopian tube.
     d. placenta.

2.   Which of these substances is associated with the process of cell respiration?
     a. ATP
     b. RNA
     c. DNA
     d. Rh factor

3.   What would be a likely result if all the bees and butterflies in an area were destroyed?
     a. Birds would have more food.
     b. More plant seeds would be produced.
     c. More flowers would bloom.
     d. Fewer plant seeds would be produced.

4.   The tiny projections in the small intestine adapted for absorption are called
     a. venules.
     b. villi.
     c. alveoli.
     d. ventricles.

5.   More energy is used in pushing a box up along an inclined plane to a height of 4 meters than in lifting the box straight up to the same height. This is because
     a. more force is needed in pushing the box than in lifting it.
     b. work is done against friction in pushing the box along the plane.
     c. the box moves a greater distance when pushed along the plane than when lifted.
     d. it takes more time to push the box along the plane than to lift it.

6.   Which of the arrows in the graph below represents the wavelength of the wave shown?

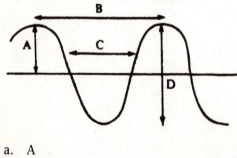

     a. A
     b. B
     c. C
     d. D

7.   What is the reading on the voltmeter scale shown below?

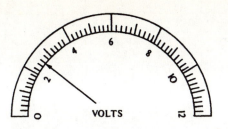

   a.   2.3 volts
   b.   2.6 volts
   c.   3 volts
   d.   23 volts

8.   Which type of circuit is shown in the diagram below?

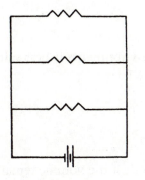

   a.   open
   b.   complex
   c.   series
   d.   parallel

9.   The device shown in the circuit diagram below consists of copper wire wrapped around an iron rod and connected to a switch and a battery.

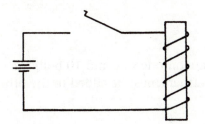

   When the switch is closed, the device could serve as
   a.   a transformer.
   b.   an electromagnet.
   c.   a motor.
   d.   a generator.

10. The following graph shows the motion of a car over a 10-second period of time.

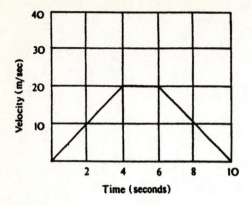

During which time interval did the car cover the greatest distance?
a. 0–2 sec
b. 2–4 sec
c. 4–6 sec
d. 8–10 sec

11. A student wants to grow a bacterial culture. Which of these environments is best suited for growing most kinds of bacteria?
a. a lighted window at 72°F
b. a refrigerator at 45°F
c. an incubator at 37°C
d. a freezer at 10°C

12. A closed container of hydrogen gas is warmed from 20°C to 25°C. If the volume remains the same, what will happen to the pressure in the container?
a. It will remain the same.
b. It will decrease.
c. It will fluctuate.
d. It will increase.

13. Most of the work done by the human kidney occurs in the
a. nephron.
b. neuron.
c. ureter.
d. alveolus.

14. An equal-arm balance is balanced when 20 washers are on one side and 10 bolts are on the other. Four bolts are added to one side. How many washers must be added to the other side to maintain balance?
a. 14
b. 8
c. 4
d. 2

15. Compounds that have different molecular structures but the same formula are called
a. isomers.
b. isobars.
c. isotonic compounds.
d. isomorphs.

16. A student wanted to test the effects different sugars have on the growth of a certain mold. The sugars to be tested were glucose, fructose, and sucrose. One gram of each sugar was placed in a tube of 10 ml of water, and a bit of the mold was put in each of the three solutions. To add a control to the experiment, the student should also have
    a. made two setups of each of the three sugars.
    b. tested ribose and galactose sugars.
    c. made one setup of just water and mold.
    d. kept the three setups in the light.

17. Vinegar is a common antidote for the ingestion of lye. What is the chemical process underlying this procedure?
    a. digestion
    b. alkalinization
    c. oxidation
    d. neutralization

18. Undisturbed layers of rock were examined. Mammal, fish, and bird fossils were found only in the upper layers. Fish were in layers beneath those, and neither fish, birds, nor mammals were in the deepest layers. This would tend to support the hypothesis that
    a. vertebrates always coexisted with invertebrates.
    b. fish were the first vertebrates to evolve.
    c. all vertebrates evolved at about the same time.
    d. birds evolved before fish.

19. Four test tubes are filled with water and placed in a test tube rack as shown in the following diagram. Three of them are covered, each with a different material.

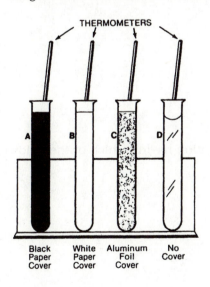

A thermometer is placed in each test tube, and the test tubes are placed in bright sunlight for 15 minutes. In which test tube will the temperature rise most rapidly?
    a. A
    b. B
    c. C
    d. D

20. In the diagram of a bean seed shown below, which letter represents stored food for the growing embryo?

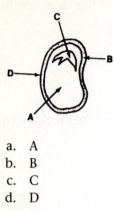

a. A
b. B
c. C
d. D

21. Objects X and Y are identical. In a laboratory, object X is dropped at the same moment that object Y is thrown horizontally. The paths followed by X and Y are shown in the diagram below.

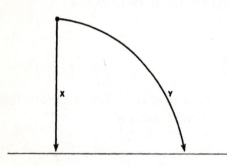

Which of these statements is true?
a. X will hit the ground first.
b. Y will hit the ground first.
c. X and Y will hit the ground simultaneously.
d. Y has a greater vertical displacement than X.

22. Blue litmus paper will turn red when placed in a solution having which of the following pH values?
a. 14
b. 12
c. 7
d. 3

23. Given the *unbalanced* equation

$$\_KClO_3 \rightarrow \_KCl + \_O_2$$

What is the coefficient of O_2 in the balanced equation?
a. 1
b. 2
c. 3
d. 4

24. The compound H_2SO_4 is an example of
    a. a salt.
    b. a base.
    c. an acid.
    d. a halogen.

25. Many people believe that some trees drop their leaves in the late fall because the temperature is near freezing. Which of the following statements would *LEAST* support this idea?
    a. Maple trees in northern Minnesota drop their leaves in late fall.
    b. Maple trees growing near city lights stay green longer than those far from the lights.
    c. Maple trees pass through a time of near freezing before they bud.
    d. Maple trees in southern Florida drop their leaves in late fall.

The next two questions refer to this chart showing approximate energy expenditure in a variety of activities.

Activity	Time (hr)	Men Rate (cal/min)	Men Total	Women Rate (cal/min)	Women Total
Sleeping	8	1.1	530	1.0	480
Sitting, driving a car, bench work	6	1.5	540	1.1	400
Standing or limited walking	6	2.5	900	1.5	540
Walking, purposeful, outdoors	2	3.0	360	2.5	300
Occupational activities involving light physical work, weekend swimming	2	4.5	540	3.0	360
	24		2870		2080

(Chart adapted from *Recommended Dietary Allowances*, 6th ed. *Report of Food and Nutrition Board* (Public 1146), National Academy of Sciences—National Research Council, Washington D.C., 1964.)

26. In which of the following do men expend energy most rapidly?
    a. light physical work
    b. walking outdoors
    c. limited walking
    d. bench work

27. Based on the data, which of these conclusions can be drawn?
    a. The number of calories used by men and women is most similar for purposeful walking activities.
    b. Men use calories as rapidly sitting as women do walking outdoors.
    c. Women use calories more quickly than men do when driving a car.
    d. Women burn calories more slowly than men do in all activities listed.

28. Which of the following is considered to be a principal ecological role of green plants in the environment?
    a. providing shade to regulate the environmental temperature
    b. using the mineral content of the soil
    c. providing nesting places for animals
    d. manufacturing food from simple materials

29. The apparatus shown in the diagram is used for what purpose?

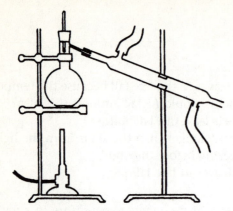

    a. electrolysis of water
    b. distillation of a solution
    c. synthesis of a salt
    d. oxidation of an organic compound

30. The diagram below shows a plant growing in the direction of its light source.

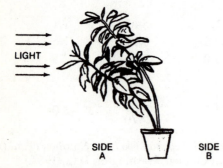

Which of the following processes best explains this phenomenon?
    a. photosynthesis
    b. geotropism
    c. hydrotropism
    d. phototropism

31. The diagram below shows four different waves traveling along the same path. Which two of these waves have the same wavelength?

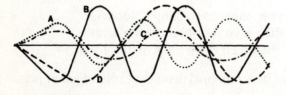

    a. A and B
    b. A and C
    c. B and D
    d. C and D

32.   The following table shows the melting and boiling points for four substances.

Substance	Melting Point	Boiling Point
W	−40°F	105°F
X	10°F	80°F
Y	105°F	1600°F
Z	115°F	280°F

Which of these substances is a liquid over the smallest temperature range?
a. W
b. X
c. Y
d. Z

33.   The diameter of the low-power field of a certain microscope is 1.6 mm. The diameter of a cell that is half the diameter of the field is
a. 500 microns.
b. 800 microns.
c. 1,000 microns.
d. 1,600 microns.

34.   There are 5 gm of salt dissolved in 25 ml of water. What percentage solution is it?
a. 5%
b. 12.5%
c. 20%
d. 25%

35.   In pea plants, plant height and seed color obey the Law of Independent Assortment. If seeds are hybrid for both of these traits, how will their offspring most likely appear?
a. all tall, with green seeds
b. all short, some with yellow and some with green seeds
c. some tall and some short, with all green seeds
d. some tall and some short, with either green or yellow seeds

Question 36 refers to the following graph of the speed of an object over a period of 10 seconds.

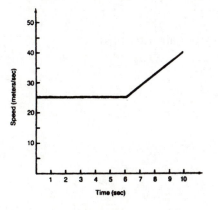

36.   This graph shows an object that is
a. at rest, and then moving at a constant speed.
b. moving at a constant speed and then accelerating.
c. at rest, and then accelerating.
d. accelerating slowly, and then accelerating rapidly.

37. During the 1930s and through the 1950s, thousands of American children received x-ray treatment for swollen tonsils and adenoids. X-rays are no longer used to treat this condition because large doses of radiation
    a. were found to stimulate excessive hair growth.
    b. are thought to cause certain types of cancer.
    c. are thought to increase the severity of acne during adolescence.
    d. were found to increase the number of cases of tonsillitis.

38. A student studies a structure microscopically and notes that it contains glandular cells. It has blood vessels entering and leaving it, but it has no duct leading out of it. The structure must be
    a. an endocrine gland.
    b. an excretory gland.
    c. a digestive gland.
    d. a tear gland.

39. Which laboratory reagent turns starch blue-black?
    a. phenolphthalein
    b. benedict's solution
    c. nitric acid
    d. iodine

40. What types of body cells are most *directly* involved when a person walks uphill?
    a. smooth muscle cells
    b. subcutaneous cells
    c. striated muscle cells
    d. epithelial cells

41. Because the body of the hydra is only two cells thick, it can absorb and give out dissolved substances by the process of
    a. peristalsis.
    b. diffusion.
    c. active transport.
    d. osmosis.

42. In the diagram shown below, a ray of light travels from air into glass.

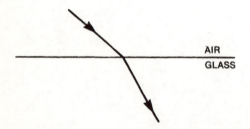

Which of these measuring instruments is needed to find the index of refraction of the glass?
    a. ruler
    b. protractor.
    c. balance
    d. thermometer

43.   Many chemical reactions occur more rapidly with platinum as a catalyst. At the end of the reaction, the platinum is found to be
   a.   increased in quantity.
   b.   unchanged in weight.
   c.   changed into another state.
   d.   combined into the final product.

44.   Which formula represents a compound containing one double bond?
   a. C_6H_6
   b. C_2H_6
   c. C_2H_2
   d. C_2H_4

45.   When looking through a microscope, a student observes centrosomes in a group of cells. The cells might be from the
   a.   root of a bean plant.
   b.   leaf of a moss.
   c.   skin of a mouse.
   d.   stem of a fern.

46.   Ohm's law is used in the study of
   a.   electricity.
   b.   mechanics.
   c.   thermodynamics.
   d.   optics.

47.   A cloud chamber is a device used for
   a.   studying the formation of weather systems.
   b.   recreating the atmosphere of the primitive earth.
   c.   treating a respiratory infection.
   d.   studying charged particles.

The diagram below represents a portion of a food web. The next three questions refer to this diagram.

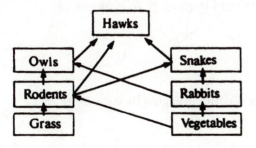

48.   The correct order of a food chain represented in this diagram is
   a.   grass → rabbit → snake → hawk
   b.   hawk → owl → rabbit → vegetable
   c.   grass → rodent → snake → hawk
   d.   grass → rodent → rabbit → snake

49.   A necessary member of an ecosystem *NOT* represented in this food web is a
        a. producer.
        b. primary consumer.
        c. decomposer.
        d. secondary consumer.

50.   If vegetables were removed from this food web, which of these results would be the most probable?
        a. The snake population would increase.
        b. The rodent population would die out.
        c. The grass would increase.
        d. The rabbit population would decrease.

51.   Which of these temperatures could *NOT* occur?
        a. $-100°$ Celsius
        b. $-10°$ Kelvin
        c. $2,000°$ Fahrenheit
        d. $10^{4°}$ Celsius

52.   Which organisms are classified as protists?
        a. protozoa, bacteria, and worms
        b. fungi, ferns, and mollusks
        c. monkeys, apes, and man
        d. slime molds, protozoa, and algae

53.   How much of 12 gm of a radioactive isotope with a half-life of 20 years will be left after 40 years?
        a. 0 gm
        b. 3 gm
        c. 6 gm
        d. 8 gm

54.   Two atoms are isotopes if they have the same atomic number but a different number of
        a. neutrons.
        b. mesons.
        c. electrons.
        d. protons.

55.   Shivering to maintain a 98.6°F temperature in cold weather is an example of
        a. homeostasis.
        b. synthesis.
        c. hydrolysis.
        d. transpiration.

56.   If a plain soda cracker is chewed slowly, after a while it begins to taste more
        a. salty.
        b. sweet.
        c. bitter.
        d. bland.

57.   An organism that contains a specialized system for distributing digested food throughout the body is the
   a.   amoeba.
   b.   paramecium.
   c.   earthworm.
   d.   hydra.

58.   The first step by which a mutation may occur is a change in the
   a.   location of a nitrogen base in DNA.
   b.   messenger RNA.
   c.   transfer RNA.
   d.   amino acid in a protein synthesis.

59.   At sea level, the pressure exerted by the atmosphere is approximately
   a.   1 pound per square inch.
   b.   15 pounds per square inch.
   c.   30 pounds per square inch.
   d.   50 pounds per square inch.

60.   A compound that can act like either an acid or a base is described as
   a.   amphoteric.
   b.   isomeric.
   c.   hydrolytic.
   d.   polymeric.

III. Science

60 Minutes

Read each question carefully, and then select the best answer. The correct answers will be found at the end of section C.

1. The diffusion of water through a semipermeable membrane is called
    a. pinocytosis.
    b. osmosis.
    c. active transport.
    d. transpiration-tension.

The next question refers to a historic experiment by Otto Loewi. He placed two fresh frog hearts still beating in separate dishes of saline solution. The first frog heart was still attached to two nerves: the accelerator, which speeds the heart, and the vagus, which slows it. When the vagus nerve of the first heart was stimulated by a mild electric current, the first heart slowed as expected. The saline solution from the first dish was then transferred to the second heart, which then also began to beat more slowly.

2. Based on these results, which of the following conclusions is most reasonable?
    a. The electric current accidentally touched the second heart.
    b. The first heart's vagus nerve accidentally touched the second heart.
    c. The second heart was dying because it was not stimulated.
    d. The first heart's vagus nerve released a chemical substance into the saline solution.

3. Bean plant seeds are germinated in a dark closet. The seedlings lack the color green. Which of the following statements is the best explanation for this?
    a. Bean plants are heterotrophs.
    b. Bean seedlings lack nitrogen in their seed leaf.
    c. The absence of an environmental factor limits the proper genetic expression.
    d. Bean plants cannot be classified as green plants.

4. An organism that has jointed legs, an exoskeleton, and a specialized segmented body belongs to the phylum
    a. mollusks.
    b. echinoderms.
    c. arthropods.
    d. chordates.

5. Nerve impulses from the retina are transmitted to the brain by the
    a. olfactory nerve.
    b. optic nerve.
    c. eustachian tube.
    d. auditory nerve.

6. In which of these structures does the normal development of a human embryo occur?
    a. ovary
    b. uterus
    c. vagina
    d. oviduct

7.   In humans, which of these blood components carries most of the oxygen?
     a.   plasma
     b.   white blood cells
     c.   platelets
     d.   red blood cells

The next question refers to the experiment described below.

   During a lecture, a group was instructed to write the letter "T" whenever the instructor said the word "write." The instructor tapped the desk every time he said the word "write." After doing this repeatedly, he stopped speaking but continued to tap. Many students continued to write the letter "T" with each tap.

8.   Which of these phenomena is demonstrated by this experiment?
     a.   conditioned behavior
     b.   use and disuse
     c.   innate behavior
     d.   habit formation

9.   Compound A reacts with Compound B to give Compound C plus Compounds D and E as shown by the following equation:

$$A + B \rightarrow C + D + E$$

   If 7 g A react with 4 g B to give 2 g C plus 3 g E, how many grams of D are produced?
     a.   5
     b.   6
     c.   11
     d.   16

10. What percentage of the reactants in the diagram shown below has been converted to products when the reaction is at equilibrium?

     a.   0%
     b.   50%
     c.   70%
     d.   100%

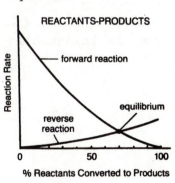

11. Which of the following statements best describes how pressure and volume will be affected as a sample of ideal gas is heated in a rigid, sealed container?
     a.   Neither pressure nor volume will increase.
     b.   Pressure will remain constant while volume will increase.
     c.   Both pressure and volume will decrease.
     d.   Pressure will increase while volume remains constant.

12. An object is traveling at a constant velocity of 100 meters per second. How far will it travel in 20 seconds?
    a. 5 meters
    b. 120 meters
    c. 200 meters
    d. 2,000 meters

13. A student placed a stone in a graduated cylinder containing 30 cm of water. She then noted that the water level rose to the 55 cm mark. What is the volume of the stone?
    a. 25 cm³
    b. 30 cm³
    c. 55 cm³
    d. 85 cm³

14. A 36-watt lamp is operated by a 9-volt battery. How many amperes of current are flowing through the lamp?
    a. .25
    b. 4
    c. 27
    d. 45

15. Which of the following terms are included in the scientific name of an organism?
    a. genus and species
    b. phylum and species
    c. family and genus
    d. kingdom and phylum

16. Which of these tissues is an example of connective tissue?
    a. striated muscle
    b. epidermis
    c. nerves
    d. tendons

17. The diagram below shows the endoplasmic reticulum of a cell as seen under the electron microscope. The structures labeled Z are the site of protein synthesis. Z represents

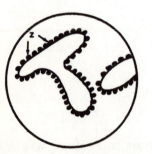

    a. mitochondria.
    b. ribosomes.
    c. chromosomes.
    d. centrosomes.

18. The entry and exit of materials in the animal cell is regulated by which of these cell organelles?
    a. nucleolus
    b. cell wall
    c. endoplasmic reticulum
    d. cell membrane

19. Which of the following structures is the functional unit of the human kidney?
    a. oviduct
    b. malpighian tubule
    c. nephron
    d. alveolus

20. Which of these substances is an end product of protein digestion?
    a. amino acids
    b. lipid
    c. fatty acids
    d. cholesterol

21. If a person's gallbladder were removed by surgery, which of the following substances would he have the most difficulty digesting?
    a. carbohydrates
    b. nucleic acids
    c. fats
    d. proteins

22. Which of the following phenomena is most likely to speed the evolutionary rate of a species?
    a. lack of environmental changes
    b. increase in mutations
    c. decrease in migration
    d. increase in death rate

23. While working in the chemistry lab, a student spills a strong acid on her hand. What is the first action the student should take?
    a. flushing the hand with water
    b. pouring a strong base on the spill to neutralize the acid
    c. notifying the instructor
    d. drying the hand with a towel

The next two questions refer to the following chart showing the vapor pressure of various substances in relation to temperature changes.

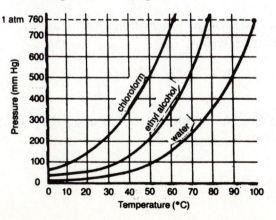

24. At 50°C, the vapor pressure of chloroform is closest to
    a. 100 mm Hg.
    b. 200 mm Hg.
    c. 350 mm Hg.
    d. 500 mm Hg.

25. As the temperature of ethyl alcohol rises from 50°C to 70°C, by approximately how many mm Hg will its vapor pressure increase?
    a. 150
    b. 200
    c. 300
    d. 500

26. Which of the following particles are contained in the nucleus of an atom?
    a. neutrons and electrons
    b. electrons, protons, and neutrons
    c. neutrons and protons
    d. electrons, photons, and neutrons

The next question refers to the indicator chart shown below.

Indicator	Color Change	pH when Color Change Occurs
Congo red	Blue to red	3.0–5.0
Methyl orange	Red to yellow	3.2–4.4
Bromothymol blue	Yellow to blue	6.0–7.6
Phenolphthalein	Colorless to pink	8.2–10.0

27. The pH of a solution in which both congo red and methyl orange produce red is
    a. 3
    b. 5
    c. 8
    d. 14

28. Quantities having both magnitude and direction are called
    a. line segments.
    b. scalars.
    c. vectors.
    d. directrixes.

29. Which of the following statements best describes the functioning of a battery?
    a. It changes chemical energy into electrical energy.
    b. It stores electricity.
    c. It creates electrons.
    d. It changes current into voltage.

30. A 4 newton and 18 newton force are acting in opposite directions upon the same point of an object. The magnitude of their resultant is
    a. 0 newtons.
    b. 14 newtons.
    c. 18 newtons.
    d. 22 newtons.

31.   Which one of the graphs shown below represents an object at rest?

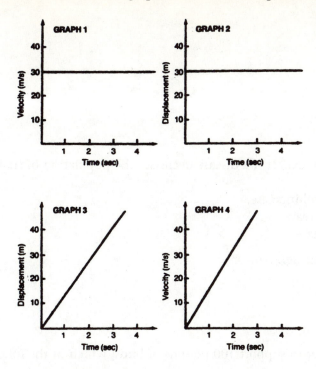

a.   Graph 1
b.   Graph 2
c.   Graph 3
d.   Graph 4

32.   Which of the following equations represents aerobic respiration?
a. $C_6H_{12}O_6 + 6O_2 \rightarrow 6CO_2 + 6H_2O + 38ATP$
b. $C_6H_{12}O_6 + C_6H_{12}O_6 \rightarrow C_{12}H_{22}O_{11} + H_2O$
c. $C_6H_{12}O_6 \rightarrow 2CO_2 + 2C_2H_5OH + 2ATP$
d. $6CO_2 + 12H_2O \rightarrow C_6H_{12}O_6 + 6O_2 + 6H_2O$

33.   An overdose of a muscle relaxant may cause a person to cease breathing because
a.   the diaphragm will be unable to contract.
b.   the lung muscles will cease to function.
c.   the muscles around the trachea will constrict.
d.   the alveoli will constrict.

34.   A decrease in acetylcholine synthesis in humans would most likely lead to
a.   an increase in protein digestion.
b.   a decrease in nerve impulse transmission.
c.   an increase in muscular activity.
d.   a decrease in white blood cells.

35.   An unknown substance is boiled with Benedict's solution. The brick-red color that results indicates the presence of
a.   protein.
b.   acid.
c.   starch.
d.   glucose.

The next three questions refer to the pyramid shown below.

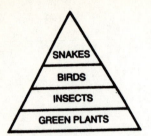

36. What first, if any, result would you expect if a disease decreases the population of snakes?
    a. No change will occur.
    b. The number of green plants will increase.
    c. The number of insects will increase.
    d. The number of birds will increase.

37. Which of these organisms represent herbivores?
    a. green plants
    b. insects
    c. birds
    d. snakes

38. According to this pyramid, in order to support 100 pounds of birds, which of the following is needed?
    a. more than 100 pounds of insects
    b. more than 100 pounds of snakes
    c. less than 100 pounds of green plants
    d. 100 pounds of insects

39. Ozone is an allotrope of
    a. hydrogen.
    b. water.
    c. oxygen.
    d. uranium.

40. Which of these values could be the pH of an acid rain sample?
    a. 12.0
    b. 8.0
    c. 7.0
    d. 4.0

41. A specific isotope has an atomic number of 51 and a mass number of 122. How many electrons are contained in the neutral atom?
    a. 51
    b. 71
    c. 122
    d. 173

42. Which of the following terms best describes a mixture of oil and water?
    a. homogeneous
    b. saturated
    c. unsaturated
    d. heterogeneous

43. Which of the following terms is the metric unit for work?
     a. joules
     b. watts
     c. amperes
     d. meters

44. A woman standing at a bus stop hears the siren of an approaching ambulance. As the ambulance passes by her, she observes a shift in frequency of the siren. The effect she observed is known as the
     a. photoelectric effect.
     b. Doppler effect.
     c. phase shift effect.
     d. Einstein effect.

45. The pitch of a vibrating string depends on all of the following *EXCEPT*
     a. the length of the string.
     b. the amplitude of the vibration.
     c. the thickness of the string.
     d. the frequency of the vibration.

46. The specific heat of water is 1 calorie/g Å C. How many calories of heat are needed to raise the temperature of 30 g of water from 25°C to 75°C?
     a. 50
     b. 750
     c. 1,500
     d. 2,250

47. As the angle of incidence of a ray of light passing from air to water increases from 0° to 90°, the angle of refraction will
     a. increase.
     b. decrease.
     c. remain the same.
     d. first increase, then remain constant.

48. The response of a plant to gravity is known as
     a. hydrotropism.
     b. phototropism.
     c. chemotropism.
     d. geotropism.

49. In a food chain, an organism that feeds on green plants is known as a
     a. decomposer.
     b. producer.
     c. first-order consumer.
     d. second-order consumer.

50. Which of the following parts of a compound microscope is used to adjust the amount of light?
     a. diaphragm
     b. objective lens
     c. eyepiece
     d. coarse adjustment knob

51.   A cell is placed in a drop of distilled water. The cell swells and bursts. The most likely reason for this is that
        a.   active transport of salts occurs.
        b.   water moves from an area of low concentration to an area of high concentration.
        c.   water moves from an area of high concentration to an area of low concentration.
        d.   salts from the distilled water enter the cell.

52.   The diameter of the field of a microscope under low power is 2 mm. The diagram below represents a long narrow cell as seen under this microscope. What is the approximate length of this cell?

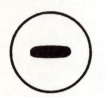

        a.   1 micron
        b.   500 microns
        c.   1000 microns
        d.   2000 microns

53.   In pea plants, tallness is dominant over shortness. If 25% of one generation of pea plants is short, what were the probable genotypes of the parents?
        a.   tt × tt
        b.   Tt × tt
        c.   TT × Tt
        d.   Tt × Tt

54.   Which of the following terms refers to the capacity of a microscope to distinguish between objects that lie very close to each other?
        a.   resolving power
        b.   staining
        c.   microdissection
        d.   magnifying power

55.   Which of the following formulas would be most probable for a compound formed from aluminum and sulfur? (Aluminum has an oxidation number of $3+$. Sulfur has an oxidation number of $2-$.)
        a.   AlS
        b. Al_3S_2
        c. Al_2S
        d. Al_2S_3

56.   Which of the following mixtures can best be separated by filtration?
        a.   oil and gasoline
        b.   table salt and gasoline
        c.   table salt and water
        d.   water and gasoline

57.   The Law of Chemical Equilibrium states that in the reversible reaction

$$N_2 + 3H_2 \rightleftarrows 2NH_3$$

the equilibrium constant is expressed as

a. $K = \dfrac{[N^2][H^2]^3}{[NH_3]^2}$

b. $K = \dfrac{[NH_3]}{[N_2][H_2]}$

c. $K = \dfrac{[N^2][H^2]^3}{[NH_3]}$

d. $K = \dfrac{[NH_3]^2}{[N_2][H_2]^3}$

58.   Which of the following elements would be classified as a nonmetal?
a.   Na (Sodium)
b.   Hg (Mercury)
c.   S (Sulfur)
d.   Mn (Manganese)

59.   Machines may be used for all of the following purposes *EXCEPT* to
a.   multiply force.
b.   increase energy.
c.   transform energy.
d.   multiply speed.

The next question refers to the following diagram showing a ray of light as it strikes a mirror at an angle of 30°.

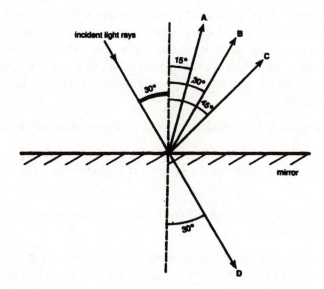

60.   Which of the rays in this diagram best represents the reflected ray?
a.   A
b.   B
c.   C
d.   D

Answers

I. Science

1.   **The answer is b.** Chloroplasts contain the green pigment chlorophyll. This pigment is necessary for the process of photosynthesis, which occurs in plants.

2.   **The answer is d.** Water molecules are polar. This is due to the fact that oxygen draws the electrons in the molecule towards itself. Thus, there is a negative charge surrounding the oxygen and a positive charge around the hydrogens. The unbalanced charges cause the water molecules to cluster together and this gives water the property called surface tension. Surface tension is the attraction between molecules at the surface of a liquid, which allows a glass to be filled above the rim without the water flowing over.

3.   **The answer is a.** An impulse travels down the axon of a neuron and reaches the terminus. There, chemicals are released in response, which travel across the synapse to the next neuron. Thus, the impulse is transmitted to the next neuron.

4.   **The answer is c.** Carbohydrates, proteins, and nucleic acids (RNA and DNA) are all very important chemicals in living things. Carbohydrates are energy sources, proteins are building matter, and nucleic acids contain our genetic information.

5.   **The answer is b.** The alimentary canal begins at the mouth and ends at the anus. In between are the pharynx, esophagus, stomach, small intestine, and large intestine.

6.   **The answer is d.** The villi in the intestine are tiny projections in the small intestine. The surface area of the villi increases the total surface area of the intestine.

7.   **The answer is c.** Refraction is the bending of light as it passes obliquely from air to water. The speed of the light wave changes when it passes between two media. When the light wave enters the second media at an oblique angle it changes direction; the light wave is bent. Diffraction refers to the spreading out of light waves as they pass through a narrow opening. Reflection occurs when light bounces off an object. The phenomenon of dispersion occurs when light is separated into its spectrum.

8.   **The answer is d.** The nucleus is surrounded by cytoplasm that provides scaffolding for the organelles of a cell.

9.   **The answer is b.** Of the choices offered, the nitrous oxide level is highest when the air-fuel ratio is 16:1.

10. **The answer is d.** The chart is showing amounts of different gases in automobile exhaust. These gases are a major cause of air pollution.

11. **The answer is b.** This graph was created to show the amount of gases released at differing air-fuel ratios. If carbon dioxide is not included, it can be inferred that this gas is not effected by the ratios.

12. **The answer is a.** Glucose, a monosaccharide, undergoes cellular respiration, which results in the production of energy in the form of ATP. Glycogen is a starch that serves as a reserve. When there are low levels of glucose available, glycogen is broken down into glucose, which can then be used by the cells.

13. **The answer is a.** A sensory neuron conveys a message to the spinal cord, which transmits the message via a motor neuron to the effector muscle.

14. **The answer is c.** Potential energy can be thought of as a function of height. Since total energy is always conserved, the kinetic energy is at a maximum when the potential is at a minimum, or at the bottom of the incline.

15. **The answer is c.** Bacteria comprise the decomposer portion of the food chain. They are responsible for recycling organic material into inorganic material that plants can use to undergo photosynthesis.

16. **The answer is a.** High pitch sounds are heard when the receptor cells closer to the oval window are stimulated, while low pitch sounds results from stimulation of those cells that are farther down the cochlea.

17. **The answer is a.** Remember that during a phase change, the temperature remains constant. This is due to the fact that all of the heat that is added is used to break the bonds and change the phase.

18. **The answer is b.** The substance would only change back to a liquid if enough heat were withdrawn.

19. **The answer is a.** Self-pollination would allow this plant to produce gametes, sperm, and eggs, that would unite, form seeds. Observing the color of the plants from these seeds would allow the planter to determine if this changed occurred at the level of the gametes.

20. **The answer is b.** A human male has one X chromosome and one Y chromosome, while human females have two X chromosomes. The Y chromosome can only come from the male.

21. **The answer is b.** Sunlight is absorbed by the chlorophyll contained in plants. The absorbed energy fuels the process of photosynthesis, which produces glucose.

22. **The answer is a.** Baking soda, or sodium bicarbonate, is often used to neutralize acids. The reaction in A illustrates sodium bicarbonate reacting with a hydrogen ion (causes acidity) to produce nonacidic products.

23. **The answer is c.** Only 5 drops of lemon juice were needed to bleach the solution, which indicates that it contains the most vitamin C of all the solutions tested.

24. **The answer is b.** After the orange juice was heated, more drops were necessary to bleach the solution. Thus, the amount of vitamin C was reduced.

25. **The answer is a.** The indophenol solution is used to test for the presence of the vitamin and thus does not intially contain it.

26. **The answer is a.** A has the tallest bar on the graph.

27. **The answer is a.** Nuts is the only protein containing food of the choices.

28. **The answer is b.** Diffusion refers to the process in which particles randomly disperse from areas of high particle concentration to areas of low particle concentration.

29. **The answer is b.** The organs of the endocrine system produce hormones, which are secreted in response to various stimuli.

30. **The answer is c.** #3 points to the parathyroid glands, which produce parathyroid hormone. Parathyroid hormone, PTH, works antagonistically with calcitonin, which is produced in the thyroid gland. When calcium levels in the blood are low, PTH causes bone cells to break down

and release calcium. When calcium levels are high, calcitonin causes calcium to deposit onto the bones.

31. **The answer is d.** The pancreas produces enzymes that take part in digestion. In addition, the pancreas produced hormones such as insulin and glucagon.

32. **The answer is c.** The formula for converting temperature in Celsius to temperature in Fahrenheit is:

$$T \text{ (Fahrenheit)} = \{\tfrac{9}{5} \times T \text{ (Celsius)}\} + 32.$$

Therefore, 5 degrees Celsius convert to 41 degrees Fahrenheit.

$$(\tfrac{9}{5} \times 5) = 9; 9 + 32 = 41$$

33. **The answer is d.** An alcohol involves is usually characterized structurally by the presence of an OH group attached to a hydrocarbon. The presence of a COOH group represents a carboxylic acid.

34. **The answer is c.** If a car's rate of change of velocity is negative, the car's acceleration is negative. This means that the car is decelerating (slowing down).

35. **The answer is b.** When balancing an equation, the number of atoms of each element must be the same on both sides of the equation.

36. **The answer is b.** II B represents the steepest part of the graph, which indicates the greatest increase in population.

37. **The answer is d.** IV D represents a decline in the population, which occurred when the carrying capacity leveled off.

38. **The answer is d.** The population of all organisms will fluctuate around the carrying capacity of the environment.

39. **The answer is a.** Examples of nucleic acids which contain 5-carbon sugars and nitrogen bases are RNA and DNA.

40. **The answer is d.** A substance with a PH between 8 and 14 is basic. The closer the substance gets to a pH of 14, the more basic it is.

41. **The answer is d.** Binary fission is an example of asexual reproduction, while conjugation is an example of sexual reproduction.

42. **The answer is a.** Magnesium hydroxide is the only base of the four choices. Thus, in water, magnesium hydroxide will form a basic, or alkaline, solution.

43. **The answer is d.** Paper chromotography is a method that uses the natural capillary action of liquids to separate out substances into their different components. In this case, the green filtrate is shown to be made up of yellow and green constituents.

44. **The answer is b.** Not knowing whether only chlorophyll was contained in the filtrate, it can be inferred that more than one type of filtrate was present.

45. **The answer is a.** The bonding between the two chlorine atoms involves a sharing of electrons. Ultimately, a molecule of chlorine is formed without a separation of charge. HBr and LiCl

are both ionic as they are combinations of metal and non-metal atoms. Ammonia, or NH_3, is covalently bonded but is polar since the nitrogen and hydrogens do not attract electrons equally.

46. **The answer is c.** Since the concentrations are so much greater in seaweed than in the surrounding water, iodine must have to move against a concentration gradient. Thus, the transport process using energy must be involved in order for the seaweed to accumulate such a great concentration of iodine.

47. **The answer is c.** In this reaction, zinc will replace hydrogen and produce zinc chloride. Thus, hydrogen gas is released.

48. **The answer is d.** Bread mold is a fungus. Fungi are unable to make their own food and are dependent on other life forms for nutrition. Of the choices offered, the fungus has the closest nutritive process to that of animals.

49. **The answer is c.** When the air holds all the water vapor that it can, it is saturated.

50. **The answer is b.** Alcohols have lower boiling points than water, usually close to 80 degrees Celsius.

51. **The answer is c.** As the pressure increases from 1 to 2 the graph line indicating the temperature increases by 20°.

52. **The answer is b.** A decrease in volume would result in an increase in pressure (Boyle's Law!) and thus exhalation.

53. **The answer is a.** Cellular respiration begins with the splitting of glucose. The products then enter the Kreb's cycle and then the electron transport chain.

54. **The answer is c.** Work done is independent of who is doing the work. Since both people do the same thing they do the same amount of work.

55. **The answer is c.** Hydronium ions, or H_3O^+, are essentially hydrogen ions combined with a nearby water molecule. In essence, acids are characterized by the presence of hydrogen or hydronium ions.

56. **The answer is b.** A similarity in amino acids suggests a similarity in the structure of the DNA and thus a close relationship between the organisms in question.

57. **The answer is d.** Einstein's equation, $E = M C$ squared, means Energy = Mass $\times$ (speed of light)^2.

58. **The answer is a.** Sublimation is the process in which a solid changes directly into a vapor or a vapor changes directly into a solid.

59. **The answer is b.** The boiling point of a solution is the temperature at which the vapor pressure is equal to the pressure of the atmosphere. At the top of a mountain, the atmospheric pressure is lower and thus the temperature it takes for the vapor pressure of a solution to reach this pressure is lowered.

60. **The answer is c.** Cube A has a volume of 1000 cm³ while cube B has a volume of 125 cm³. Cube A has 6 times the volume of cube B.

II. Science

1. **The answer is d.** The placenta is a highly vascular organ through which the fetus absorbs nutrients and excretes wastes.

2. **The answer is a.** Cellular respiration is an energy yielding process that releases ATP (adenosine triphosphate) from organic molecules.

3. **The answer is d.** Fewer bees and butterflies, which are excellent pollinators, would result in a decline in the dispersal of pollen and thus fewer plant seeds would be produced.

4. **The answer is b.** Villi are tiny projections that are barely visible to the naked eye. They are clustered over the entire mucous surface of the small intestine. The villi diffuse and transport fluids and nutrients.

5. **The answer is b.** Whenever a box is pulled along a surface, energy goes into counteracting friction. The amount of energy required is determined by the coefficient of friction.

6. **The answer is b.** The wavelength of a wave is defined as the distance between two successive crests.

7. **The answer is b.** Each small marking on the voltmeter represents 0.2 volts.

8. **The answer is d.** A parallel circuit is defined as a circuit with the same voltage across all of its resistors.

9. **The answer is b.** Whenever a wire is wrapped around a rod and connected across a power source like a battery, the device will act as an electromagnet.

10. **The answer is c.** During the 4–6 second interval the car travels at the constant maximum velocity. In all other possibilities the average velocities over the given time periods are less then 20m/s

11. **The answer is c.** The optimal temperature at which bacteria grows is 37° Celsius.

12. **The answer is d.** According to Gay-Lussac's law of gases, as temperature increases at constant volume, pressure increases proportionally. The pressure will increase. Boyle's Law ($PV = RT$) states that if temperature increases while volume remains the same, pressure must increase as well.

13. **The answer is a.** The functional unit of the kidney is the nephron. Urine is formed in the nephron by the processes of filtration, reabsorption, and secretion.

14. **The answer is b.** Since the equal-arm balance is balanced at a ratio of 20 washers to 10 bolts, the weight of the bolts must be double the washers. Two washers are equivalent in mass to one bolt. Thus, four bolts are equivalent in mass to eight washers. An increase of 4 bolts on one side will require 8 washers on the other side to maintain the balance.

15. **The answer is a.** Isomers are compounds that have the same formula but different molecular structure.

16. **The answer is c.** A control for this experiment would be to grow the mold in just water so that the results of the mold growth with sugar can be compared to the mold growth without sugar.

17. **The answer is d.** Vinegar, an acid, would neutralize lye, a base.

18.   **The answer is b.** New layers of sediment cover old ones and provide a record of emergence of flora and fauna. The fish were the only fossils found in the layers beneath the upper layers, which indicates that they evolved first.

19.   **The answer is a.** The tube with the black cover will have the most rapid temperature rise.

20.   **The answer is a.** A points to the endosperm, which provides the growing embryo with nutrients.

21.   **The answer is c.** Any horizontal motion such as that of object Y is irrelevant because it will not effect the time taken to drop that amount.

22.   **The answer is d.** Blue litmus paper turns red when placed in an acid solution.

23.   **The answer is c.** A balanced equation contains the same number of atoms of each element on both sides of the written reaction.

24.   **The answer is c.** H_2SO_4 is sulfuric acid. Acidic solutions are characterized by the presence of hydrogen ions. Thus, acids such as sulfuric acid or hydrochloric acid (HCl) contain hydrogen atoms that they "donate" to a solution.

25.   **The answer is d.** The statement in D least supports the idea that the leaves are dropped due to the temperature since the temperature in southern Florida in late fall is not freezing, yet the leaves are dropping. The key word in the question is LEAST.

26.   **The answer is b.** Walking outdoors expends the greatest number of calories per minute according to the data chart.

27.   **The answer is d.** The rate of calorie expenditure is greater for men than women in all the listed activities. None of the other choices are supported by the data on the chart.

28.   **The answer is d.** Plants undergo photosynthesis, which allows them to make glucose from the simple materials carbon dioxide and water.

29.   **The answer is b.** This apparatus allows for two solvents to be separated from each other. For instance, assume the flask contains water and alcohol. Alcohol will boil first since it has a lower boiling point, and the gas will be collected in the long tube, recondense, and collect in a second flask that is not shown. Thus, the alcohol can be separated from the water.

30.   **The answer is d.** Tropism refers to the response of a plant to external stimuli such as light.

31.   **The answer is a.** The wavelength is the distance between two successive crests. Waves A and B have all their crests at the same distance along the line.

32.   **The answer is b.** The melting point is the temperature at which a substance changes from a solid to a liquid. The boiling point is the temperature at which a substance changes from a liquid to a gas. Thus, the substance with the smallest difference between its melting and boiling points is a liquid over the smallest temperature range. Substance X is liquid over a 70 degree range. W has a 145 degree-range, Y has a 1495-degree range, and Z has a 165-degree range.

33.   **The answer is b.** 1mm = 1000 microns. 1.6 mm = 1600 microns. One half of the field $\frac{1600}{2}$ = 800 microns.

34.   **The answer is c.** $\frac{5 \text{ grams}}{25 \text{ mL}}$ = 20% solution

35.   **The answer is d.** The Law of Independent Assortment states that traits are passed onto offspring independently of each other. Thus, a seed may contain either of the height alleles and either of the color alleles.

36.   **The answer is b.** The flat part of the velocity vs. time graph is the part where velocity is constant. The sloped part is where velocity is increasing. It starts out moving at a constant velocity and then accelerates.

37.   **The answer is b.** Radiation exposure has been linked to cancer.

38.   **The answer is a.** Endocrine glands are ductless glands with blood vessel associations. Exocrine glands, such as digestive and tear glands, empty their secretions via ducts.

39.   **The answer is d.** Iodine is an indicator that turns blue-black in the presence of starch.

40.   **The answer is c.** Muscles are the tissues mostly involved when a person is exercising. Smooth muscle is found in the lining of organs such as the uterus. Skeletal muscle, such as found in the muscles of the legs and arms, is striated.

41.   **The answer is b.** Diffusion is the spontanous dispersion of particles from areas of high concentration to areas of low concentration. Since the body of the hydra involves very few membranes, and thus few barriers, diffusion is the means of transport. Osmosis is a special type of diffusion and specifically refers to the diffusion of water.

42.   **The answer is b.** The refraction of a ray is determined by Snell's law. $N1 \sin\theta1 = N2 \sin\theta2$. If we can measure the angles and then find $\sin\theta1$ and $\sin\theta2$, we can determine the index of refraction of the glass, since N (air) $= 1$. The device used to measure an angle is a protractor.

43.   **The answer is b.** A catalyst only effects the rate of a reaction and is not changed or consumed during a reaction.

44.   **The answer is d.**

45.   **The answer is c.** A centrosome is an organelle found in animal cells.

46.   **The answer is a.** Ohm's law applies to the study of electricity, it states that voltage is proportional to current and resistance ($V = IR$).

47.   **The answer is d.** A cloud chamber makes the paths of ionizing radiation rays visible. The device reveals the paths of high-speed charged particles.

48.   **The answer is c.** Follow the arrows!

49.   **The answer is c.** Decomposers, such as bacteria, are not represented here.

50.   **The answer is d.** According to the diagram, rabbits are solely dependent on vegetables. Thus, if the vegetables were removed, the rabbit population would diminish. The rodent population would not be as affected by the removal of vegetables since the rodents also depend upon grasses.

51.   **The answer is b.** Zero° Kelvin is absolute zero, which is the lowest possible temperature; therefore, -10 Kelvin does not exist.

52.   **The answer is d.** Bacteria are in the kingdom *Monera;* worms, mollusks, humans, apes, and monkeys are in the kingdom *Animalia;* ferns in the kingdom *Plantae;* and fungus in the kingdom *Fungi.*

53.   **The answer is b.** Half-life is the amount of time it takes for one-half of the mass of a sample of a radioactive substance to decay. In 20 years a 12 gm isotope with a half-life of 20 years will be 6 gm. Twenty years after that, the isotope will be 3 gm.

54.   **The answer is a.** An example of isotopes are carbon-12 and carbon-14. Both have the same atomic number (number of protons), but while carbon-12 contains 6 neutrons, carbon-14 contains 8 neutrons.

	Carbon-12	Carbon-14
#protons	6	6
#electrons	6	6
#neutrons	6	8

55.   **The answer is a.** Homeostasis refers to the maintenance of a stable internal environment.

56.   **The answer is b.** The enzyme amylase, which is found in saliva, breaks down the starches present in food, such as crackers, into simple sugars.

57.   **The answer is c.** Of these four organisms, only the earthworm has two openings to its digestive tract. The other, more primitive, organisms have one opening and less specialized means of transporting food throughout the body.

58.   **The answer is a.** The sequence of messenger RNA, transfer RNA, and amino acids in protein synthesis all depend on the sequence of DNA found in the nucleus. Thus, the first step in which a mutation may occur is at the level of the DNA, which is made up of a specific sequence of bases.

59.   **The answer is b.** The atmospheric pressure at sea level is approximately 15 pounds per square inch. As the altitude increases the pressure decreases.

60.   **The answer is a.** An amphoteric substance can behave either as an acid or a base. Water is an example of an amphoteric substance because it can act as an acid by furnishing a proton, or it can act as a base by accepting a proton.

III. Science

1.   **The answer is b.** Osmosis refers to the diffusion of water from areas that contain a high concentration of water to areas that contain a low concentration of water.

2.   **The answer is d.** The saline solution contained acetylcholine released by the first heart's vagus nerve, which is a neurotransmitter that has the inhibitory effect of slowing down heart rate.

3.   **The answer is c.** The seedlings lacked light which, interfered with their development.

4.   **The answer is c.** An example of an arthropod is a lobster.

5.   **The answer is b.** The eustachian tube and auditory tubes are involved in hearing, while the olfactory nerve is involved with the sense of smell.

6.   **The answer is b.** The ovary releases the egg into the oviduct, or fallopian tube, where it is fertilized. If fertilization occurs, the zygote travels to the uterus where it implants and develops.

7. **The answer is d.** Red blood cells contain hemoglobin, which binds, transports, and delivers oxygen throughout the body.

8. **The answer is a.** Conditioned behavior refers to the association of behavior with a specific stimulus.

9. **The answer is b.** The law of conservation of mass says that mass may neither be created nor destroyed. Therefore, the mass of the reactants must be equal to the mass of the products of a reaction.

10. **The answer is c.** Find the point on the graph that indicates equilibrium. That point is over the 70% point on the horizontal line.

11. **The answer is d.** A "rigid" container implies no change in volume. According to Gay-Lussac's gas law, at constant volume an increase in temperature causes an increase in pressure and vice-versa.

12. **The answer is d.** Distance traveled is directly proportional to velocity and time.

    Distance = velocity × time
    Distance = 100 × 20
    2,000 = 100 × 20
    Distance = 2,000 meters

13. **The answer is a.** The stone causes the volume in the cylinder to increase by 25 cm cubed. The volume of a liquid displaced by a submerged object is equal to the volume of the object itself; Therefore, the volume of the stone is 25 cm cubed.

14. **The answer is b.**
    Power = Voltage × Current
    36 watts = 9 volts × (current) amperes
    Current = 4

15. **The answer is a.** Genus and species are used in the scientific name of an organism.

16. **The answer is d.** Connective tissue binds and supports other tissues. For example, tendons attach muscle to bone.

17. **The answer is b.** There are two types of endoplasmic reticulum: rough and smooth. Rough endoplasmic reticulum is studded with ribosomes, which are the sites of protein synthesis in a cell.

18. **The answer is d.** The plasma membrane, which is made of carbohydrates, lipids, and proteins, is selectively permeable and regulates traffic into and out of a cell.

19. **The answer is c.** The oviduct, or fallopian tube, conveys the released egg to the uterus. Malpighian tubules are excretory organs found in insects while alveoli are the functional units of lungs.

20. **The answer is a.** Proteins are made up of chains of amino acids.

21. **The answer is c.** The gallbladder stores bile, which is the substance produced by the liver. Bile contains bile salts, which aid in the digestion and absorption of fats.

22. **The answer is b.** Mutations of DNA are the original source of variation and alter the gene pool in a population. An increase in the number of mutations would increase the variation in the gene pool and thus speed up the evolutionary rate of a species.

23. **The answer is a.** The first action to take with any spill in a laboratory is to flush the substance off the body.

24. **The answer is d.** Find 50°C on the graph's horizontal line. Follow the vertical line above 50°C up to the point where it intersects with the chloroform line. Follow the horizontal line over to the vertical line that indicates vapor pressure; the reading is 500 mm Hg.

25. **The answer is c.** Locate the ethyl alcohol line and follow it from 50°C to 70°C. At the 50°C point the pressure is 200 mm hg. At the 70°C point the vapor pressure is 500 mm Hg. The vapor pressure has risen 300 mm Hg.

26. **The answer is c.** Neutrons and protons are contained in the nucleus of an atom while the electrons reside outside the nucleus.

27. **The answer is b.** Congo Red and Methyl Orange are indicators which both indicate the presence of acids. Congo Red begins to turn red between the pH's of 3–5 and remains red as the pH approaches zero.

28. **The answer is c.** By definition vectors are quantities with magnitude and direction.

29. **The answer is a.** In an electrochemical cell, which makes up a battery, chemical energy is converted into current.

30. **The answer is b.** When two forces act in opposite directions, the total force is determined by subtracting the smaller force from the larger one.

31. **The answer is b.** Displacement is the distance that an object is from some starting point. Graph 2 shows an object with constant displacement. It is not moving.

32. **The answer is a.** Aerobic respiration refers to the breakdown of glucose and the formation of energy. The reaction shown in D is the reverse of aerobic respiration and is photosynthesis.

33. **The answer is a.** The diaphragm must contract in order for the process of inhalation to occur.

34. **The answer is b.** Acetylcholine is a common neurotransmitter. Neurotransmitters act as chemical messengers and spread information from one neuron to the next.

35. **The answer is d.** Benedict's solution is used to indicate the presence of monosaccharides, glucose.

36. **The answer is d.** The diagram shows a food chain in which snakes feed on birds. If the number of snakes declined, then the number of birds will increase.

37. **The answer is b.** Herbivores are animals that feed on plants. Thus, insects are herbivores because they consume green plants.

38. **The answer is a.** The diagram increases in size in the direction of birds to insects indicating that more insects are required to support a certain amount of birds. Thus, 100 pounds of birds will consume an amount of insects exceeding 100 pounds.

39. **The answer is c.** Ozone, or O_3, is an allotrope of oxygen. It is a molecule made up of more than two atoms of the same element.

40. **The answer is d.** Acid rain has an acidic pH. A substance with a pH between 0 and 7 is an acid.

41. **The answer is a.** The mass number is the sum of the number of protons and neutrons. The atomic number is the number of protons, which is always equal to the number of electrons in a neutral atom.

42. **The answer is d.** Oil and water do not mix and thus from a heterogenous solution. A homogenous solution is one in which the concentration of the substances are constant throughout.

43. **The answer is a.** The joule is the unit of energy equal to the work done by a force of one newton acting over a distance of one meter.

44. **The answer is b.** The Doppler effect occurs whenever there is relative motion between the source of the sound waves and the observer. The pitch of a siren will be higher as it approaches you and lower as it drives away. The siren has not changed its frequency but the motion of the siren towards you increases the frequency of the sound waves you hear.

45. **The answer is b.** Observed pitch is independent of the amplitude of the vibration. The amplitude is related to the loudness of the sound.

46. **The answer is c.** The specific heat capacity of a substance is the heat required to raise the temperature of 1 gram of a specific substance by 1° Celsius. In the case of water the specific heat capacity is 1 calorie/gram C. The formula for specific heat capacity is:

$$\text{Specific Heat Capacity} = \frac{\text{Heat}}{\text{Mass} \times \text{Change in Temperature}}$$

47. **The answer is a.** As the angle of incidence of a light wave passing from one medium to another increases, the angle of refraction increases.

48. **The answer is d.**

49. **The answer is c.** Green plants are producers since they produce their own food via the process of photosynthesis. Consumers depend on other organisms for their food sources. A first-order consumer is a herbivore and eats plants and algae. A second-order consumer is a carnivore and eats herbivores.

50. **The answer is a.** The diaphragm adjusts the amount of light in a microscope.

51. **The answer is b.** Osmosis refers to the diffusion of water from areas that contain a high concentration of water and low concentration of solute (outside the cell) to areas that contain a low concentration of water and high concentration of solute (inside the cell).

52. **The answer is c.** The field is 2mm, which equals 2000 microns. The cell takes up half of the fields, therefore, the approximate length of the cell is 1mm or 1000 microns.

53. **The answer is d.** A cross in which both of the parents are heterozygotes yields 25% TT, 50% Tt, and 25% tt.

54. **The answer is a.** Resolving power refers to the capacity to distinguish between objects that lie very close to each other.

55. **The answer is d.** The ions that make up a compound form in such a ratio to produce a neutral compound. Thus, 2 aluminum atoms (+3 each) are needed for 3 sulfur atoms (−2 each).

56. **The answer is b.** Filtration involves passing a mixture through a membrane which separates out the insoluble substances. Salt is insoluble in gasoline and can thus be extracted via this mechanism.

57.   **The answer is d.** Equilibrium constants are expressed as the product of the concentrations of the products over product of the concentration of the reactants. The concentrations are raised to the coefficient:

$$aA + bB \rightarrow cC + dD$$

$$Keq = \frac{[C]^c[D]^d}{[A]^a[B]^b}$$

58.   **The answer is c.** Sulfur is the only element listed that is not a metal.

59.   **The answer is b.** Conservation of energy forbids a machine from increasing energy. Machines are designed to use energy efficiently. Machines cannot be designed to increase energy; they use energy for the purpose of doing work.

60.   **The answer is b.** Reflection is the bouncing back of a wave after it strikes a surface that does not absorb its energy. According to the law of reflection, the angle of incidence equals the angle of reflection. This ray struck a mirror at a 30° angle. Therefore, the reflected ray will be 30°.

Comprehensive Practice Tests

Comprehensive Practice Test 1

Verbal Ability:
Word Knowledge and Reading Comprehension

60 Minutes

WORD KNOWLEDGE: Read each sentence carefully. Then, *on the basis of what is stated in the sentence*, select the correct completion of the incomplete statement. The correct answers will be found at the end of this test.

1. The baby tried to *invert* the drinking cup. She wanted to
    a. turn it upside down.
    b. twist it around.
    c. throw it down.
    d. lift it up.

2. He was voted the most popular boy that year, because his classmates found him so
    a. edible.
    b. amiable.
    c. economic.
    d. haughty.

3. When the woman found out that the diamond she had bought wasn't real, she realized that she had been
    a. impersonated.
    b. hoodwinked.
    c. dejected.
    d. reprimanded.

4. A person who allays her fears and anxieties appears to be
    a. hysterical.
    b. hilarious.
    c. calm.
    d. somber.

5. A person who steals small articles of little value is considered a
    a. pilferer.
    b. confiscator.
    c. spendthrift.
    d. benefactor.

6. The carpenter drilled several holes in the wooden board. These holes are
    a. indentations.
    b. omissions.
    c. blemishes.
    d. perforations.

7.   According to the law, young men must register for the draft when they reach eighteen years of age. Such registration is
       a. impulsive.
       b. superfluous.
       c. compulsory.
       d. obsolete.

8.   The physician was remunerated for his services.
       Remunerated means
       a. belittled.
       b. compensated.
       c. praised.
       d. swindled.

9.   While studying the mixture, the scientist noticed a trace of red stain. The scientist saw
       a. a combination.
       b. a tincture.
       c. an adage.
       d. a fissure.

10.   A person who is constantly talking in a pointless fashion is said to be
       a. garrulous.
       b. stoical.
       c. cosmopolitan.
       d. jovial.

11.   When someone has eccentric ideas and presents them suddenly in a fanciful way, such behavior is characterized as
       a. pugnacious.
       b. cosmopolitan.
       c. literal.
       d. whimsical.

12.   A file of papers containing detailed information about a particular subject is called a
       a. dossier.
       b. glossary.
       c. synthesis.
       d. testament.

13.   The sentence was written in a complex code that made the meaning difficult for the translator to
       a. construe.
       b. exacerbate.
       c. variegate.
       d. transmute.

14.   The coven of witches attempted to communicate with the dead. They practiced
       a. misogyny.
       b. chicanery.
       c. necromancy.
       d. declamation.

15. The actress continued to take acting classes in the hope that the quality of her performance would be
    a. augmented.
    b. ensconced.
    c. pervaded.
    d. usurped.

16. Jane thought that the conversation at the party was banal; she felt that such talk was
    a. trite.
    b. obscene.
    c. lively.
    d. affected.

17. The gossamer fabric made a beautiful gown.
    Gossamer means

    a. sequined.
    b. synthetic.
    c. colorful.
    d. sheer.

18. In a special ceremony, Joe was presented with the key to the city and named honorary assistant mayor. This position is considered to be
    a. retractable.
    b. obligatory.
    c. temporary.
    d. titular.

19. The couple arranged to meet in secret. Such meetings are known as
    a. carousals.
    b. trysts.
    c. parleys.
    d. sequels.

20. The police officer made every effort to help the waif.
    A *waif* is a

    a. homeless citizen.
    b. stray child.
    c. handicapped person.
    d. crime victim.

21. The guest speaker addressed the assembly with a loud, ranting speech. The speech was
    a. a recrimination.
    b. a harangue.
    c. an edict.
    d. a dogma.

22. The style of a house decorated with furniture of many periods can be described as
    a. eclectic.
    b. reverent.
    c. calamitous.
    d. sumptuous.

23. A good debater should be steadfast about his opinions. He must not
     a. circumnavigate.
     b. vacillate.
     c. oust.
     d. broach.

24. The many acres of wheat in the fields would yield a supply of food that was
     a. copious.
     b. equable.
     c. voracious.
     d. salubrious.

25. The reporter questioned the wealthy man about his philanthropy.
     Philanthropy means

     a. affectation.
     b. benevolence.
     c. idealism.
     d. fervor.

26. The young boy heeded the sagacious counsel of his grandfather.
     Sagacious means

     a. altruistic.
     b. resilient.
     c. nebulous.
     d. discerning.

27. The members of a church are called its
     a. hierarchy.
     b. laity.
     c. partisans.
     d. zealots.

28. In her will, Aunt Edna left her books to cousin Charles. Such a gift is called
     a. a legacy.
     b. an heirloom.
     c. an artifact.
     d. a profit.

29. Many of the founding fathers of the United States originally advocated government by a small
     group. This kind of government is called
     a. a theocracy.
     b. a monarchy.
     c. an oligarchy.
     d. an anarchy.

30. The stand upon which a coffin rests is called a
     a. bier.
     b. pall.
     c. chalice.
     d. mausoleum.

READING COMPREHENSION: There are five reading passages in this section. Read each passage carefully. Then, *on the basis of what you have read in the passage*, select the best answer for each question.

I

When Vincent van Gogh took a knife to himself in 1888, he did more than just cut off part of his ear; he carved a permanent place for himself in the psychiatric hall of fame. Over the years, art historians and physicians have been trying to deduce what malady drove van Gogh to such bizarre acts as lopping off an earlobe, drinking kerosene, and eating paint. Explanations have ranged from schizophrenia to digitalis toxicity (*Discover*, April 1981). Now, in a speech before a gathering of neurologists in Boston, Shahram Khoshbin, an assistant professor of neurology at Harvard Medical School, has offered yet another theory for van Gogh's wildly aberrant behavior.

According to Khoshbin, van Gogh was a victim of temporal lobe epilepsy and a personality disorder called Geschwind's syndrome, which is often—but not exclusively—associated with epilepsy. Named after Norman Geschwind, the late Harvard neurologist who described the link between temporal lobe epilepsy and the personality disorder, the syndrome is characterized by hypergraphia, a compulsion to write or produce graphic material, an obsession with religion, a change in sexual behavior, and a certain "stickiness," a tendency to be fixated—for instance, refusing to let a conversation end.

Khoshbin, who has been studying van Gogh for 15 years, backs his theory with plenty of historical evidence. In his famous 15-month stay in Arles, which ended shortly after he cut off his earlobe, van Gogh produced some 200 paintings, more than 100 drawings and watercolors, and 200 letters, the shortest of which was six pages long. He also had a life-long obsession with religion: in his youth, he wanted to be a Lutheran priest, and Khoshbin emphasizes the religious imagery in such paintings as the *Resurrection of Lazarus* and the *Pieta*.

Khoshbin speculates that van Gogh's sexual orientation changed when Paul Gauguin joined him at Arles, and that their relationship "went beyond just friendship." And, says Khoshbin, Gauguin's letters about van Gogh frequently make mention of van Gogh's tendency to be obsessed about a topic of conversation; he would refuse either to change or to terminate it, even hours after it was introduced.

From "A New Portrait of Van Gogh." Copyright © *Discover* magazine, August 1985, Time, Inc.

31.   The main idea of this passage is that
  a.   van Gogh has been studied by many experts.
  b.   van Gogh was a prolific artist.
  c.   van Gogh suffered from a psychobiological disorder.
  d.   van Gogh wanted to be a Lutheran priest.

32.   According to Khoshbin, association with Gauguin affected van Gogh's
  a.   artistic expression.
  b.   religious beliefs.
  c.   sexual inclination.
  d.   conversational style.

33. How many works of art did van Gogh produce during his stay at Arles?
    a. 500
    b. 300
    c. 200
    d. 100

34. Khoshbin's conclusions about van Gogh are based upon
    a. biographical evidence about van Gogh.
    b. the findings of physicians who treated van Gogh.
    c. the memoirs of van Gogh.
    d. studies of van Gogh's work by art historians.

35. The "graphic material" mentioned in this passage is material that is
    a. extremely colorful and artistic.
    b. similar to graphite.
    c. geometric in design.
    d. drawn or written.

36. One conclusion we can draw about epilepsy after reading this passage is that
    a. it results in bizarre eating habits.
    b. it is accompanied by Geschwind's syndrome.
    c. it has more than one form.
    d. it is caused by brain damage.

II

No one has ever seen the solid surface of Venus, at least not by eye, even with a big telescope. Venus is always covered by its thick cloud layers. So why not send a spacecraft down underneath the clouds? A Russian spacecraft tried that and actually landed on the surface. But it managed to send back only one or two pictures before it quit working at the scorching temperature of the surface—900°F. You can see the problem. Underneath the clouds it is too hot to use anything like a camera. Above the clouds all you can see is clouds.

I had not thought about that problem until I saw a map of Venus. . . . The map comes from measurements made by the spacecraft Pioneer Venus Orbiter, which has been orbiting Venus since 1978.

How can you make a map of a surface you can't see? It was done by radar, which goes right through the clouds. The spacecraft carries a radar altimeter.

. . . A radar beam is sent straight down toward the surface. A receiver catches a reflection of the beam and keeps track of the time it took for the beam to go down and back. We know how fast the beam travels (the same as the speed of light). So a computer can easily figure out how far the beam travels . . . that gives the altitude, the distance down to the surface. . . . Altitudes have been measured over more than a thousand paths of the spacecraft across the surface. All those measurements were put together to make a map.

. . . The mapping of Venus is done much the same way that we map the ocean floors. We bounce a beam of sound off the ocean floor and measure how long it takes to hear the echo. This is called sonar. It uses sound waves instead of the radio waves of radar. . . .

The maps show big things on the surface, but they are not good enough to show much detail. They show mountains that look like volcanoes but not whether any lava is spilling out.

To learn more about Venus, both Russia and the United States are getting better radar systems ready for mapping. The new system is called imaging radar. Its beam will go down at an angle instead of straight down. That way the beam will be reflected by the sides of mountains and valleys. It will show more details and give us much better maps. All this is planned for a new spacecraft called Venus Radar Mapper, which will be sent up by NASA in 1988. Someday we may have maps of Venus as good as those of earth, even if no one has been there to see it.

From, "Venus, Mapping a Planet You Can't See" by Jack Myers, *Highlights for Children,* February 1985. Copyright © 1985 Highlights for Children, Inc. Columbus, Ohio.

37. The passage is mainly about
   a. launching a spacecraft to Venus.
   b. how a radar altimeter works.
   c. measuring surfaces of invisible celestial bodies.
   d. using an imaging radar technique.

38. Which of these conditions hinders telescopic viewing of Venus's surface?
   a. the thick clouds surrounding Venus
   b. the scorching surface temperature of Venus
   c. the path of Venus's orbit
   d. the limited power of telescopes

39. One might infer from the first paragraph that the reason the Russian spacecraft took only one or two pictures was that it
   a. left the planet.
   b. started to melt.
   c. ran out of film.
   d. was hit by a meteor.

40. A radar altimeter is used to
   a. guide a spacecraft to the proper altitude.
   b. compute the speed of a radar beam.
   c. make an outline of a land mass.
   d. measure the distance down to the surface.

41. According to the passage, which of the following would produce the most detailed map?
   a. imaging radar
   b. radar altimeter
   c. sonar
   d. reflection receiver

42. A map transmitted by the Venus Radar Mapper might be expected to indicate
   a. areas of intense heat.
   b. the number of Venusian craters.
   c. the occurrence of lava spilling from volcanoes.
   d. colorful, spiraling cloud patterns.

III

A California researcher has accomplished what most scientists had thought was impossible. He has turned laboratory rats into alcoholics. The secret, according to UCLA psychologist Gaylord Ellison, is to provide the rats with a lounge where they can go to drink.

Ellison's findings run counter to the theory that rats will not drink enough alcohol to alter their behavior if provided with other sources of food and water.

In previous alcohol research with animals, the subjects were studied for a few months while isolated in small cages and did not become problem drinkers. But human alcoholism develops over a period of time, so Ellison designed studies that would simulate human conditions.

He studied ten colonies of 27 rats for six or seven months each. The animals' habitat included a park-like recreational area where they could socialize. Nearby was a lounge where the rats could drink from six spouts, three dispensing water and three offering a 10-percent alcohol solution flavored with anise.

Most of the rats drank alcohol in moderation, but two or three rats (about 9 percent) in each colony developed an extreme preference for alcohol, about the same percentage of people who become problem drinkers in society.

Ellison says the heavy drinkers ate less than other rats, were much less active, spent more time in their burrows, and ranked low in dominance in social situations. The alcoholic rats tended to drink on a regular schedule, sipping alcohol before feeding and again before they went to sleep. When alcohol was withheld, the drinkers became more active but remained low in dominance.

Ellison hopes to find out whether the rats become socially subordinate because of their heavy drinking or if they become alcoholics because of an initial inferior social status. He also hopes to be able to predict which rats in a colony will become alcoholics.

From "Lounge Rats" by Joel Schwarz, *Omni,* September 1984. Copyright © Omni Publications Int., Ltd.

43. The main idea of this passage is that
    a. studies with rats now prove that we can predict who will become alcoholic.
    b. under certain conditions alcoholism develops in rats at a faster rate than in humans.
    c. under certain conditions rats develop problems with alcohol at the same rate as humans.
    d. studies now prove that rats have a social environment similar to that of humans.

44. The study described in this passage differs from similar studies conducted in the past in that it
    a. studied a larger number of subjects.
    b. placed its subjects in social situations.
    c. disguised alcohol with flavoring.
    d. included social and antisocial subjects.

45. Ellison's study is different from others in that it took into account
    a. the sleep patterns of alcoholics.
    b. the nutritional habits of prospective alcoholics.
    c. the social problems resulting from alcoholism.
    d. the progressive nature of alcoholism.

46.   One can infer from this passage that in future studies, Ellison probably intends to
   a. increase the percentage of alcohol in the solution.
   b. observe the rats for a longer period of time.
   c. observe the rats before they are offered alcohol.
   d. offer alcohol with various flavorings.

47.   The total number of rats that Ellison studied was
   a. 10.
   b. 27.
   c. 100.
   d. 270.

48.   The passage states that the alcoholic rats were "socially subordinate."
   Subordinate means
   a. low in rank.
   b. deprived of privileges.
   c. passive.
   d. unacceptable.

IV

Shortly after she arrived from Japan to begin graduate school at San Francisco State University, Shoko Araki began to notice cultural differences in complimenting behavior. For one thing, her friends reacted differently to her new haircut. Comments from Americans were "frequent, explicit, direct and extreme." "Fantastic! You look great!" one told her. "I love your short hair!" Most of her Japanese friends did not mention the haircut at all. Those who did took a more tentative approach: "Your short hair is nice, but I like it long too."

Intrigued by this experience and encouraged by her communication professor, Dean Barnlund, Araki undertook a systematic comparison of compliments as they occur in Japan and the United States.

One difference between these two cultures, Araki and Barnlund report, is that Americans give more compliments. When they asked American students to recall the most recent compliments they had given and received, the average student recalled ones that had occurred within a few hours or even minutes. Japanese students, in contrast, had to go back 13 days on the average to come up with such compliments. Some reported incidents as old as a month or a year. Araki and Barnlund suggest that Japanese and Americans living in the other country find the relative abundance or paucity of compliments troubling.

These differences seem consistent with what we know about the two cultures' differing emphasis on the individual and the group. Since compliments reveal perceptions of individual differences, it is not surprising that in Japan, a society which promotes group rather than individual values and stresses harmony over confrontation, people give fewer compliments.

Perhaps some of the differences in the reported frequency of compliments in Japan and the United States are rooted in what we expect to hear. Americans regard almost all favorable comments as compliments, Araki and Barnlund say, whereas the Japanese regard most favorable comments, especially direct compliments, as flattery rather than true admiration.

In our study, we found that most American compliments are direct: "You are invaluable to me." The Japanese in Araki and Barnlund's study typically used indirect forms, which imply praise but do not directly state the value of the person or act described: "I'd hate to lose you."

So far there are no reports of a culture without compliments, but our knowledge of compliments in cultures around the world is sparse and largely anecdotal. Preliminary reports highlight obvious and possibly superficial differences, but linguist Nessa Wolfson, who has collected compliments from students throughout the world, suggests that Americans may have difficulty recognizing compliments by people from different cultures because the forms are so different from those commonly used here.

From "Compliments and Culture" by Mark L. Knapp, Robert Hopper, and Robert A. Bell. Reprinted with permission from *Psychology Today* magazine. Copyright © 1985 (APA).

49. The main idea of this passage is that
    a. the use of compliments differs among cultures.
    b. all cultures contain compliments.
    c. the Japanese have difficulty adjusting to American life.
    d. the Japanese are more polite than Americans.

50. According to this passage Americans and Japanese have in common that they both
    a. value compliments greatly.
    b. have difficulty adjusting to the other's compliments.
    c. admire physical beauty.
    d. have a tentative approach to compliments.

51. According to this passage, Japanese culture emphasizes
    a. assertiveness.
    b. individualism.
    c. flattery.
    d. harmony.

52. Araki and Barnlund drew data on complimenting behavior from a population of
    a. friends of Araki and Barnlund.
    b. Japanese students acclimated to American culture.
    c. students from Japan and America.
    d. Japanese and American citizens residing in Japan.

53. According to this passage, most of our knowledge about the compliments of other cultures has been derived from
    a. scholarly research.
    b. casual observance.
    c. documentary evidence.
    d. personal stories.

54. The passage discusses "the relative abundance or paucity of compliments" in Japan and the United States.
    Paucity means
    a. amplitude.
    b. candor.
    c. dearth.
    d. extremity.

V

It seems clear that a jubilant home crowd can lead athletes to perform poorly. What is not clear is when it does and when it doesn't. Will it make any difference, for example, if the crowd expects a win rather than a loss? To see, we examined the results of every game 6 played in the World Series we studied. Only in that game does one team (the team trailing three games to two) face final defeat in the series, while the other can wrap up the series in that game or get another crack at it in the seventh game. Under those circumstances, home teams with a shot at the series lost more than 60 percent of the games. But when home teams faced elimination, they did quite well, winning more than 70 percent of the time. The home team's tendency to choke, then, seems to be due to the prospect of winning, not losing, the championship. Perhaps the harmful effects of home audiences depend on whether they expect the home team to win.

A laboratory study by James Hamilton, Dianne Tice and me supported that reasoning. Undergraduates were led by one of us to expect either success or failure in deciphering a series of anagrams. Some of the students were also told that they were expected to do well by one of us who was present through the test. The results were dramatic. Those who were privately led to expect success did well, while those who knew that the experimenter (essentially, the audience) expected success tended to choke. Supportive home fans, then, may boost an underdog but also add pressure when they expect a win.

This seemed to be the case during the summer Olympics in Los Angeles. No experts had expected the United States team to win a gold medal in gymnastics. On the last night of the men's team competition however, the Americans staged a dramatic upset victory. In the final of the women's competition the following night, the Americans again were within striking distance. The women, however, performed below their usual level of excellence and ended up losing ground to the eventual winner. On the balance beam, three of the six American athletes completely lost their balance. Two even fell to the floor.

Consider their situation. Privately, realistically, they had no reason to expect a win, but they were suddenly faced with an audience with precisely that expectation—exactly the worst psychological situation for good performance.

From "Choking to Win . . . Or Lose?" by Ray F. Baumeister. Reprinted with permission from *Psychology Today* magazine. Copyright © 1985 (APA).

55.   The main idea of this passage is that
   a.   women are more affected by audiences than men.
   b.   an audience that expects a win can cause a loss.
   c.   home teams usually lose in the World Series.
   d.   teams perform better without an audience.

56.   The students were asked to decipher anagrams. The students' task was to
   a.   make a word from a group of letters.
   b.   match geometric shapes to a pattern.
   c.   discover the key to an encoded phrase.
   d.   perceive a mathematical pattern in a series of numbers.

57. When home teams in the World Series faced elimination, they
    a. tended to ignore the audience.
    b. lost more often than they won.
    c. won 10% more often than when they had a better chance.
    d. lost less than 30% of the games.

58. The author describes a study of every game 6 of the World Series. The sixth game was chosen because in that game
    a. the outcome can decide the championship.
    b. the winning team wins the championship.
    c. the home team has a greater chance of winning.
    d. the home audience expects the home team to win.

59. The author describes the case of the Olympic gymnastic team in order to illustrate
    a. the influence of the ordinal position on performance.
    b. the unique tension under which gold medalists compete.
    c. the difference between American men and women gymnasts.
    d. the validity of the results of the two studies.

60. One might infer from this passage that those who might be less inclined to choke are those who are less
    a. self-conscious.
    b. skilled.
    c. experienced.
    d. educated.

Mathematics

45 Minutes

Work each problem carefully. Use scrap paper to do your calculations. The correct answers will be found at the end of the test.

1. If A > 9, could equal
   a. 10.
   b. 9.
   c. 8.
   d. 0.

2. $47.2 - 3.86 =$
   a. 0.86
   b. 43.34
   c. 43.46
   d. 44.44

3. An area of 1500 square feet must be painted. The painters use three gallons of paint to cover the first 950 square feet. How many *more* gallons will be needed to complete the job? (round up to the next full gallon.)
   a. 5 gal
   b. 4 gal
   c. 3 gal
   d. 2 gal

4. An automobile was driven 408 miles in 8.5 hours. What was the average speed in miles per hour?
   a. 45 mi/hr
   b. 48 mi/hr
   c. 51 mi/hr
   d. 55 mi/hr

5. $48.41 \div 0.47 =$
   a. 103
   b. 10.3
   c. 1.03
   d. 0.97

6. The diagram below illustrates which of the following processes?

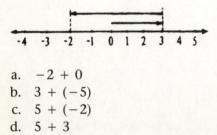

   a. $-2 + 0$
   b. $3 + (-5)$
   c. $5 + (-2)$
   d. $5 + 3$

238

7. $2\sqrt{25} =$
      a. 7
      b. 10
      c. 25
      d. 50

8.   In a school, the first class begins at 8:00 AM and the sixth class ends at 2:30 PM. A total of 1½ hours is allotted for lunch and for time between classes. How long is each class session, if all sessions are of equal length?
      a. 30 min
      b. 50 min
      c. 55 min
      d. 60 min

9. $23 - 5(7) + [-6(-2)] =$
      a. -24
      b. -1
      c. 0
      d. 7

10. $|-7| =$
      a. 7
      b. 1
      c. 0
      d. -7

11.   If 65% of a student body of 2000 students passed a mathematics examination, how many students did not pass?
      a. 1300
      b. 1200
      c. 900
      d. 700

12. $(2½) \div ⅔ =$
      a. 1⅔
      b. 2⅚
      c. 3¾
      d. 4¼

13.   37½% of 65 =
      a. 2.4376
      b. 24.375
      c. 24.39
      d. 243.75

14.   For every 7 people exposed to a virus, 3 will become infected. If 273 people were exposed to the virus, how many will probably be infected?
      a. 156
      b. 117
      c. 112
      d. 78

15. If two different lines have equal slopes, the lines
    a. coincide.
    b. are parallel.
    c. are perpendicular.
    d. intersect.

16. Solve the following equation for x.

$$\frac{2x}{9} = \frac{24}{27}$$

    a. 4
    b. 8
    c. 12
    d. 54

17. Solve the following equation for x.

$$2\frac{1}{2} = \frac{x}{5}$$

    a. 5
    b. 12½
    c. 24½
    d. 25

18. A baseball player has 91 hits out of 250 times at bat. To the nearest tenth of a percent, what percent of the time was the batter successful?
    a. 36.4%
    b. 37.0%
    c. 60.4%
    d. 63.6%

19. A particular breed of dog has a life expectancy of 12 years. After 9 years, what percentage of the expected life span remains?
    a. 20%
    b. 25%
    c. 33%
    d. 40%

20. A rectangle is 9 feet wide and 9½ feet long. Find the perimeter.
    a. 18½ ft
    b. 36 ft
    c. 37 ft
    d. 85.5 ft

21. A particular operation is successful 90% of the time. If 30 such operations are performed, how many unsuccessful results can be expected?
    a. 2
    b. 3
    c. 10
    d. 27

22. An individual's health insurance premiums increased from $280 per year to $310 per year. What was the percent of increase (to the nearest tenth of a percent)?
    a. 110.7%
    b. 90.3%
    c. 11.0%
    d. 10.7%

23. If you spend ¼ of your annual income for housing, ⅕ for transportation, ¹⁄₁₀ for clothing, and ³⁄₂₀ for food, what fractional part is left for all other uses?
    a. ⁹⁄₂₀
    b. ⁷⁄₂₀
    c. ⅓
    d. ³⁄₁₀

24. The circle graph below shows the percent of time devoted to various activities during a teacher's 7-hour day.

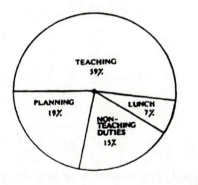

How much time is spent teaching?
    a. 3.7 hrs
    b. 4.13 hrs
    c. 4.6 hrs
    d. 5 hrs

25. A rectangle is 7 feet long and 5 feet wide. If 1 foot is approximately equal to .304 meters, what is the perimeter of the rectangle in meters?
    a. 5.346 m
    b. 7.296 m
    c. 8.33 m
    d. 10.64 m

26. 36 is 120% of what number?
    a. 45
    b. 43.20
    c. 30
    d. .03

27. $3(-¾) + (-1⅔) =$
    a. ²⁵⁄₄
    b. 3½
    c. −6¼
    d. −7½

28. A tablet contains 2 grains of a particular drug. The maximum dosage is not to exceed 1 gram of the drug. If 1 gram is approximately 15.432 grains, how many tablets are needed for maximum dosage?
    a. 9 tablets
    b. 8 tablets
    c. 7 tablets
    d. 6 tablets

29. 6 out of 10 =
    a. 4
    b. ⅔
    c. ⅗
    d. .06

30. In the figure below, what is the length of AB + BC?

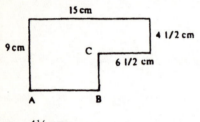

    a. 4½ cm
    b. 8½ cm
    c. 11 cm
    d. 13 cm

31. In the health screening of 270 elementary school pupils, 160 were free of any defect. The remainder represent what percent (to the nearest whole percent) of the total number examined?
    a. 40%
    b. 41%
    c. 59%
    d. 60%

32. Twenty-eight students received passing grades on a test. One fifth of the class did not pass. How many students were in the class?
    a. 7 students
    b. 33 students
    c. 35 students
    d. 40 students

33. .375 equals what fraction in simplest terms?
    a. ⅕
    b. 3/7
    c. ⅜
    d. 375/1000

34. One meter equals approximately 1.09 yards. How many meters are there in 100 yards?
    a. 91.7 m
    b. 108.73 m
    c. 109 m
    d. 110 m

35. A cake recipe calls for 1¼ cups of sugar. To make 9 of these cakes, how many pounds of sugar will be required?

    (2¼ cups = 1 pound)

    a. 4 lb
    b. 5 lb
    c. 5.5 lb
    d. 20.25 lb

36. A central angle of a circle measures 60 degrees. This is equal to what fraction of the circle?
    a. ⅜
    b. ⅓
    c. ¼
    d. ⅙

37. What is the length of diagonal c?

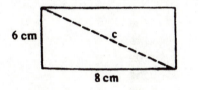

    a. 10 cm
    b. 14 cm
    c. 24 cm
    d. 48 cm

38. A measurement is given as .31 ± .03 cm. What is the permitted range of measure?
    a. from .03 to .31 cm
    b. from .28 to .31 cm
    c. from .28 to .34 cm
    d. from .31 to .34 cm

39. Triangle ABC is the same shape as triangle DEF. Find x.

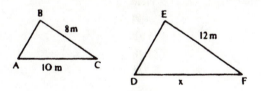

    a. 16 m
    b. 15 m
    b. 14 m
    d. 13 m

40. What is the area of a circle whose radius is 7 inches? (Use 3.14 for π)
    a. 21.98 sq in
    b. 49 sq in
    c. 150 sq in
    d. 153.86 sq in

Science

60 Minutes

Read each question carefully, and then select the correct answer. The correct answers will be found at the end of the test.

1. Some young clams attach themselves to the gills of fish. The clams harm the fish by feeding on their blood. This illustrates the ecological interrelationship known as
   a. parasitism.
   b. mutualism.
   c. commensalism.
   d. saphrophytism.

2. What is the temperature reading on the thermometer shown below?

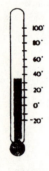

   a. 23°
   b. 25°
   c. 30°
   d. 34°

3. All of the following organs remove metabolic wastes from the human body. Which one excretes carbon dioxide as a primary function?
   a. skin
   b. lungs
   c. kidneys
   d. liver

4. Fats are esters of organic acids and
   a. ethanol.
   b. ethylene glycol.
   c. glycerol.
   d. methyl ether.

5. The movement of molecules from an area of high molecular concentration to an area of low molecular concentration is called
   a. active transport.
   b. pinocytosis.
   c. phagocytosis.
   d. diffusion.

6.   Which of these organs of the human digestive system secretes hydrochloric acid?
      a. esophagus
      b. stomach
      c. liver
      d. pancreas

7.   Which of these properties of an object will change if the object is moved from the earth to the moon?
      a. its mass
      b. its weight
      c. its volume
      d. its density

8.   Which of these diagrams correctly shows a water wave passing through a small opening in a barrier?

      a. A
      b. B
      c. C
      d. D

The next two questions refer to the chart below.

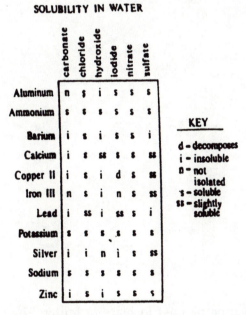

9.   Which of these compounds is most soluble?
      a. lead chloride
      b. lead hydroxide
      c. lead iodide
      d. lead nitrate

10.   Which of these compounds reacts with water?
      a. aluminum carbonate
      b. barium hydroxide
      c. copper II iodide
      d. lead chloride

11. The following table show the melting and boiling points for four substances.

Substance	Melting Point	Boiling Point
W	−40°F	105°F
X	10°F	80°F
Y	105°F	1600°F
Z	115°F	280°F

Which of these substances is a liquid over the smallest temperature range?
a. W
b. X
c. Y
d. Z

12. A baseball player ducks out of the way of a wild pitch. In which order would the impulses travel through the player's system?
a. motor neuron → interneuron → sensory neuron
b. sensory neuron → motor neuron → interneuron
c. sensory neuron → interneuron → motor neuron
d. interneuron → motor neuron → sensory neuron

13. For what purpose is the instrument shown in the diagram usually used?

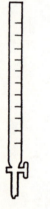

a. dissolving a gas in a liquid
b. separating a solid from a liquid
c. measuring the volume of a liquid
d. filtering a solution

14. Nutritionists recommend that corn oil margarine be used in place of butter. The primary reason for this is that corn oil margarine
a. supplies fewer calories than butter.
b. has more vitamin A than butter.
c. has more saturated fat than butter.
d. has less saturated fat than butter.

15. In which of these forms is sugar most soluble?
a. powdered
b. rock candy
c. cubes
d. granulated

The next three questions refer to this graph of the absorption spectrum of chlorophyll in alcohol.

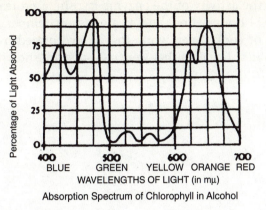

Absorption Spectrum of Chlorophyll in Alcohol

16.   Which of these wavelength of light is most completely absorbed by the chlorophyll in alcohol?
       a.   400 mμ
       b.   475 mμ
       c.   550 mμ
       d.   625 mμ

17.   At a wavelength of 625 mμ the percentage of light absorbed is approximately
       a.   5%
       b.   20%
       c.   70%
       d.   88%

18.   If you were to do an experiment testing the effect of various wavelengths of light on the growth of a green plant, which wavelength would cause the least amount of growth?
       a.   425 mμ
       b.   675 mμ
       c.   550 mμ
       d.   650 mμ

19.   High concentrations of lactic acid are produced during periods of
       a.   strenuous exercise.
       b.   overeating.
       c.   high fever.
       d.   hyperventilation.

20.   A substance that increases the rate at which a chemical reaction occurs is called
       a.   an oxidizing agent.
       b.   a reducing agent.
       c.   an emulsion.
       d.   a catalyst.

21.   Which of these substances is a carbohydrate?
       a. C_6H_6
       b. $C_6H_{12}O_6$
       c. $C_6H_{11}OH$
       d. CH_2NH_2COOH

The next two questions refer to the experiment and the data.

A student is studying the effect of pH on the activity of the enzyme trypsin, a protease that functions in the small intestine. Over a 24-hour period, and at a constant temperature of 37°C, the student measures the amount of cooked egg white that is hydrolyzed by equal amounts of trypsin at five different pH values. The data that were collected are shown in the following table.

pH	Amount of Hydrolysis (mm)
4	0.0
6	2.8
8	7.0
10	1.8
12	0.0

22. The student decides to repeat the experiment with the identical conditions of the first experiment but with a pH value of 5. What amount of hydrolysis might be expected?
    a. more than 7.0
    b. between 0.0 and 2.8
    c. between 2.8 and 7.0
    d. exactly 7.0

23. From the data, the student assumes that trypsin would be ineffective in the human stomach. This assumption is most likely based on the fact that
    a. food will not remain in the stomach for 24 hours.
    b. the temperature of the stomach is much greater than 37°C.
    c. the stomach does not hydrolyze protein.
    d. the pH in the stomach is less than 4.

24. It is known that during photosynthesis green plants liberate free oxygen. The source of this oxygen could be CO_2 or H_2O or both. To determine the source of the oxygen, which of these techniques would you use?
    a. heavy oxygen used as a tracer in H_2O, but not CO_2
    b. heavy oxygen used as a tracer in CO_2, but not H_2O
    c. heavy oxygen used as a tracer first in CO_2, and then in H_2O
    d. radioactive carbon used as a tracer in CO_2, along with heavy water

25. An increase in the pressure on a gas contained in a cylinder with a piston may cause a decrease in which of these properties of the gas?
    a. volume
    b. temperature
    c. mass
    d. energy

The following 2 questions refer to this diagram of the human eye.

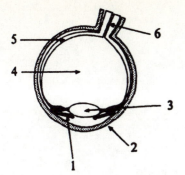

26. Rods and cones would be found in the structure labeled
    a. 1
    b. 2
    c. 5
    d. 6

27. Light entering the eye is normally fine-focused for near vision by the action of the structure numbered
    a. 2
    b. 3
    c. 4
    d. 6

28. The tissue depicted below is composed of striated multinucleated cells.

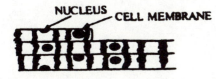

    In which of these structures would these cells be found?
    a. the heart
    b. the stomach
    c. the brain
    d. the arm muscle

29. The graph below shows the relationship between volume and temperature for an ideal gas.

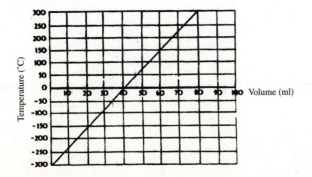

As the temperature changes from − 50°C to 50°C the volume changes by about
a. 14 mL
b. 20 mL
c. 33 mL
d. 47 mL

30. Which of these terms refers to a unit of force?
a. newton
b. joule
c. calorie
d. watt

31. In an ecosystem, decomposers are necessary in order to recycle
a. light energy.
b. oxygen.
c. water.
d. nitrogen.

32. The structure in the human ear that helps to establish the sense of equilibrium is the
a. middle ear.
b. cochlea.
c. semicircular canal.
d. tympanic membrane.

33. The DNA (deoxyribonucleic acid) molecule is composed of smaller units called
a. nucleotides.
b. monosaccharides.
c. amino acids.
d. polypeptides.

34. Organic compounds must contain
a. oxygen.
b. carbon.
c. nitrogen.
d. hydrogen.

35. Which of these equations show the neutralization of an acid with a base?
a. $H_2SO_4 + 2NaNO_3 \rightarrow 2HNO_3 + Na_2SO_4$
b. $H_2SO_4 + 2 NaOH \rightarrow Na_2SO_4 + 2H_2O$
c. $H_2SO_4 + BaCl_2 \rightarrow BaSO_4 + HCl$
d. $H_2SO_4 + Zn \rightarrow ZnSO_4 + H_2$

36. The term that refers to the disorder of the molecules of a substance is
a. entropy.
b. enthalpy.
c. free energy.
d. phase.

37. The scientific principle that explains why a drop of red dye spreads evenly throughout a beaker of water is called the law of
a. transpiration.
b. osmosis.
c. diffusion.
d. hydrolysis.

38. If the label on a bottle reads "Shake well before using," the substance contained in that bottle will most likely be a
    a. solution.
    b. suspension.
    c. tincture.
    d. compound.

39. Whole grains, raw fruits, and vegetables are important to the diet because they supply large amounts of
    a. protein.
    b. thiamin.
    c. fiber.
    d. amino acids.

40. Which of these diagrams correctly shows the shape of the magnetic field in the vicinity of two magnets whose north poles are facing each other?

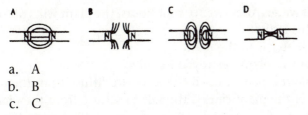

    a. A
    b. B
    c. C
    d. D

41. The diagram below shows four general areas on the periodic table.

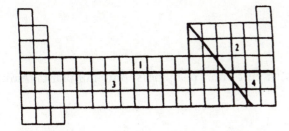

    Which of these areas contain the metals?
    a. 1 and 2
    b. 1 and 3
    c. 2 and 4
    d. 3 and 4

42. Four people each move a 1-kg load from A to B as shown.

    Which person did the most work?
    a. A
    b. B
    c. C
    d. D

43. When the positively charged rod approaches the positively charged electroscope shown in the diagram, what will happen?

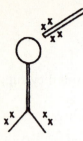

   a. The leaves will fall.
   b. The leaves will spread further apart.
   c. Nothing will happen unless the rod touches the ball of the electroscope.
   d. Nothing will happen even if the rod touches the ball of the electroscope.

44. The roots of a plant are placed in salt water. After twenty-four hours, the plant wilts noticeably. The most logical explanation for this is that
   a. the salt blocked the passage of water into the plant.
   b. the diffusion of salt throughout the plant destroyed its cells.
   c. the concentration of salt outside the plant caused the water to diffuse from the plant.
   d. the concentration of salt outside the plant caused the salt to diffuse from the plant.

45. Which of these parts of the plant would most likely have the greatest number of mitochondria per cell?
   a. mature stem
   b. growing root tip
   c. xylem cell
   d. epithelial cells of the leaf

46. When pure tall pea plants are crossed with pure short pea plants, only tall plants result. This illustrates Mendel's
   a. law of segregation.
   b. law of independent assortment.
   c. concept of unit characters.
   d. principle of dominance.

47. In the human nervous system, which of these parts of the neuron transmits impulses to other cells of the body?
   a. nucleus
   b. cytoplasm
   c. dendrite
   d. axon

48. A function of the endocrine glands is to
   a. increase the rate of oxygen transport by erythrocytes.
   b. regulate muscle tone.
   c. regulate the growth of the bones.
   d. decrease cellular transpiration.

49. If a concentrated solution of KNO_3 is able to dissolve additional crystals of KNO_3, then the solution is
   a. saturated.
   b. unsaturated.

    c. supersaturated.

    d. dilute.

50.   Which of these substances, if injected subcutaneously into the human body, would trigger an immunological reaction?

    a. antibody

    b. sucrose

    c. antigen

    d. adrenalin

The next two questions are based on this graph, which shows the velocity of a car over a period of 10 seconds.

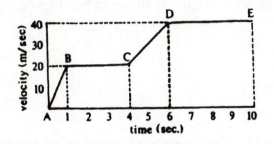

51.   During which of these time intervals will the car have the greatest acceleration?

    a. AB

    b. BC

    c. CD

    d. DE

52.   How far will the car travel during interval BC?

    a. 20 m

    b. 40 m

    c. 60 m

    d. 80 m

53.   Two forces of 10N each are exerted on an object. Which of these diagrams shows the greatest resultant force acting on the object?

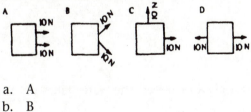

    a. A

    b. B

    c. C

    d. D

54.   The intensity of visible light is most closely related to which of these characteristics of the light wave?

    a. its amplitude

    b. its length

    c. its frequency

    d. its period

55. When we compare the mass of the reactants in a chemical reaction with the mass of the products, we find
    a. a greater mass at the end of the reaction.
    b. a greater mass at the beginning of the reaction.
    c. the same mass before and after the reaction.
    d. sometimes the mass increases and sometimes the mass decreases during the reaction.

56. The compound formed by the ions X^{+2} and Y^{-1} has the formula
    a. XY
    b. X_2Y
    c. XY_2
    d. X_2Y_2

57. A wire is placed between two poles of a horseshoe magnet as shown in the diagram.

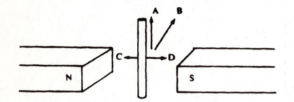

    In which direction would the wire have to be moved in order to induce an electric current in it?
    a. A
    b. B
    c. C
    d. D

58. A student observed a series of slides depicting various stages of mitotic division in the cells of an organism. The student determined that this organism is a plant. Which of these statements is the best reason for this decision?
    a. The nuclear membrane is not present during metaphase.
    b. A cell plate is formed during telophase.
    c. Spindle fibers appear during metaphase.
    d. New daughter cells are formed by the mother cell pinching in half.

59. The structures of a neuron that receive stimuli from sense organs and other neurons are called
    a. dendrites.
    b. axons.
    c. myelin sheaths.
    d. terminal branches.

60. A short time after a drop of ink is placed in a glass of water, the water takes on a uniform color. This illustrates the process of
    a. osmosis.
    b. diffusion.
    c. active transport.
    d. pinocytosis.

Answers Comprehensive Practice Test 1

Verbal Ability: Word Knowledge and Reading Comprehension

1.	a		31.	c
2.	b		32.	c
3.	b		33.	b
4.	c		34.	a
5.	a		35.	d
6.	d		36.	c
7.	c		37.	c
8.	b		38.	a
9.	b		39.	b
10.	a		40.	d
11.	d		41.	a
12.	a		42.	b
13.	a		43.	c
14.	c		44.	b
15.	a		45.	d
16.	a		46.	b
17.	d		47.	d
18.	d		48.	a
19.	b		49.	a
20.	b		50.	b
21.	b		51.	d
22.	a		52.	c
23.	b		53.	a
24.	a		54.	c
25.	b		55.	b
26.	d		56.	a
27.	b		57.	d
28.	b		58.	a
29.	c		59.	d
30.	a		60.	a

Mathematics

1. **The answer is a.** If A > 9, it means that all values of A are greater than 9. Therefore, the only choice for A is 10.

2. **The answer is b.**

$$\begin{array}{r} 47.20 \\ -\ 3.86 \\ \hline 43.34 \end{array}$$ (It's ok to add a zero to the right of the decimal point.)

3.   **The answer is d.** You may use a proportion to view the problem this way: If it takes 3 gallons to paint 950 square feet, how many gallons does it take to paint 1500 square feet? Be sure to align the units correctly: gallons across from gallons, and square feet across from square feet.

$$\frac{3\ g}{950\ sq.\ ft.} = \frac{x}{1500\ sq.\ ft.} \qquad \text{Cross multiply.}$$

$$950\ x = 4500 \qquad \text{Divide both sides by 950 to solve for x.}$$

$$x = \frac{4500}{950} = \frac{450}{95} = \frac{90}{19} = 4\frac{14}{19} \qquad \text{Round this up to 5 gallons}$$

Thus, it takes 5 gallons to paint the entire 1500 square feet. *But don't be fooled!* This is not the answer. The question asks for how many more gallons of paint are needed. If it takes 5 gallons for the entire job, and 3 have already been used, then only 2 more gallons are required. Your answer is 2 gallons.

4.   **The answer is b.** To find the average speed (or the rate of travel), divide 408 miles by 8.5 hours. Recall that a rate is a ratio of two different amounts.

$$\frac{408\ miles}{8.5\ hours} \qquad \text{Divide.}$$

$$\frac{408\ miles}{8.5\ hours} = 8.5\overline{)408} \qquad \text{Multiply both divisor and dividend by 10.}$$

$$\overset{48}{85\overline{)4080}} \qquad \text{48 miles per hour is your answer.}$$

5.   **The answer is a.**

$$0.47\overline{)48.41} \qquad \text{Multiply both the divisor and the dividend by 100.}$$

$$\overset{103}{47\overline{)4841}} \qquad \text{Divide. 103 is your answer.}$$

6.   **The answer is b.** The diagram illustrates starting at zero and moving 3 spaces to the right. This is represented by a positive 3. Next, the diagram illustrates moving 5 spaces to the left. This is represented by -5. Thus, you have $3 + (-5)$.

7.   **The answer is b.** $\sqrt{25} = 2 \cdot 5 = 10$

8.   **The answer is b.** First, determine how many total hours are in the school day. From 8:00 AM to 2:30 PM there are **6.5 hours.**
Next, subtract from the total the 1.5 hours set aside for lunch and for time between classes. $6.5 - 1.5$ leaves **5 hours.**
Next, change 5 hours to minutes by multiplying 60 by 5 (there 60 minutes in each hour). Thus, 5 hours = **300 minutes.**
Finally, divide the 300 minutes of class time by the number of classes: 6.
$300 \div 6 = $ **50 minutes** in each class period.

9.   **The answer is c.** Follow the order of operations to simplify this expression.

$$23 - 5(7) + [-6(-2)] =$$
$$23 - 5(7) + [12] =$$
$$23 - 35 + 12 =$$
$$-12 + 12 = 0$$

10.   **The answer is a.** Here is the problem again: $|-7|$
The two vertical bars around -7 mean *absolute value*. The simplest and most direct definition of absolute value is: the distance from zero. In this sense, it does not matter if the number is positive or negative; absolute value is only concerned with the distance away from zero. In this case, -7 is 7 units away from zero. Therefore, $|-7| = 7$.

11.   **The answer is d.** *Don't be tricked!* The question asks for the number of students who *did not pass* the examination. If 65% of a student body of 2000 passed the examination, then the rest did not pass. Since the total student body is 100%, then "the rest" must be 35%.

$$35\% \text{ of } 2000 =$$
$$0.35 \cdot 2000 = 700 \quad \text{This is your answer.}$$

12.   **The answer is c.**

$$\left(2\frac{1}{2}\right) \div \frac{2}{3} = \qquad \text{Change the mixed number to an improper fraction.}$$

$$\frac{5}{2} \div \frac{2}{3} = \qquad \text{Invert the divisor and multiply.}$$

$$\frac{5}{2} \cdot \frac{3}{2} = \frac{15}{4} = 3\frac{3}{4} \quad \text{Your answer is } 3\frac{3}{4}.$$

13.   **The answer is b.** Change to 37½% to 37.5%, and then into a decimal by dividing by 100: 0.375.

Now multiply 0.375 by 65:

$$
\begin{array}{rl}
0.375 & \text{3 decimal places} \\
\times\ 65 & \text{0 decimal places} \\
\hline
1875 & \\
+\ 22500 & \\
\hline
24.375 & \text{3 decimal places}
\end{array}
$$

14.   **The answer is b.** You may use a proportion to solve this problem. As always, be sure to align the units correctly: people exposed across from people exposed, and people infected across from people infected.

$$\frac{7}{3} = \frac{273}{x} \quad \text{Cross multiply.}$$

$$7x = 819 \quad \text{Divide both sides by 7 to solve for x.}$$

$$x = 117 \quad \text{This is your answer.}$$

15.   **The answer is b.** Two different lines, in the same plane, with the same slope will never meet. They are called parallel lines.

16.   **The answer is a.** A proportion! You know how to solve this!

$$\frac{2x}{9} = \frac{24}{27}$$ Cross multiply.

$54x = 216$ Divide both sides by 54 to solve for x.

$x = 4$ This is your answer.

It is worth mentioning that you could also reduce the fraction ²⁴/₂₇ before cross multiplying: $\frac{2x}{9} = \frac{8}{9}$. Once you have this, you will see that denominators are equal. This means that the numerators must also be equal. Stated another way:

$2x = 8$
$x = 4$

17.   **The answer is b.** You may set up a proportion to solve this problem. The only tricky part is recognizing that the mixed number must be made into a complex fraction. The entire mixed number goes into the numerator, and gets a denominator of 1.

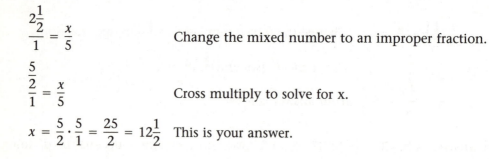

$$\frac{2\frac{1}{2}}{1} = \frac{x}{5}$$ Change the mixed number to an improper fraction.

$$\frac{\frac{5}{2}}{1} = \frac{x}{5}$$ Cross multiply to solve for x.

$$x = \frac{5}{2} \cdot \frac{5}{1} = \frac{25}{2} = 12\frac{1}{2}$$ This is your answer.

18.   **The answer is a.** To find the percent of successful hits, make a fraction out of the information, and divide.

$$\frac{91}{250} = 250\overline{)91}$$

$$250\overline{)91.000} \quad .364$$ Multiply 0.364 by 100 to find your percent: 36.4%

19.   **The answer is b.** After 9 years, only 3 years remain. The problem now becomes one of 3 types of common percent problems: 3 is what percent of 12? You can solve this easily by making a fraction out of the information.

$$\frac{3}{12} = \frac{1}{4} = 0.25 = 25\%$$

This is an excellent example of why it pays to be familiar with the common fraction–decimal-percent equivalencies.

20. **The answer is c.** Use the following formula to find the perimeter of a rectangle.

$$2L + 2W = P \quad \text{Substitute 9.5 for L and 9 for W.}$$
$$2(9.5) + 2(9) = P \quad \text{Simplify.}$$
$$19 + 18 = P \quad \text{Combine like terms.}$$
$$37 = P \quad \text{This is your answer.}$$

21. **The answer is b.** A 90% success rate means a 10% failure rate. If 30 operations are performed, then 10% will be unsuccessful.

$$10\% \text{ of } 30 =$$
$$0.1 \cdot 30 = 3 \text{ unsuccessful attempts}$$

22. **The answer is d.** To find the percent increase, make a fraction out of the information. Put the amount of increase (in dollars) in the numerator, and the original amount (in dollars) in the denominator.

$$\frac{30}{280} \qquad \text{Change this fraction to a decimal by dividing.}$$

$$280\overline{)30.00000} \quad \substack{.1071...} \qquad \text{The quotient is a repeating decimal, but we are only}$$

interested in the first four decimal places.

$$0.1071 \cdot 100 = 10.71\% \quad \text{Multiply by 100 to change the decimal to a percent.}$$
$$10.7\% \qquad \text{Round the nearest tenth of a percent.}$$

23. **The answer is d.** Find a common denominator for all of the fractions, and convert them to equivalent fractions.

$$\frac{1}{4} = \frac{5}{20}, \ \frac{1}{5} = \frac{4}{20}, \ \frac{1}{20} = \frac{2}{20}, \ \frac{3}{20}$$

Now add them all together:

$$\frac{5}{20} + \frac{4}{20} + \frac{2}{20} + \frac{3}{20} = \frac{14}{20}$$

If $^{14}/_{20}$ of the annual income is spent, then $^6/_{20} = ^3/_{10}$ remains.

24. **The answer is b.** The circle represents the teacher's total day: 7 hours. If 59% of that time is spent teaching, then 59% of 7 hours = the time spent teaching.
Change 59% to a decimal by dividing by 100: 59% ÷ 100 = 0.59.

Multiply 0.59 by 7: 0.59 · 7 = 4.13 hours. This is your answer.

25. **The answer is b.** Use the following formula to find the perimeter of the rectangle in feet.

$$P = 2L + 2W \qquad \text{Substitute 7 for L and 5 for W.}$$
$$P = 2(7) + 2(5) \qquad \text{Simplify and add.}$$
$$P = 14 + 10 = 24 \text{ ft.} \quad \text{This is the perimeter in feet.}$$

Since one foot is approximately 0.304 meters, multiply 24 by 0.304 to find the perimeter in meters. 0.304 · 24 = 7.296 meters. This is your answer.

26. **The answer is c.** This is one of three common types of percent problems.

> 36 is 120% of what number? Change the problem to an equation.
> $36 = 1.2 \cdot x$
> $36 = 1.2x$ Divide both sides by 1.2 to solve for x.
> $30 = x$ This is your answer.

27. **The answer is c.** Follow the order of operations to simplify this expression.

$$3\left(-\frac{3}{4}\right) + \left(-\frac{12}{3}\right) =$$ Multiply by 3, and simplify $-\frac{12}{3}$.

$$-\frac{9}{4} - \frac{4}{1}$$ Change $-\frac{4}{1}$ to an equivalent fraction

with a denominator of 4.

$$-\frac{9}{4} - \frac{16}{4} = -\frac{25}{4} = -6\frac{1}{4}$$ This is your answer.

28. **The answer is b.** Use proportions to solve this problem. First, note the following relationships between the information, expressed as ratios.

$$\frac{1\ tablet}{2\ grams} \quad \text{and} \quad \frac{1\ gram}{15.432\ grains}$$

Now the proportion:

$$\frac{1\ tablet}{2\ grains} = \frac{x}{15.432\ grains}$$ When you solve for x, you will know how many

tablets needed for 15.432 grains, or 1 gram (the maximum dosage).

$$\frac{1\ tablet}{2\ grains} = \frac{x}{15.432\ grains}$$ Cross multiply.

$2x = 15.432$ Divide both sides by 2 to solve for x.

$x = 7.716$ This is how many tablets are needed for the maximum dosage.

To get the maximum dosage, you will need *more* than 7 tablets. Thus, your answer is 8 tablets.

29. **The answer is c.** 6 out of 10 can be expressed as a ratio and reduced: $\frac{6}{10} = \frac{3}{5}$

30. **The answer is d.** The length of AB can be found by subtracting 6.5 cm from 15 cm, because both sides are parallel to each other. Thus, AB = 8.5. Similarly, the length of BC can be found by subtracting 4.5 cm from 9 cm. Thus, BC = 4.5. Therefore, AB + BC = 8.5 + 4.5 = 13 cm.

31. **The answer is b.** If 160 of 270 pupils are found free of defect, then the remainder is 270 − 160 = 110. To find what percent 110 is of 270, make a fraction out of the information.

$$\frac{110}{270} = 270\overline{)110}$$ Divide to find the decimal equivalent.

$$.40\overline{7407}$$
$$270\overline{)110.000000}$$ Change the repeating decimal to a percent by multiplying by 100.

$.40\overline{7407} \cdot 100 = 40.7\overline{407}\%$ Round this off to the nearest whole percent.
$40.7\overline{407}\% \approx 41\%$ This is your answer.

32. **The answer is c.** Twenty-eight students received passing grades. If one-fifth did not pass, then four-fifths must have passed. This means that twenty-eight out of the total number of students equals four-fifths of the class. This sounds like a proportion.

$$\frac{28}{x} = \frac{4}{5}$$ Cross multiply.

$4x = 140$ Divide both sides by 4 to solve for x.

$x = 35$ This is your answer, the total number of students in the class.

33. **The answer is c.** Once again, knowing your decimal-to-fraction equivalents comes in handy. However, if you are not yet familiar with them, here is what to do.
You need to know the names of the decimal places. In this case, 0.375 ends in the thousandths place, so place 375 over 1000, and reduce the fraction.

$$0.375 = \frac{375}{1000} = \frac{3}{8}$$

34. **The answer is a.** You may use a proportion to solve this problem. As always, be sure to align the units correctly: meters across from meters, and yards across from yards.

$$\frac{1\ meter}{1.09\ yards} = \frac{x}{100\ yards}$$ Cross multiply.

$1.09\ x = 100$ Divide both sides by 1.09 to solve for x.

$x = 91.743 \ldots \approx 91.7$ This is your answer.

35. **The answer is b.** If one cake requires 1¼ cups of sugar, then nine cakes will require 9 · 1¼ cups of sugar.

$$9 \cdot 1\frac{1}{4} =$$

$$\frac{9}{1} \cdot \frac{5}{4} = \frac{45}{4}\ \text{cups of sugar.}$$

To convert $^{45}\!/_4$ cups of sugar to pounds, divide by 2¼, the number of cups in 1 pound.

$$\frac{45}{4} \div 2\frac{1}{4} =$$ Change the mixed number to an improper fraction.

$$\frac{45}{4} \div \frac{9}{4} =$$ Invert the divisor and multiply the fractions.

$$\frac{45}{4} \cdot \frac{4}{9} = \frac{45}{9} = 5$$ 5 is your answer. Note that you can cross cancel the 4's in this multiplication problem.

36.   **The answer is d.** To find what fraction 60 is of the entire circle, recall that the entire circle is made up of 360 degrees. Make a fraction of this information, and reduce it.

$$\frac{60}{360} = \frac{6}{36} = \frac{1}{6}$$

37.   **The answer is a.** The *Pythagorean Theorem* comes in handy in this problem. You must recognize that in the rectangle, diagonal c forms the hypotenuse of a right triangle, with legs 6 cm and 8 cm. Once you see this, use the theorem.

$a^2 + b^2 = c^2$ Substitute 6 for a and 8 for b.
$6^2 + 8^2 = c^2$ Simplify.
$36 + 64 = c^2$ Combine like terms.
$100 = c^2$
$\sqrt{100} = \sqrt{c^2}$ Take the square root of both sides of the equation.
$10 = c$ This is your answer.

38.   **The answer is c.** The symbol "±" means plus or minus. In our problem, it means that the measurement can be 0.03 cm greater or less than 0.31. Thus, add 0.03 to 0.31 to find the upper limit (0.34), and subtract 0.03 from 0.31 to find the lower limit (0.28).

39.   **The answer is b.** The two triangles are the same shape, or similar. Similar triangles have their corresponding sides in proportion.

$\dfrac{8}{10} = \dfrac{12}{x}$ Cross multiply.
$8x = 120$ Divide both sides by 8 to solve for x.
$x = 15$ This is your answer.

You could also use the following proportion:

$\dfrac{8}{12} = \dfrac{10}{x}$ When you cross multiply, you find the same equation as above.
$8x = 120$ Wow! Therefore, the answer is the same: 15.

40.   **The answer is d.** Use the following formula to find the area of a circle.

$A = \pi r^2$ Substitute 3.14 for π and 7 for r^2.
$A = (3.14) \cdot 7^2$ Simplify.
$A = 3.14 \cdot 49$ Multiply.
$A = 153.86$ sq. in.   This is your answer.

Science

1.   **The answer is a.** Parasitism refers to the symbiotic relationship in which one organism benefits from the relationship whereas the other organism is harmed. Mutualism describes a symbiotic relationship where both organisms benefit. In commensalism, one organism benefits while the other is neither harmed nor benefits from the relationship.

2.   **The answer is d.** Since the top of the mercury column lies somewhere between 30 degrees and 40 degrees the closest answer is 34 degrees.

3.   **The answer is b.** The lungs take in oxygen with each inhalation and release carbon dioxide with each exhalation.

4.   **The answer is c.** Three fatty acids and one glycerol molecule make up one molecule of fat.

5.   **The answer is d.** Diffusion refers to a process in which molecules randomly disperse from areas of high concentration towards areas of low concentration.

6.   **The answer is b.** Cells in the lining of the stomach release gastric juice, which contains hydrochloric acid. The pH of the hydrochloric acid is very low (acidic!), and the acidity aids in the digestion of proteins and also activitates other enzymes necessary for digestion.

7.   **The answer is b.** Mass, volume, and density are properties of an object that remain unchanged on the moon. The weight of an object is the magnitude of the force of gravity acting on the object. The force of gravity on the moon is less than that of earth, so when an object moves to the moon the force of gravity decreases and its weight will change.

8.   **The answer is b.** When a wave passes through a small opening in a barrier it spreads at the same rate in all directions. The only diagram that fits this description is choice B.

9.   **The answer is d.** According to the table, lead chloride and lead iodide are slightly soluble (able to dissolve in water) while lead hydroxide is insoluble. Lead nitrate on the other hand is soluble in water.

10.   **The answer is c.** According to the key, "d" represents a substance that will decompose in water. Decomposition is a reaction in which one reactant produces more than one product. Of the four choices, only copper II iodide decomposes in water.

11.   **The answer is b.** The melting point is the temperature at which a substance will change from a solid to a liquid while the boiling point refers to the temperature at which the substance changes from a liquid to a gas. The chart indicates that substance X is a liquid over the shortest range since it turns into a liquid at 10 degrees Fahrenheit and becomes a gas at 80 degrees Fahrenheit. Thus, it remains a liquid for a span of 70 degrees unlike the other substances that remain in this phase for a much longer period.

12.   **The answer is c.** Sensory neurons triggered by the observation that a baseball is coming in the player's direction convey this information to a motor neuron. The motor neuron sends

the signal to the muscles that allow the baseball player to duck. Interneurons mediate the message as it travels from the sensory to the motor neurons.

13. **The answer is c.** A burette is often used to determine the concentration on an acid or a base. This is accomplished by filling the burette with an unknown acid and observing the volume needed to neutralize a known volume of a base with a known concentration. The small handle allows one to release small amounts of the unknown solution to be released slowly to a flask placed beneath the burette containing the known solution and thus accurate volume measurements can be made.

14. **The answer is d.** Corn oil has less saturated fat than butter.

15. **The answer is a.** Increasing the surface area of a solute, the substance being dissolved, increases its solubility, or ability to be dissolved.

16. **The answer is b.** From the graph it is clear that almost 90% of the light is absorbed at 475mμ, which is the highest value of absorption on the graph.

17. **The answer is c.** At 625 mμ the amount of light absorbed is just below 75%. The best answer is 70%.

18. **The answer is c.** Light of wavelength 550 mμ is hardly absorbed at all, almost 0%. All other options have much higher rates of light absorption.

19. **The answer is a.** Lactic acid is produced during anaerobic respiration (respiration without oxygen). During strenuous exercise, reserves of oxygen in the muscles have been depleted, which cause the build up of lactic acid.

20. **The answer is d.** A catalyst increases the rate of a reaction by lowering the amount of energy needed for the reaction to proceed.

21. **The answer is b.** Carbohydrates are composed of sugars that contain carbon, hydrogen, and oxygen and are characterized by a ratio of twice as much hydrogen as oxygen.

22. **The answer is b.** Trypsin is an enzyme that hydrolyzes or breaks down protein. This experiment measures the rate at which this digestive enzyme breaks down the protein in egg white at different pH's.

23. **The answer is d.** The pH in the stomach is close to 2 due to the presence of hydrochloric acid.

24. **The answer is c.** Heavy oxygen refers to using an isotope of oxygen that has a higher atomic mass. Thus, it can be characterized by chemical techniques from normal oxygen. In this case, labeling carbon dioxide with this special oxygen and then allowing the reaction of photosynthesis to proceed would allow a researcher to see if the oxygen produced is heavy or normal. If it is heavy, this indicates that the oxygen does come from carbon dioxide. Next, labeling the water with heavy oxygen and studying the oxygen produced would tell the researcher whether some of the oxygen produced was originally present in the water molecule.

25. **The answer is a.** Boyle's Law states that the volume of a fixed amount of gas varies inversely with the pressure of the gas. If the volume of the gas is decreased, the number of particle collisions will increase and the pressure of the gas will increase. If the volume of the gas is increased, the pressure of the gas will decrease.

26. **The answer is c.** #5 points to the retina that contains the rods and cones, which are structures which respond to light and send messages to the brain, which result in vision.

27. **The answer is b.** #3 points to the lens which focuses light on the retina.

28. **The answer is d.** Skeletal muscle cells are multinucleated and form in layers (striated). The heart contains cardiac muscle cells, while the stomach contains smooth muscle cells.

29. **The answer is a.** According to the graph, the volume changes from approximately 34 ml to 48 ml as the temperature changes from $-50°$ Celsius to $50°$ Celsius.

30. **The answer is a.** A newton is a unit of force defined as the force required to accelerate a 1 kg block at 1 m/s².

31. **The answer is d.** Decomposers, such as bacteria, are able to "fix" nitrogen, or make it nutritionally available to consumers, by converting it to N_2 from NH_3 or ammonia.

32. **The answer is c.** The semicircular canals of the inner ear sense changes in position or rates of rotation of the head and help to maintain balance.

33. **The answer is a.** Monosaccharides make up sugars, and amino acids and polypeptides make up proteins.

34. **The answer is b.** By definition, compounds containing carbon are called "organic" compounds.

35. **The answer is b.** A strong acid reacting with a strong base produces a salt and water, which are neutral products.

36. **The answer is b.** Entropy is the measure of the disorder of a system.

37. **The answer is c.** Diffusion refers to a process in which molecules randomly disperse from areas of high concentration towards areas of low concentration.

38. **The answer is b.** A suspension is a heterogenous mixture that contains large solute particles that remain suspended in the solvent. Thus, suspensions must be shaken to distribute the solute particles throughout the solvent.

39. **The answer is c.** All of these nutrients supply dietary fiber.

40. **The answer is b.** Magnetic field lines must point away from the nearest north pole.

41. **The answer is b.** Areas 1 and 3 represent the transition metals.

42. **The answer is c.** Work done by each person is force times distance moved in the vertical direction.

43. **The answer is b.** As the rod approaches the electroscope more positive charge gets forced onto the leaves. They will then repel each other more, and so they will separate more.

44. **The answer is c.** Osmosis refers to the diffusion of water from areas of high water concentration to areas of low water concentration.

45. **The answer is b.** The growing root tip requires a great deal of energy and thus contains the most amount of mitochondria, which are responsible for the production of ATP.

46. **The answer is d.** Since all of the offspring are tall, the trait of being tall must be dominant over the trait of being short, which is recessive.

47. **The answer is d.** Dendrites receive a signal and conduct that signal to the cell body, which contains the nucleus. From here, the axon transmits the signal down the length of the neuron to the end, or synaptic terminal. This portion of the neuron makes contact with other neurons or target organs.

48. **The answer is c.** Endocrine cells that are formed in endocrine glands secrete hormones. Hormones are chemical messengers that play many important roles in the body; for instance, growth hormone, parathyroid hormone, and calcitonin all work to regulate the growth of bones.

49. **The answer is b.** If the crystals settle then the solution is saturated, meaning the solvent contains as much solute as it can possible hold. If the crystals dissolve this means the solution is unsaturated meaning the solvent can hold more crystals than it does.

50. **The answer is c.** An antigen is a foreign substance that triggers an immune response. Antibodies are specific proteins induced by the immune system in response to an antigen.

51. **The answer is a.** The acceleration is the slope of the velocity graph. The velocity graph is the steepest over the interval AB.

52. **The answer is a.** Over the interval BC the velocity is constant at 20 m/s, and the interval lasts for 3 seconds. The distance traveled is 20 m/s $\times$ 3 s = 60 m

53. **The answer is a.** Since all forces are the same magnitude, the greatest resultant force occurs when both forces point in the same direction.

54. **The answer is a.** Frequency, period, and wavelength all determine the type of light we see. The amplitude determines the intensity of the light.

55. **The answer is c.** The law of conservation of mass states that mass cannot be created or destroyed.

56. **The answer is c.** Ions of opposite charge are attracted to each other and compounds formed from ions form in such a manner that the charge is zero. Thus, one X and two Y ions will combine to form XY_2, a neutral compound.

57. **The answer is b.** The magnetic field points from the North Pole to the South Pole. The direction the rod must be moved in order to induce a current in it, is determined by the right-hand rule.

58. **The answer is b.** In plant cells, cytokinesis (division of the cytoplasm) is characterized by the formation of a cell plate, which extends from the middle of the cell to the cell wall. In animal cells, cytokinesis is characterized by a "pinching" of the cell into two new cells of equal size.

59. **The answer is a.** Axons transmit the messages down the length of a neuron, myelin sheaths surround the neuron, and increase the efficiency of conduction, and terminal branches transmit the message received by the dendrites to the next neuron or target organ.

60. **The answer is b.** Diffusion is the random dispersal of particles from areas of high particle concentration to areas of low particle concentration.

Comprehensive Practice Test 2

Verbal Ability
Word Knowledge and Reading Comprehension

60 Minutes

WORD KNOWLEDGE: Read each sentence carefully. Then, *on the basis of what is stated in the sentence,* select the correct completion of the incomplete statement. The correct answers will be found at the end of this test.

1. When machine oil is used to reduce friction, it is used as
   a. a catalyst.
   b. a fuel.
   c. a lubricant.
   d. an igniter.

2. A person who wanders from place to place is called a
   a. nomad.
   b. native.
   c. mutant.
   d. surrogate.

3. The diplomats hoped that they had established a durable agreement.
   Durable means

   a. economical.
   b. efficient.
   c. acceptable.
   d. long lasting.

4. Sandstone is a very porous material.
   Porous means

   a. common.
   b. permeable.
   c. thin.
   d. inexpensive.

5. The altar of the church was ornate.
   Ornate means

   a. rustic.
   b. holy.
   c. decorated.
   d. destroyed.

6. The patient was ravenous, so the nurse brought him a
   a. pill.
   b. meal.
   c. bandage.
   d. book.

7. A person who spends a great deal of money in a short time is
   a. ingenious.
   b. extravagant.
   c. fastidious.
   d. admonitory.

8. If she loses her financial assistance, she will be
   a. depreciated.
   b. impoverished
   c. accentuated.
   d. bolstered.

9. The child's intense dislike of vegetables amounted to an
   a. audit.
   b. aversion.
   c. exultation.
   d. acquisition.

10. A raconteur is a good
    a. storyteller.
    b. tennis player.
    c. musician.
    d. doctor.

11. The woman bought a bauble from the street vendor. She bought a
    a. dessert.
    b. beverage.
    c. figurine.
    d. trinket.

12. When the will was read, we were stunned by the aggregate wealth of my uncle.
    Aggregate means
    a. monetary.
    b. inherited.
    c. total.
    d. undisclosed.

13. The funds were allocated to various organizations.
    Allocated means
    a. donated.
    b. promised.
    c. conveyed.
    d. assigned.

14. The critic made some stinging remarks about the film. The remarks were
    a. caustic.
    b. arduous.
    c. salutary.
    d. tertiary.

15. The highest point in his career was when he was elected senator; he had reached his
    a. gauntlet.
    b. conception.
    c. zenith.
    d. dynasty.

16. If a play has an epilogue, it is placed
    a. at the beginning.
    b. in the middle.
    c. at the end.
    d. between acts.

17. The woman had the audacity to push to the front of the line.
    Audacity means

    a. impudence.
    b. courage.
    c. animosity.
    d. amenity.

18. The people rebelled against the despotism of the king. The king was guilty of
    a. unruliness.
    b. incompetence.
    c. tyranny.
    d. assassination.

19. The patient had a penchant for rare meat.
    Penchant means

    a. addiction.
    b. order.
    c. need.
    d. partiality.

20. Compared to today's x-ray machines, the machines used in the 1950s seem
    a. antediluvian.
    b. autonomous.
    c. contiguous.
    d. reticulated.

21. When you behave in a pleasant and polite manner, you are being
    a. brusque.
    b. candid.
    c. affable.
    d. complacent.

22. Unlike the volunteer jobs that the student had held in the past, this job would provide a
    a. stipend.
    b. paroxysm.
    c. montage.
    d. matrix.

23. The author of the book was clearly a charlatan.
    Charlatan means
    a. genius.
    b. impostor.
    c. autobiographer.
    d. aesthete.

24. A vivacious person is one whose manner is
    a. animated.
    b. demure.
    c. celestial.
    d. eccentric.

25. A fetish is an object that is believed to be
    a. costly.
    b. decorative.
    c. fragile.
    d. magical.

26. Someone who lacks sophistication and maturity could be described as
    a. recondite.
    b. rapacious.
    c. callow.
    d. omniscient.

27. An area of the country that is unspoiled can be said to be
    a. intemperate.
    b. pristine.
    c. prolific.
    d. impervious.

28. Applying butter to the burnt skin of the woman's hand will exacerbate the wound.
    Exacerbate means
    a. aggravate.
    b. soothe.
    c. protect.
    d. inflame.

29. The face in the drawing had a jocund look. It looked
    a. remorseful.
    b. assured.
    c. displeased.
    d. mirthful.

30. Each member of the group investigated the topic and worked with the other members to pull all the information together. The resulting report was
    a. an analogy.
    b. a synthesis.
    c. a hypothesis.
    d. a cavalcade.

READING: There are five reading passages in this section. Read each passage carefully. Then, *on the basis of what you have read in the passage*, select the best answer for each question.

I

Artifacts found in a bay near Rio de Janeiro may mark the wreck of a Roman ship that could have reached Brazil 17 centuries before Portugese adventurers discovered the region, according to a leading underwater archeologist.

A large accumulation of amphoras, or tall jars, of the type carried by Roman ships in the second century B.C., has been found in Guanabara Bay, 15 miles from Rio de Janeiro, according to the archeologist, Robert Marx, who is a well-known hunter of sunken treasure . . .

Amphoras are tall jars tapering to the bottom and usually fitted with twin handles . . . They were used to carry wine, oil, water or grain on long voyages.

Mr. Marx, the author of many books and articles on early exploration and underwater archaeology, believes the amphoras were carried to Brazil on a Roman ship that was blown off course. It may have anchored off Rio, then been driven by a storm onto the reef near where the amphoras now lie.

To reach the harbor, he said, it had to be navigated and therefore could not have been an unmanned derelict.

According to Dr. Harold E. Edgerton of the Massachusetts Institute of Technology, a pioneer in underwater photography who has worked extensively with Mr. Marx, the amphoras are definitive, both as to the age in which they were used and the identity of the users. . . . Dr. Edgerton said of Mr. Marx's qualifications, "For my money he is as reliable as they come."

Mr. Marx . . . said he suspected a hoax when he first heard of the amphoras, but was convinced . . . when he dived at the site and saw an area comparable to three tennis courts strewn with jars, most of them broken. He brought some to the surface and plans to have their age and origin authenticated by specialists.

The amphoras could not have been planted there, he said. Four intact amphoras and parts of at least 50 more are on the surface. Digging with his hands into the mud he encountered some as much as five feet down. The jars are barnacle-encrusted and some long ago became enclosed in coral. Mr. Marx believes all coral in that area was killed by pollution 30 or 40 years ago.

For years he has sought to prove that Europeans reached the Americas long before Columbus. Because of his well-known interest in this subject, . . . he was suspicious when informants sought him out to report the Brazilian finds . . .

Divers in search of lobsters in the area . . . brought up some jars as souvenirs . . .

Six years ago a diver named Jose Roberto Teixeira located the site and recovered two complete amphoras. It was he who led Mr. Marx to the site.

Mr. Marx has formed a company with Mr. Teixeira to excavate the site and, if granted permission to do so, has offered to donate all finds to the Brazilian Government. Mapping the site will be difficult because the water is so polluted that one can see only a few feet, if at all.

Mr. Marx hopes with sonar or other devices to probe the mud in which he believes some of the vessel's wood may be preserved. Recovery of weapons, tools and other relics of Roman type would leave no doubt about the nature of the ship.

"If we only find amphoras," Mr. Marx added, "then I'm in trouble."

31. Which of these titles is most appropriate for this passage?
    a. "Robert Marx, Famous Archeologist, Digs for Amphoras"
    b. "Second-Century Roman Ships"
    c. "Artifacts in Rio May Mean Roman Visit"
    d. "Diving in Ruins"

32. If one were to look inside an amphora, the bottom would appear
    a. flat.
    b. pointed.
    c. rounded.
    d. grooved.

33. Marx believes that the amphoras found at the site indicate that
    a. an abandoned ship floated into the bay.
    b. Romans sailed into the bay.
    c. a wrecked ship was towed into the bay.
    d. a Brazilian ship carried the artifacts into the bay.

34. Dr. Edgerton has helped the project by
    a. investing in the excavation company.
    b. photographing the amphoras.
    c. confirming the authenticity of the amphoras.
    d. solving the mysteries of the artifacts.

35. From the passage, it can be inferred that Rio de Janeiro has a problem with
    a. waste disposal.
    b. food shortage.
    c. severe storms.
    d. coral reefs.

36. According to the passage, Mr. Marx cannot begin serious excavation of the site until he
    a. gets the lobster divers to agree to help him.
    b. guarantees the donation of any treasure to the Brazilian government.
    c. draws a map of the complete area.
    d. receives authorization from the Brazilian government.

II

Interested in joining [the French Foreign Legion]? First you must get to France. There, present yourself to one of the 16 recruiting offices or to the French national police in any town, airport or bus station; they will take you in charge. If you are younger than 17 or older than 40, you need not apply. The French Foreign Legion wants only strong men who are willing to give up their past lives. If you have images of a *Beau Geste* life-style, put them aside.

Be prepared to be thoroughly investigated. In the past, the Legion served as a haven for those on the lam from criminal or political problems. Today, most of the recruits are young men who are simply looking for work. A petty crime such as theft is no impediment, but even the Legion cannot overlook a murder. You will undergo three weeks of intensive physical and psychological testing. If you pass you go to boot camp, and if you pass again, the Legion may invite you to enlist. The enlistment contract will bind you for the next five years, with a starting monthly salary of nearly 2,000 francs—about $250.

You are now part of a family of nearly 10,000 men of 125 nationalities. The Legion gives you a new name for which you can invent a past, and, after your five-year stint, make a future. (About 12 percent of legionnaires are fleeing "social obligations," such as alimony.) If you are married, it is not acknowledged for three years. If you are single at the time of enlistment, you must wait five years to marry. French law grants you the right of asylum, and you can later become a citizen of France. You have no credit cards and no passport—no identity other than that of a legionnaire.

. . . [The Legion was] founded by King Louis-Philippe in 1831 as a haven for Europeans fleeing the various revolutions of 1830. . . .

After the Spanish Civil War of 1936–39, it was the defeated Communists and Socialists, fleeing Franco's wrath, who flocked to the Legion. Then after World War II came the Germans and Italians, including scores of SS officers escaping war-crime trials.

In 1956, after Russia's invasion of Budapest, most of the new legionnaires were Hungarian. In 1968 they were Czech. After the independence of Angola they were Portugese. "We reflect the troubles of the world," said Colonel Robert Devouges, a Legion veteran. . . .

From the "The French Foreign Legion" by John Gerassi. First printed in *GEO* magazine. Copyright © 1983, Knapp Communications Corporation.

37. The passage is mainly about
    a. the history of the Legion.
    b. a legionnaire's training.
    c. the investigation of Legion candidates.
    d. enlistment in the Legion.

38. A legionnaire's name must
    a. be French.
    b. indicate his marital status.
    c. reflect his country of origin.
    d. be changed.

39. A legionnaire's monthly salary is
    a. 250 francs.
    b. 2,000 francs.
    c. 2,000 dollars.
    d. 125 dollars.

40. A woman who seeks alimony from a former husband who has joined the Legion can expect the Legion to
    a. turn the legionnaire over to the authorities.
    b. make deductions from the legionnaire's salary.
    c. provide protection for the legionnaire.
    d. expel the legionnaire.

41.   The remark "We reflect the troubles of the world" refers to the
   a. hardships of the lives of the legionnaires.
   b. conditions in the places the legionnaires came from.
   c. standard of living in France.
   d. economic troubles in the world.

42.   The passage states that a petty crime such as theft is not an impediment.
   Impediment means

   a. a requirement.
   b. a hindrance.
   c. a punishable offense.
   d. an option.

III

In demographic terms, there are deaf people and deaf people. Of the 2 million Americans who can't hear speech, about a quarter lost that ability before the age of 19, and roughly one in eight either was born without it or lost it before the age of 3. Possibly half the deaf are elderly, and many more are approaching old age. But deafness has social as well as physical consequences; when it strikes early and hard, it has educational ones as well.

Americans who lose their hearing early in life do form a distinctive social and cultural group, a society strongly cohesive. This is especially true for sign-language users, but even among those who communicate largely in oral language, relying more or less on hearing aids, or lipreading, four out of five marry a deaf spouse rather than a hearing one. And most prevocationally deaf spend nearly all their leisure time and find their basic personal identity in the company of others like themselves.

Overwhelmingly, they find employment in industries engaged in manufacture of nondurable goods and in trades such as printing and sewing, where they can get by with stereotyped, and thus reasonably predictable, oral communication. It's no surprise, therefore, that the prevocationally deaf earn much less than the hearing. Deaf people average a bit more than 70 percent of the earnings of the nondeaf. It might seem, at first innocent glance, that a person is deaf who cannot hear. If one can hear imperfectly, but well enough for many purposes, then he or she is probably hard-of-hearing. And probably anyone with hearing defective to any degree is hearing-impaired. But logic rarely helps when dealing with belief, and the field of hearing impairment has been rent for centuries by a conflict as fierce as any that ever sundered a party cell or a religious denomination. . . .

The plain truth is that "deaf" and "hearing-impaired," when used by people in the field, usually do not describe physiological conditions but signal loyalties in a continuing war over communication and, ultimately, over the place of the hearing-handicapped in society. Those who favor manual communication tend to describe people with serious hearing losses as "deaf"; those who oppose it tend to call them "hearing-impaired."

43. A *demographer* is one who
    a. measures hearing loss.
    b. compiles statistics on populations.
    c. runs for political office.
    d. teaches sign language.

44. According to this passage, how many Americans lost their hearing before they were 19 years old?
    a. two million
    b. one million
    c. a half million
    d. a quarter million

45. According to the passage, people who have been deaf since an early age
    a. earn less money than non-deaf people.
    b. often cannot communicate at all.
    c. are often highly successful in business.
    d. usually develop other physical problems.

46. In the phrase "the field of hearing impairment has been rent for centuries," the word *rent* means
    a. occupied.
    b. split.
    c. involved.
    d. dormant.

47. The usage of the terms "deaf" and "hearing-impaired" by people in the field reflects a conflict over whether deaf people should
    a. be paid higher wages.
    b. form a political action group.
    c. use sign language.
    d. learn lipreading.

48. We can infer from this passage that the *prevocationally* deaf are those who
    a. were fired from their jobs when they lost their hearing.
    b. lost their hearing before they were regularly employed.
    c. can work only with other deaf people.
    d. are unable to work because of their deafness.

IV

A computer without mass storage is like an employee who needs retraining after lunch. Mass storage is any medium that lets you save the computer's memory contents in a form that the computer can read back directly. As a result, you don't have to retype the programs and data each time you restart the computer.

The premium mass storage system for today's popular computers is the floppy disk, a . . . circle of plastic film coated with iron oxide.

A floppy disk is made of materials similar to cassette tape but has magnetic coatings on both sides and is shaped like a disk. Instead of being protected by a hard plastic shell, the disk is encased in a flexible plastic envelope, the jacket. Like the cassette's shell, the jacket has a slot through which the drive's read/write (play/record) head can reach the magnetic surface, a hole through which the drive can engage and move the magnetic medium, and a notch to indicate whether or not the disk can be recorded.

The disk's shape is one reason for its greater speed. With cassette tape, getting from the first program or data block to the very last means winding past hundreds of feet of tape. With a floppy disk, getting from one "end" to the other means moving the head an inch or two across the disk.

Another reason for its extra speed is that a floppy disk is designed to record digital impulses directly. With an audio cassette tape, the data flow must be slowed enough to allow encoding into audio tones that can be recorded accurately.

. . . Speeds differ among makes and models. On [one] . . . model . . . , [a] program can be found and loaded into memory from disk in about four to eight seconds. The same program on cassette could require about four to eight minutes to load, not counting the time required to find that program. . . .

Data on floppy disks is recorded in concentric *tracks* which are divided into *sectors.* When a disk is initialized or "formatted," codes are recorded on it to identify each track and sector, and a directory of the disk's contents is recorded on a specified sector and track. The disk-controller circuits and disk-operating-system (DOS) program read the directory to find where programs and data files are recorded on the disk and move directly to them.

49. The main subject of the passage is
     a. the storage capacity of cassette and disk systems.
     b. the comparison between cassette and disk storage systems.
     c. the comparison between human memory and computer memory.
     d. the making of a floppy disk system.

50. Which of these features is used to indicate whether a disk can be recorded?
     a. a slot
     b. a drive
     c. a notch
     d. a hole

51. One reason the floppy disk system is faster than the cassette system is that
     a. the shape of the disk allows for rapid access.
     b. the disk spins faster.
     c. the magnetic coating is on both sides of the disk.
     d. the cassette heads move slowly.

52. If you want to go from the first to the last program on a floppy disk, it is necessary for the system to
     a. wind past each program.
     b. move the head to the program.
     c. move the needle to the program.
     d. decode the audio tones of each program.

53. The information on floppy disks is recorded in
     a. concentric tracks.
     b. formats.
     c. straight lines.
     d. audio tones.

54. We can infer from the passage that a disk system can load a program about how many times
     faster than a cassette?
     a. sixty times
     a. ten times
     c. eight times
     d. two times

V

For years, Disneyland was an object of scorn in architectural circles. Many people who had never visited the park deplored its vulgarity and its disregard of textbook precepts. Those who did take the trouble to experience it at first hand were often surprised to discover that Disneyland worked—worked at the very basic level of being a compact architectural complex which could efficiently handle up to fifty thousand people a day. While they paid grudging tribute to Disney's multilayer transportation system, and admitted that the park was rather innovative, the most that the majority of city planners and architects were prepared to say was that Disneyland was a happy accident.

Walt Disney World proved less easy to dismiss, and in fact rapidly attracted a good deal of favorable interest. Taking advantage of the experience gained in developing the first park, and able to plan the entire complex from start to finish, the Disney organization came up with solutions to urban-planning problems that were remarkably similar to those that had been proposed in architectural schools and publications around the world, but had never been put into practice. Disney and his assistants were in a position to implement them. Other planners, hobbled by more conservative clients, watched with considerable envy.

The first difficulty the Disney team had to face was that of turning swamps into building sites without falling back on the expedient of draining the entire area—an unfortunate practice, commonplace in Florida for fifty years or more, that had disastrous effects on the equilibrium of nature. Disney insisted that his planners find a way of creating adequate sites without upsetting the ecological balance.

From the outset one large area—7,500 acres—was set aside as a nature preserve. This tract of swamp and hardwood forest has been kept in its virgin state (only a few poachers have ever ventured into it, hunting for alligators, which are plentiful enough), and it is the home of a variety of rare native wildlife, including what are believed to be the last surviving Florida black bears. It is closed to the public, and its untouched character is carefully protected by a team of resident scientists, aided by such organizations as the Audubon Society.

Had Disney decided to follow common practice and drain his entire property, such a preserve would have been impossible, because the change in water level would have altered the terrain irrevocably. Instead, he listened to the best advice and made use of existing high ground wherever possible. A certain amount of drainage was still necessary, but it was kept to a minimum and the water table of the remainder of the forty-three square miles was protected by an elaborate system of levees and sluice gates.

Within this overall framework, extraordinary individual feats of engineering were undertaken. Without disturbing the surrounding landscape, a 200-acre lake was pumped dry, enough white sand from its bed was moved up to the shoreline to provide beautiful beaches, and islands were constructed and planted with palm trees. Then the lake was refilled with clear water free of the dense concentration of tannic acid that had discolored the original water. Thus, a murky Central Florida lake was transformed into something that looked more like a Micronesian lagoon.

Reprinted from *The Art of Walt Disney* by Christopher Finch, copyright © 1973 by Walt Disney Productions, published by Harry N. Abrams, Inc., New York. All rights reserved.

55.   The main idea of this passage is that Disneyland and Disney World used innovative
a.   managerial practices.
b.   agricultural designs.
c.   construction techniques.
d.   buying strategies.

56.   According to the passage, the practice of draining Florida's swampland resulted in
a.   the enhancement of the land's natural beauty.
b.   the creation of land that could be developed fully.
c.   the depletion of mineral resources.
d.   the destruction of the balance between plants and animals.

57.   It can be inferred from this passage that little concern is given to the actions of
a.   alligator poachers.
b.   city planners.
c.   Disney staff.
d.   mechanical engineers.

58.   According to the passage, the game preserve is being used to
a.   conduct scientific experiments.
b.   protect endangered species.
c.   allow people to see animals in their natural habitat.
d.   create an ecosystem for wildlife.

59.   When the natural lake was being improved, the Disney engineers were able to use the original
a.   water.
b.   trees.
c.   sand.
d.   wildlife.

60.   The general attitude toward Disneyland's architecture was one of
a.   bitterness.
b.   surprise.
c.   admiration.
d.   criticism.

Mathematics

45 Minutes

Work each problem carefully. Use scrap paper to do your calculations. The correct answers will be found at the end of this test.

1. If 78% of a hospital's patients are discharged within a week after being admitted, what percent remain longer than a week?
    a. 20%
    b. 22%
    c. 25%
    d. 30%

2. A patient is to be given a medication for 84 hours. How many days does this time period cover?
    a. 3 days
    b. 3½ days
    c. 3⅔ days
    d. 4 days

3. What is the area of the square in the diagram below?

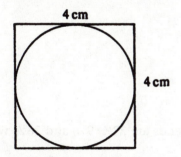

4 cm

4 cm

    a. 32 cm²
    b. 20 cm²
    c. 16 cm²
    d. 8 cm²

4. If there are 14 pulse beats in ⅙ of a minute, how many beats will there be in one minute?
    a. 78
    b. 80
    c. 84
    d. 93

5. A person is 58 inches tall. What would this measurement be if expressed in feet and inches?
    a. 4 ft 6 in
    b. 4 ft 8 in
    c. 4 ft 10 in
    d. 5 ft 2 in

6.   A salesperson earns a salary of $250 for a 5-day week plus a percentage of the total sales for each day. If the percentages of sales earnings during one week were $83, $116, $49, $94, and $67, what was the salesperson's total income that week?
  a. $750
  b. $659
  c. $409
  d. $250

7.   If x = 4, x^3 =
  a. 12
  b. 16
  c. 64
  d. 256

8. $(3)\sqrt{64}$ =
  a. 11
  b. 24
  c. 66
  d. 192

9.   Your 37½ hour work week includes a daily ¼ hour rest period and a ½ hour lunch break. How many duty-free hours are included in your 5-day work week?
  a. 3½
  b. 3¾
  c. 4
  d. 5

10.   If x = 43, which of the following statements is correct?
  a. 40 < x < 43
  b. 40 < x ≤ 43
  c. 40 ≤ x < 43
  d. 40 > x ≥ 43

11.   If the sum of four numbers is 120, and three of the addends are 23½, 9⅔, and 78¾, what is the fourth addend?
  a. 1¹¹⁄₁₂
  b. 7¹⁄₃₀
  c. 8¹⁄₁₂
  d. 11½

12.   You have $1200 to live on for a month. If ½ is spent for rent, and ¼ is spent for food, how much is left for other expenses?
  a. $450
  b. $400
  c. $300
  d. $275

13.   What is the prime number that immediately precedes 19?
  a. 18
  b. 17
  c. 15
  d. 13

14. How many seconds are there in 3⅓ minutes?
    a. 200 sec
    b. 188 sec
    c. 180.33 sec
    d. 80 sec

15. $6(.83) + .3(100) - 29.09 =$
    a. -23.81
    b. 5.89
    c. 34.37
    d. 64.07

16. If 10 ml of a blood specimen contain 1.2 g of hemoglobin, how many g of hemoglobin would 15 ml of the same blood contain?
    a. 1.35 g
    b. 1.5 g
    c. 1.8 g
    d. 2 g

17. A fraction equals ⅚. Its numerator is 7 less than its denominator. Find the numerator of this fraction.
    a. 24
    b. 29
    c. 40
    d. 56

18. The triangles below are similar, with the sides of lengths 3m and 5m corresponding and those of lengths 9m and x corresponding. Find x.

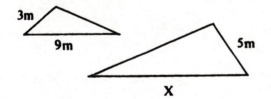

    a. 12 m
    b. 15 m
    c. 18 m
    d. 20 m

19. The winner of a 100-meter dash was .32 of a second ahead of the second-place runner. If the time for second place was 10.72 seconds, what was the time for first place?
    a. 11.04 sec
    b. 11.00 sec
    c. 10.40 sec
    d. 10.32 sec

20. If 3 inches on a map represents 20 miles, find the mileage between two towns that are 5½ inches apart on the map.
    a. 40 mi
    b. 36⅔ mi
    c. 32⅓ mi
    d. 29½ mi

21. $3 \times 4 \times 5 \times 0 =$
    a.   60
    b.   35
    c.   17
    d.   0

22. $625 \div .25 =$
    a.   2500
    b.   250
    c.   25
    d.   2.5

23.   If your annual salary of $17,200 were increased by 5½%, what would your new annual salary be, to the nearest dollar?
    a. $17,209
    b. $17,295
    c. $18,146
    d. $18,150

24.   A patient's caloric intake is to be increased each day by 10% of his caloric intake on the previous day. If his caloric intake was 950 on the first day, how many calories (to the nearest calorie) will he consume on the third day?
    a.   190 cal
    b.   200 cal
    c.   1140 cal
    d.   1150 cal

25.   What fraction is equal to .88?
    a. $^{8}/_{11}$
    b. $^{22}/_{25}$
    c. $^{8}/_{9}$
    d. $^{5}/_{7}$

26.   A prescription costs $6.85 for 15 capsules. To the nearest penny, what does each capsule cost?
    a.   45¢
    b.   45.6¢
    c.   45.7¢
    d.   46¢

Use the following diagram to answer the next 2 questions.

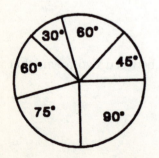

27. The central angle of 45° represents what percent of the circle? (to the nearest whole percent)
    a. 7%
    b. 13%
    c. 15%
    d. 20%

28. If $\frac{1}{12}$ of your monthly budget is for transportation, which central angle would represent this budget item?
    a. 30°
    b. 45°
    c. 60°
    d. 75°

29. $(\frac{2}{5})x - (\frac{1}{6})y + (\frac{3}{10})x + (\frac{3}{4})y =$
    a. $(\frac{7}{10})x + (\frac{7}{12})y$
    b. $(\frac{7}{20})x - (\frac{7}{24})y$
    c. $(\frac{7}{10})x - (\frac{7}{12})y$
    d. $(\frac{1}{3})x + (\frac{1}{5})y$

30. $4\frac{1}{2} \times 3\frac{5}{6} =$
    a. $12\frac{5}{12}$
    b. $12\frac{5}{8}$
    c. $13\frac{2}{3}$
    d. $17\frac{1}{4}$

31. One quart equals 0.9 liters. How many quarts are there in 12 liters?
    a. 10.8 qt
    b. $11\frac{2}{3}$ qt
    c. 12.5 qt
    d. $13\frac{1}{3}$ qt

32. $\frac{2}{3} + 7(\frac{1}{2}) - \frac{6}{5} =$
    a. $2\frac{5}{6}$
    b. $2\frac{8}{15}$
    c. $2\frac{29}{30}$
    d. $5\frac{11}{30}$

33. The length of a rectangle is 3 times the width, and the area is 147 cm². What is the length?
    a. 21 cm
    b. 15 cm
    c. 9 cm
    d. 7 cm

34. 5 is 3% of what number?
    a. $166\frac{2}{3}$
    b. 16.67
    c. 1.5
    d. .15

35. Increase the number $\frac{1}{5}$ by $\frac{2}{3}$ of itself. What decimal number, to the nearest thousandth place, is equivalent to the resulting fraction?
    a. .867
    b. .667
    c. .333
    d. .133

36. $13x^2y \div {}^{-}\frac{1}{2}x$
   a. $26y^2$
   b. $26x^3y$
   c. $-26xy$
   d. $-26x^3y$

37. $9 - \frac{3}{4}n = 45$. Find n.
   a. $n = -48$
   b. $n = -72$
   c. $n = 48$
   d. $n = 72$

38.   In the figure below, find the length of side AB.

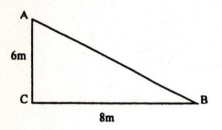

   a.   17 m
   b.   14 m
   c.   12 m
   d.   10 m

39.   The use of tobacco among a student population decreased by 350 students compared to the previous year. This represented a 20% decline in users. If the student population remains the same, how many students still use tobacco?
   a.   1400
   b.   1750
   c.   2100
   d.   2800

40.   .5% of what number is 25?
   a.   .125
   b.   12.5
   c.   500
   d.   5000

Science

60 Minutes

Read each question carefully, and then select the correct answer. The correct answers will be found at the end of this test.

1. If a microscope under high power has an eye-piece of $10\times$, an object would be magnified 430 times. What is the magnification of the high-power objective?
    a. $10\times$
    b. $43\times$
    c. $420\times$
    d. $430\times$

2. Which of the following processes is represented by this equation?

    $$6CO_2 \overset{light}{+} 6H_2O \rightarrow C_6H_{12}O_6 + 6O_2$$

    a. respiration
    b. dehydration synthesis
    c. hydrolysis
    d. photosynthesis

3. In a normal rabbit, the cells carry on the chemical reaction represented below:

    $$\text{phenylalanine} \overset{\text{enzyme x}}{\rightarrow} \text{tyrosine enzyme y} \overset{\text{enzyme y}}{\rightarrow} \text{melanin}$$

    An albino rabbit can produce tyrosine but not melanin, due to a mutation. This mutation was most likely the result of a change in the gene that codes for
    a. enzyme x.
    b. enzyme y.
    c. phenylalanine.
    d. tyrosine.

4. Which of these elements of an ecosystem would be the first to be affected by the removal of decomposers?
    a. photosynthesis
    b. predator-prey relationships
    c. the return of inorganic nutrients to the ecosystem
    d. the number of primary consumers in the ecosystem

5. Which of these organelles would *NOT* be as essential to the ameba if the ameba had evolved in salt water rather than fresh water?
    a. mitochondrion
    b. nucleus
    c. contractile vacuole
    d. cell membrane

6. Which organ of a green plant is adapted for sexual reproduction?
    a. flower
    b. cambium
    c. stem
    d. root

7. The failure of homologous chromosomes to separate during meiosis is known as
    a. nondisjunction.
    b. synapsis.
    c. crossing-over.
    d. translocation.

8. Which of these substances is a carbohydrate that is associated with the cells of a strawberry plant but not with the cells of an earthworm?
    a. fatty acid
    b. hemoglobin
    c. lactose
    d. cellulose

9. Which of these organic compounds determine the "blueprint" for human life?
    a. enzymes
    b. nucleic acids
    c. carbohydrates
    d. lipids

The diagram below represents a portion of a food web. The next 3 questions refer to this diagram.

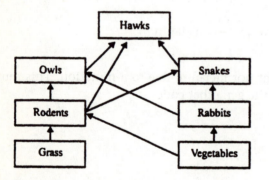

10. The correct order of a food chain represented in this diagram is
    a. grass → rabbit → snake → hawk
    b. hawk → owl → rabbit → vegetable
    c. grass → rodent → snake → hawk
    d. grass → rodent → rabbit → snake

11. If vegetables were removed from this food web, which of these results would be the most probable?
    a. The snake population would increase.
    b. The rodent population would die out.
    c. The grass would increase.
    d. The rabbit population would decrease.

12. A necessary member of an ecosystem *NOT* represented in this food web is a
    a. producer.
    b. primary consumer.
    c. decomposer.
    d. secondary consumer.

The next 3 questions refer to this experiment:

Hans Spemann wanted to see if cells in an embryo were different from the time they started to divide or whether they were alike until they got to a certain stage. He worked with very young salamander embryos. He knew which part normally develops into nerve cells and which into skin cells. He cut these parts out and reversed their positions. They grew into cells like the areas around them: skin cells became nerve cells and nerve cells became skin cells. Then he tried the experiment again with older embryos. This time the skin cells remained skin cells and the nerve cells remained nerve cells.

13. Spemann might have repeated the procedure with the older salamander embryos for which of these reasons?
    a. To find out if nerve and skin cells were larger in older embryos.
    b. The older and larger embryos were easier to work on.
    c. It was easier to identify nerve and skin cells in the older embryos.
    d. To determine if age had an effect on the cells' ability to change.

14. The results of Spemann's experiments support which of these conclusions?
    a. Very young salamander embryo cells are all alike and can develop into any tissue.
    b. Young salamander embryo cells are specialized from the beginning.
    c. Very young salamander embryo cells all resemble nerve cells.
    d. Older salamander embryo nerve cells can become skin cells.

15. Before the experiment began, the salamander eggs must have undergone
    a. fertilization.
    b. meiosis.
    c. pollination.
    d. regeneration.

The next 2 questions refer to the experiment and the data.

A student is studying the effect of pH on the activity of the enzyme trypsin, a protease that functions in the small intestine. Over a 24-hour period, and at a constant temperature of 37°C, the student measures the amount of cooked egg white that is hydrolyzed by equal amounts of trypsin at five different pH values. The data that were collected are shown in the following table.

pH	Amount of Hydrolysis (ml)
4	0.0
6	2.8
8	7.0
10	1.8
12	0.0

16.   Which of these factors is a variable in this experiment?
       a.   temperature
       b.   time
       c.   pH
       d.   volume of trypsin

17.   If the student were to plot a graph of the data, it would most likely resemble which of these
       graphs?

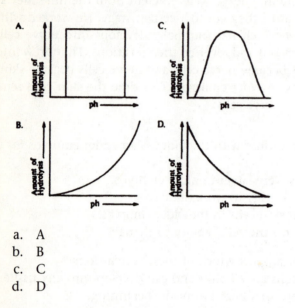

       a.   A
       b.   B
       c.   C
       d.   D

The following 3 questions refer to the diagrams below, representing different human cells.

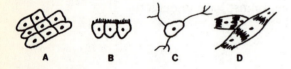

18.   Which cell would relay a message to other parts of the body?
       a.   A
       b.   B
       c.   C
       d.   D

19.   Which of these cells would most likely be found lining the inside of the cheek?
       a.   A
       b.   B
       c.   C
       d.   D

20.   Which of these cells would most likely sense a change in temperature?
       a.   A
       b.   B
       c.   C
       d.   D

21. Tubules for transport of materials within the cytoplasm of the cell are called
    a. endoplasmic reticula.
    b. ribosomes.
    c. lysosomes.
    d. mitochondria.

Carbohydrates, proteins, and fats are chemically digested as food passes through the human alimentary canal. The chart below shows the percentage of undigested food in each organ of the canal. The next 2 questions relate to this chart.

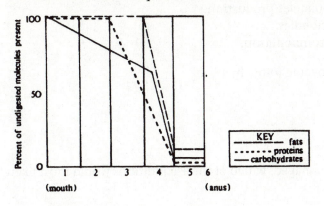

22. Proteins are digested in which of these organs as represented by numbers?
    a. 1 only
    b. 1, 2, and 3 only
    c. 3 and 4 only
    d. 4 only

23. Based on the net change in the percentage of undigested molecules present, the organ represented by 4 is most likely the
    a. stomach.
    b. small intestine.
    c. large intestine.
    d. esophagus.

24. Damage to the semicircular canals of the inner ear may result in
    a. loss of hearing.
    b. an inability to distinguish between tastes.
    c. loss of color vision.
    d. loss of balance.

25. The production of urine by the kidney involves which of these processes?
    a. peristalsis and hydrolysis
    b. filtration and hydrolysis
    c. synthesis and resorption
    d. filtration and resorption

26. The mitotic cell division in a rose bush differs from the mitotic cell division in a snake. One difference is that in the rose bush
    a. homologous chromosomes are paired.
    b. centrioles are replicated.
    c. spindle fibers are produced.
    d. cell plates are synthesized.

27.   The shrinkage of cell volume due to the outward flow of water is termed
    a.   cyclosis.
    b.   plasmolysis.
    c.   pinocytosis.
    d.   turgor.

28.   A person who was in an auto accident suffers an injury that affects the circulatory system. A blood clot forms at the site of the injury. The formation of a blood clot usually happens when
    a.   red blood cells release hemoglobin.
    b.   bone marrow cells decrease platelet production.
    c.   white blood cells release antibodies.
    d.   ruptured platelets release thromboplastin.

29.   Bones are held in position at movable joints by
    a.   cartilage.
    b.   ligament.
    c.   tendon.
    d.   muscle.

30.   If the medulla of a human were damaged, which of these conditions would most likely result?
    a.   difficulty in breathing
    b.   inability to remember
    c.   inability to control muscle movement
    d.   difficulty in saying words

31.   Proteins are synthesized from smaller molecules called
    a.   amino acids.
    b.   monosaccharides.
    c.   lipids.
    d.   nucleic acids.

32.   The table below shows the specific gravity of four substances.

Substance	Specific Gravity
A	0.75
B	1.21
C	1.80
D	6.32

    Which substance will float in water?
    a.   A
    b.   B
    c.   C
    d.   D

33.   A substance that increases the rate of a chemical reaction without itself being changed is called
    a.   an electrolyte.
    b.   an oxidant.
    c.   a catalyst.
    d.   an activator.

34. Which of these substances has a fixed shape and volume at standard temperature and pressure?
    a. NaCl solid
    b. NaCl solution
    c. O_2 gas
    d. H_2O liquid

35. The apparatus shown in the diagram is used for what purpose?

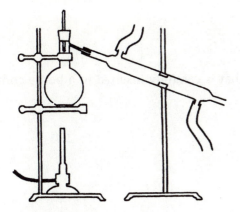

    a. electrolysis of water
    b. distillation of a solution
    c. synthesis of a salt
    d. oxidation of an organic compound

36. Water is decomposed by passing an electric current through it. Compared to the volume of hydrogen generated, the volume of oxygen generated is
    a. the same.
    b. half as much.
    c. twice as much.
    d. sixteen times as much.

37. A tincture is a solution in which the solvent is
    a. alcohol.
    b. water.
    c. oil.
    d. hydrochloric acid.

38. This diagram shows a single substance that can exist in all three states of matter. The state of a substance depends upon the particular combination of temperature and pressure.

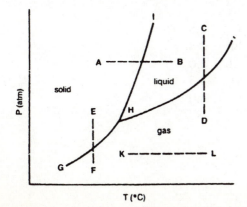

Which dashed line segment corresponds to the evaporation of a liquid?
a.   AB
b.   CD
c.   EF
d.   KL

39.   Which of these reactions is a neutralization reaction?
a. $HCl + H_2O \rightarrow H_3O^+ + Cl^-$
b. $HCl + NaOH \rightarrow NaCl + H_2O$
c. $H_2SO_4 + 2NaCl \rightarrow 2HCl + Na_2SO_4$
d. $2HCl \rightarrow H_2 + Cl_2$

40.   Colorless solution A is placed in a test tube that is carefully inserted in a bottle containing colorless solution B, as shown in the diagram.

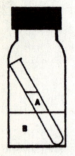

The entire apparatus is weighed. The bottle is then inverted, allowing the two solutions to mix, forming a yellow precipitate. The apparatus is reweighed. Which of these statements best predicts the outcome of this experiment?
a.   The weight of the apparatus after the solutions are mixed will be the same as before.
b.   The weight of the apparatus after the solutions are mixed will be greater than before.
c.   The weight of the apparatus after the solutions are mixed will be less than before.
d.   It is not possible to predict whether the weight will change as a result of this experiment.

41.   A substance with a pH of 8 is
a.   strong acid.
b.   weak acid.
c.   strong base.
d.   weak base.

42.   The greater the difference in electronegativity between two elements, the greater the ionic character of a compound between them. The chart below lists the electronegativities of some elements.

K	0.8		I	2.5
Na	0.9		Br	2.8
Li	1.0		Cl	3.0
Mg	1.2		O	3.5
H	2.1		F	4.0

Which of these compounds is most ionic?
a.   NaI
b.   HF
c.   KCl
d.   ICl

43. The following diagram shows a graduated cylinder partially filled with water, before and after the addition of a lead sinker. What is the volume of the lead sinker?

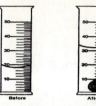

a. 14 ml
b. 18 ml
c. 32 ml
d. 50 ml

44. The diagram below shows four sealed containers partially filled with water at various temperatures. In which of these containers is the vapor pressure the greatest?

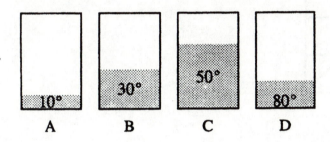

a. A
b. B
c. C
d. D

45. A sodium atom (Na) can become a sodium ion (Na^{+1}) by
a. gaining a proton.
b. losing a proton.
c. gaining an electron.
d. losing an electron.

46. 100 g of a radioactive substance disintegrates to 25 g after 8 days. What is the half-life of the substance?
a. 2 days
b. 4 days
c. 8 days
d. 25 days

47. The chart below shows the energy levels for a hydrogen atom.

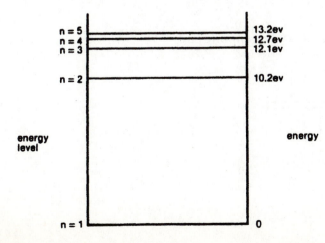

How much energy will an electron emit if it jumps from level n = 4 to level n = 2?
a. 12.7 ev
b. 12.1 ev
c. 10.2 ev
d. 2.5 ev

48. The graph below shows the velocity of an object during a 10-second period.

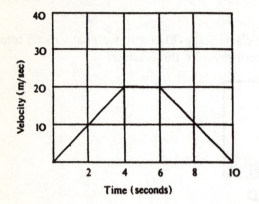

At which of these times does the object have no acceleration?
a. 0 sec
b. 2 sec
c. 5 sec
d. 8 sec

49. Four beakers containing different amounts of water at different temperatures are shown below.

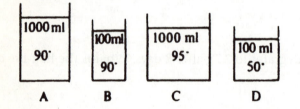

Which one requires the smallest amount of heat to come to a boil?
a. A
b. B
c. C
d. D

50. The diagram shows a lever with a heavy box on one end.

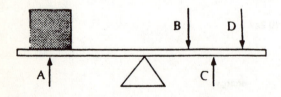

The arrows show the location and direction of four possible forces applied to the lever. Which one will require the least effort to lift the box if the force is applied as shown by the arrow?
a. A
b. B
c. C
d. D

51.   Which of the arrows in the graph below represents the wavelength of the wave shown?

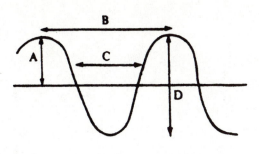

a. A
b. B
c. C
d. D

52.   More energy is used in pushing a box up along an inclined plane to a height of 4 meters than in lifting the box straight up to the same height. This is because
a.   more force is needed to push the box than to lift it.
b.   work is done against friction in pushing the box along the plane.
c.   the box moves a greater distance when pushed along the plane than when lifted.
d.   it takes more time to push the box along the plane than to lift it.

53.   Which of these rays are *NOT* considered to be radiation from radioactive materials?
a.   Alpha rays.
b.   Ultraviolet rays.
c.   Gamma rays.
d.   Beta rays.

54.   A variety of subatomic particles are shot between two oppositely charged plates as shown in the diagram.

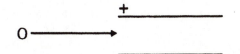

Which particles will not be deflected?
a.   protons
b.   neutrons
c.   electrons
d.   alpha particles

55.   Which type of circuit is shown in the diagram below?

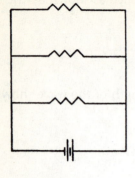

a.   open
b.   complex
c.   series
d.   parallel

56.   The device shown in the circuit diagram below consists of copper wire wrapped around an iron rod and connected to a switch and a battery.

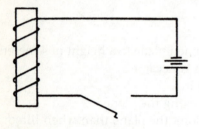

When the switch is closed, the device could serve as
a.   a transformer.
b.   an electromagnet.
c.   a motor.
d.   a generator.

57.   Two forces act on an object as shown in the diagram.

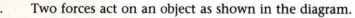

4N   6N

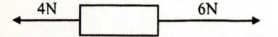

The magnitude of the net force on the object is
a.   2 newtons
b.   6 newtons
c.   10 newtons
d.   24 newtons

58.   Which of the following graphs best indicates the relationship between time and the velocity of a freely falling object?

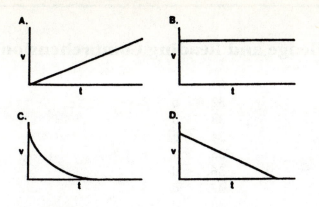

   a.   graph A
   b.   graph B
   c.   graph C
   d.   graph D

59.   The diagram below shows an object at rest on an inclined plane.

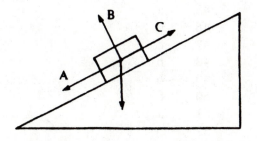

Which of these arrows correctly shows the direction of the frictional force?
   a.   A
   b.   B
   c.   C
   d.   D

60.   Four copper wires are shown below.

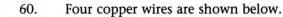
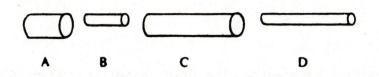

Which one has the lowest resistance?
   a.   A
   b.   B
   c.   C
   d.   D

Answers Comprehensive Practice Test 2

Verbal Ability: Word Knowledge and Reading Comprehension

1.	c		31.	c
2.	a		32.	b
3.	d		33.	b
4.	b		34.	c
5.	c		35.	a
6.	b		36.	d
7.	b		37.	d
8.	b		38.	d
9.	b		39.	b
10.	a		40.	c
11.	d		41.	b
12.	c		42.	b
13.	d		43.	b
14.	a		44.	c
15.	c		45.	a
16.	c		46.	b
17.	a		47.	c
18.	c		48.	b
19.	d		49.	b
20.	a		50.	c
21.	c		51.	a
22.	a		52.	b
23.	b		53.	a
24.	a		54.	a
25.	d		55.	c
26.	c		56.	d
27.	b		57.	d
28.	a		58.	b
29.	d		59.	c
30.	b		60.	a

Mathematics

1. **The answer is b.** The patients discharged plus the patients remaining make up all of the patients, or 100% of the patients. Therefore, if 78% are discharged within a week, then the remaining percent must be 100% − 78%, or 22%.

2. **The answer is b.** To convert hours to days, divide the number of hours by 24 (24 hours in one day).

$$\frac{84}{24} = \frac{7}{2} = 3\frac{1}{2}$$

3. **The answer is c.** Use this formula to find the area of a square: $A = s^2$.
    Substitute 4 for s in the formula and simplify: $A = 4^2 = 16$

4. **The answer is c.** You may set up a proportion to solve this problem. Be sure to align the units correctly: beats across from beats, and minutes across from minutes.

    $$\frac{14\ beats}{\frac{1}{6}\ min} = \frac{x}{1\ min}$$ Cross multiply.

    $$\frac{1}{6}x = 14$$ Multiply both sides by 6 to solve for x.

    $$x = 84$$ This is your answer.

5. **The answer is c.** To convert inches to feet, divide the number of inches by 12 (12 inches in a foot).

    $$\frac{58}{12} = 4\frac{10}{12}$$ In this case, express the remainder (10) in inches.

    So, 58 inches = 4 feet 10 inches.

6. **The answer is b.** Total the five percentages of sales for each day, and add this sum to the salesperson's base salary of $250.

    First: $83 + 116 + 49 + 94 + 67 = 409$
    Second: $409 + 250$
    Answer: $659

7. **The answer is c.** The equation x = 4 means that x and 4 are equivalent. Wherever you see x, you may substitute 4. Therefore:

    $$x^3 = 4^3 = 4 \cdot 4 \cdot 4 = 64.$$

8. **The answer is b.** Follow the order of operations to simplify this expression:

    $$(3)\sqrt{64} =$$
    $$(3) \cdot 8 = 24$$

9. **The answer is b.** If you have a ¼ hour rest period each day, and a ½ hour lunch break each day, then you have $5 \cdot \frac{1}{4}$ hours of rest and $5 \cdot \frac{1}{2}$ hours of lunch each week.

    $$5 \cdot \frac{1}{4} = \frac{5}{4} \quad 5 \cdot \frac{1}{2} = \frac{5}{2}$$

    Add these two totals together to get the grand total of duty-free hours each week:

    $$\frac{5}{4} = \frac{5}{4}$$
    $$+\ \frac{5}{2} = \frac{10}{4}$$
    $$\overline{\quad\frac{15}{4} = 3\frac{3}{4}\quad}$$

10. **The answer is b.** If x = 43, then of the four choices, only choice B is correct. Neither choice A or C allow for x to equal 43, and choice D requires x to be smaller than 40 and greater than or equal to 43—an impossibility.

11. **The answer is c.** To find the missing addend, add up the 3 addends, and subtract their sum from 120. You need to find equivalent fractions for the mixed numbers in order to add them.

$$
\begin{aligned}
23\tfrac{1}{2} &= \; 23\tfrac{6}{12} \\
9\tfrac{2}{3} &= \quad 9\tfrac{8}{12} \\
+\;78\tfrac{3}{4} &= \; 78\tfrac{9}{12} \\
\hline
&\quad 110\tfrac{23}{12} \;=\; 111\tfrac{11}{12}
\end{aligned}
$$

Now subtract $111^{11}\!/_{12}$ from 120 to find the missing addend.

$$
\begin{aligned}
120 &= 119\tfrac{12}{12} \\
-\;111\tfrac{11}{12} &= 111\tfrac{11}{12} \\
\hline
&\quad\; 8\tfrac{1}{12} \quad \text{This is your answer.}
\end{aligned}
$$

12. **The answer is c.** Beginning with $1200,

Subtract $\tfrac{1}{2}$ of $1200 for rent: $1200 − 600 = $600

Subtract $\tfrac{1}{4}$ of $1200 *from $600* for food: $600 − $300 = **$300**

13. **The answer is b.** A prime number has exactly two factors: 1 and the number itself. Choice A is not a prime number, and choices C and D do not immediately precede 19. The only choice is B.

14. **The answer is a.** To calculate how many seconds there are in 3⅓ minutes, multiply 3⅓ by 60 (because there are 60 seconds in each minute).

$$
\begin{aligned}
3\tfrac{1}{3} \cdot 60 &= &&\text{Change 60 to an improper fraction.} \\
\tfrac{10}{3} \cdot \tfrac{60}{1} &= &&\text{Multiply.} \\
\tfrac{600}{3} &= 200 \text{ seconds} &&\text{This is your answer.}
\end{aligned}
$$

15.   **The answer is b.** Following the order of operations, multiply first, and then work from left to right.

  6(.83) + .3(100) − 29.09 =
  4.98 + 30 − 29.09 =
  34.98 − 29.09 = **5.89**

16.   **The answer is c.** You may use a proportion to solve this problem. As always, remember to align the units correctly: milliliters across from milliliters, and grams across from grams.

$$\frac{10\ ml}{1.2\ g} = \frac{15\ ml}{x}$$ Cross multiply.

10 x = 18   Divide both sides by 10 to solve for x.
x = 1.8   This is your answer.

17.   **The answer is d.** This problem screams out for algebra! In the fraction that is equal to %, the numerator is *7 less than* the denominator. In algebraic terms:

The denominator = x, the numerator = $x − 7$, and the fraction = $\frac{x - 7}{x}$.

Since the fraction equals %, we have the following equation (a proportion!):

$$\frac{x - 7}{x} = \frac{8}{9}$$ Cross multiply.

9(x − 7) = 8x Simplify.
9 x − 63 = 8x Subtract 9x from both sides of the equation.
−63 = −x Multiply both sides by −1 to solve for x.
63 = x This is the numerator. Subtract 7 from 63 to find the
          denominator: 63 − 7 = 56.

18.   **The answer is b.** Similar polygons have their sides in proportion. This means the ratio of corresponding sides is constant. Set up a proportion according to the relationship in the problem.

The first ratio is → 3 cm side of first triangle : 5 cm side of second triangle

The second ratio is → 9 cm side of first triangle : x cm side of second triangle

Here is the proportion: $\frac{3}{5} = \frac{9}{x}$ Cross multiply.
                3x = 45   Divide both sides by 3 to solve for x.
                x = 15   This is your answer.

19.   **The answer is c.** The winner of the race finished ahead of, or earlier than, the second place runner. This means the winner's time must be *less than* the second place runner's time.

To find the winner's time, subtract 0.32 from 10.72: $\begin{array}{r} 10.72 \\ -\ 0.32 \\ \hline 10.40 \end{array}$

20.   **The answer is b.** You may set up a proportion to solve this problem. As always, make sure you align the units correctly: inches across from inches, and miles across from miles (or in this case, mileage).

$$\frac{3\ in}{20\ mi} = \frac{5\frac{1}{2}\ in}{x}$$ Cross multiply.

$$3x = \frac{20}{1} \cdot \frac{11}{2}$$ Simplify.

$$3x = \frac{220}{2}$$ Simplify.

$$3x = 110$$ Divide both sides by 3 to solve for x.

$$x = \frac{110}{3} = 36\frac{2}{3}$$ This is your answer.

21.   **The answer is d.** The multiplication property of zero says that if, in a multiplication problem, one of the factors is zero, than the product must be zero. This is the case in this problem. No matter what $3 \cdot 4 \cdot 5$ is, that product times 0 will equal 0.

22.   **The answer is a.**

$$0.25\overline{)625} =$$ Multiply the divisor and the dividend by 100.

$$25\overline{)62500} =$$ If you know your perfect squares, you know that $25 \cdot 25 = 625$.

$$25\overline{)62500}^{2500}$$ 2500 is your answer.

23.   **The answer is c.** This problem involves percent increase. Solve this problem in three steps:

Change $5\frac{1}{2}$%, or 5.5% into a decimal by dividing by 100:   5.5% = 0.055

Calculate 5.5% of $17,200 by multiplying:

17,200	no decimal places
× 0.055	3 decimal places
946.000	3 decimal places

Add this amount to the original price to find the new price: $17,200 + $946 = **$18,146**

24.   **The answer is d.** On the first day, the patient's caloric intake is 950. On the second day, the patient's caloric intake is increased by 10%.

950 + 10% of 950 =
950 + (0.1)(950) =
950 + 95 = 1045   This is the caloric intake on the second day.

On the third day, the increase is 10% of what the intake was on the *second day.*

1045 + 10% of 1045 =
1045 + (.1)(1045) =
1045 + 104.5 = 1149.5   This is the caloric intake on the third day.

Rounded to the nearest calorie, the patient's caloric intake on the third day is **1150**.

25. **The answer is b.** To change 0.88 to a fraction, you must know the name of the decimal. This decimal is 88 hundredths. To write it as a fraction, put 88 over 100, and reduce:

$$\frac{88}{100} = \frac{22}{25}$$

26. **The answer is d.** To find the cost for each capsule (the unit rate), divide the cost of 15 capsules by the number of capsules:

$$6.86 \div 15 = 0.45666\ldots$$

The question asks for the cost to the nearest penny. Round to the hundredths place.

$$0.45666\ldots \approx 0.46 \quad \text{Your answer is 46¢.}$$

27. **The answer is b.** Recall that all circles contain 360 degrees. (If you had forgotten this, you could have added up all of the angles and found the total.) Write a fraction of the information.

$\frac{45}{360} = \frac{1}{8}$ Change the fraction into a decimal.

$\frac{1}{8} = 0.125$ Change the decimal into a percent.

$0.125 = 12.5\%$ Finally, round to the nearest whole percent.

$12.5\% \approx 13\%$

28. **The answer is a.** To find which central angle represents $\frac{1}{12}$, calculate $\frac{1}{12}$ of 360 (total degrees in a circle).

$$\frac{1}{12} \cdot \frac{360}{1} = \frac{360}{12} = 30 \quad \text{This is your answer.}$$

29. **The answer is a.** This problem involves variables, but it is really about adding fractions. You may only add like terms, in this case, x-terms and y-terms.

$$\frac{2}{5}x + \frac{3}{10}x = \frac{4}{10}x + \frac{3}{10}x = \frac{7}{10}x$$

$$-\frac{1}{6}y + \frac{3}{4}y = -\frac{2}{12}y + \frac{9}{12}y = \frac{7}{12}y$$

$$\frac{7}{10}x + \frac{7}{12}y \qquad \text{This is your answer.}$$

30.   **The answer is d.**

$$4\frac{1}{2} \cdot 3\frac{5}{6} =$$ Change each mixed number to an improper fraction.

$$\frac{9}{2} \cdot \frac{23}{6} =$$ Multiply.

$$\frac{207}{12} = 17\frac{3}{12} = 17\frac{1}{4}$$ Remember to reduce your answer.

31.   **The answer is d.** You may set up a proportion to solve this problem. As usual, make sure you align the units properly: quarts across from quarts, and liters across from liters.

$$\frac{1 \; quart}{0.9 \; liters} = \frac{x}{12 \; liters}$$ Cross multiply.

$$0.9x = 12$$ Divide both sides by 0.9 to solve for x.

$$x = \frac{12}{0.9} = \frac{120}{9} = 13\frac{3}{9} = 13\frac{1}{3}$$ **Remember to simplify your answer.**

32.   **The answer is c.**

$$\frac{2}{3} + 7\left(\frac{1}{2}\right) - \frac{6}{5} =$$ First, multiply 7 by $\frac{1}{2}$.

$$\frac{2}{3} + \frac{7}{2} - \frac{6}{5} =$$ Find a common denominator and change

these fractions to their equivalent fractions.

$$\frac{2}{3} = \frac{20}{30} \quad \frac{7}{2} = \frac{105}{30} \quad \frac{6}{5} = \frac{36}{30}$$

$$\frac{20}{30} + \frac{105}{30} - \frac{36}{30} - \frac{89}{30} = 2\frac{29}{30}$$

33.   **The answer is a.** This geometry problem requires algebra to solve it. Begin by defining the length and width with variables.

width = w length = $3w$ (because the length is 3 times the width)

The area is 147 cm², so use the formula for area of a rectangle.

A = LW
147 = 3w · w   Substitute 147 for A and 3w for L.
147 = 3w²   Multiply 3w and w².
49 = w²   Divide both sides by 3.
7 = w   Take the square root of both sides to solve for w.

Finally, multiply 7 by 3 to find the length of the rectangle: 21.

34.   **The answer is a.** This is one of three basic types of percent problems.

5 is 3% of what number?   Turn the problem into an equation.

$5 = 3\% \cdot x$

$5 = 0.03x$ Divide both sides by 0.03 to solve for x.

$0.03\overline{)5} = x$

$3\overline{)500} = x$ Multiply divisor and dividend by 100.

$\dfrac{166.\overline{6}}{3\overline{)500.0}}$ Your answer is $166.\overline{6}$, or $166\dfrac{2}{3}$.

35.   **The answer is c.** This problem calls for you to add something to ⅕, so we begin with:

$\dfrac{1}{5} + \underline{\hspace{2cm}}.$

Now, what do you put in the blank? You put ⅔ of the number itself.

$\dfrac{1}{5} + \dfrac{2}{3}\left(\dfrac{1}{5}\right)$ Simplify this expression.

$\dfrac{1}{5} + \dfrac{2}{15}$ To add these fractions, find an equivalent fraction for $\dfrac{1}{5}$.

$\dfrac{3}{15} + \dfrac{2}{15} = \dfrac{5}{15} = \dfrac{1}{3}$ Change $\dfrac{1}{3}$ to a decimal, and round to the thousandths place.

$\dfrac{1}{3} = 0.333$ This is your answer.

36.   **The answer is d.**

$13\,x^2y \div \dfrac{-1}{2\,x} =$ Invert the divisor and multiply.

$\dfrac{13\,x^2y}{1} \cdot \dfrac{2x}{-1} =$ Multiply.

$-26\,x^3y$ Recall when multiplying like bases, you ADD exponents.

37.   **The answer is a.**

$9 - \dfrac{3}{4}n = 45$ Subtract 9 from both sides of the equation.

$-\dfrac{3}{4}n = 36$ Multiply both sides by $-\dfrac{4}{3}$ to solve for n.

$n = \dfrac{36}{1} \cdot -\dfrac{4}{3}$ Multiply.

$n = -\dfrac{144}{3}$ Simply.

$n = -4$ This is your answer.

38.   **The answer is d.** Recall the *Pythagorean Theorem*: $a^2 + b^2 = c^2$ Use this to solve for side AB (*c*).

$6^2 + 8^2 = c^2$ Simplify.

$36 + 64 = c^2$

$100 = c^2$ Take the square root of both sides.

$10 = c$ This is your answer.

39.   **The answer is a.** Solve this percentage decrease problem by making a fraction of the information. Write the *amount of decrease* as the numerator, and write the *original amount* as the denominator.

The number of students using tobacco decreased from some unknown amount (x) by 350. The amount of change is 350. The original amount is x:

$$\frac{350}{x}$$

This is a decrease of 20%. Use this information to write a proportion.

$\dfrac{350}{x} = \dfrac{20}{100}$ Cross multiply.

$20x = 35,000$ Divide both sides by 20 to solve for x.

$x = \dfrac{35,000}{20}$ Reduce the fraction before you divide.

$x = \dfrac{3500}{2}$ Divide.

$x = 1750$ This is NOT your answer. This is the number of students who used tobacco before the decrease in usage.

This question asks: "How many students still use tobacco?" Tricky! Once you find the original number of users, subtract 350 (the decrease) from 1750, to get 1400, the number of students still using tobacco. 1400 is your answer.

40.   **The answer is d.** This is one of 3 basic types of percent problems.

0.5% of what number is 25?   Turn the problem into an equation.

$0.005 \cdot x = 25$

$0.005x = 25$ Divide both sides by 0.005 to solve for x.

$x = 0.005\overline{)25}$ Multiply divisor and dividend by 1000.

$x = 5\overline{)25000}$ Divide.

$x = \dfrac{5000}{5\overline{)25000}}$ 5000 is your answer.

Science

1. **The answer is b.** Object magnification is equal to the product of the eye piece magnification and the high power objective magnification. If an object is magnified 430 times by a microscope that has an eyepiece of $10\times$, the magnification of the high-power objective must be 43.

    $$10 \times \text{(high-power objective magnification)} = 430$$

    $$10 \times 43 = 430$$

2. **The answer is d.** Plants are autotrophs, which means that they make their own food. Plants accomplish this via the process of photosynthesis.

3. **The answer is b.** If the rabbit is able to produce tyrosine, then it can be assumed that enzyme x is functioning properly. Since melanin is not produced, it is reasonable that a mutation is present in the enzyme necessary for the production of melanin.

4. **The answer is c.** Decomposers are necessary for the recycling of inorganic nutrients, which then allows for plants to photosynthesize.

5. **The answer is c.** Contractile vacuoles collect extra water that has entered the cell via osmosis and periodically expels it out of the cell. If an amoeba had evolved in salt water, water would not be entering the cell (remember how osmosis works: water moves from areas of low particle concentration to high particle concentration), rather the cell might have to create mechanisms to counter dehydration.

6. **The answer is a.** Flowers contain male and female structures that allow for fertilization to occur in the absence of an aquatic environment.

7. **The answer is a.** Nondisjunction occurs during cell division and can cause the production of gametes that either lack a chromosome or have an additional copy. For instance, Down's syndrome is caused by the presence of an extra copy of chromosome 21.

8. **The answer is d.** Cellulose is found in the cell walls of plant cells. Animal cells do not have cell walls.

9. **The answer is b.** Nucleic acids are composed of strings of nucleotides. DNA is a nucleic acid, and its specific sequences of nucleotides represents the genetic make up of an individual.

10. **The answer is c.** Follow the arrows!

11. **The answer is d.** Since rabbits are solely dependent upon vegetables according to the diagram of this food web, the removal of vegetables would cause the rabbit population to decline. Rodent populations eat vegetables, however, they also use grass as a food source and thus they would not be as effected as rabbits by the removal of vegetables.

12. **The answer is c.** Vegetables are grass are producers since they photosynthesize, rabbits, and rodents are primary consumers since they eat producers, and hawks, snakes, and owls are secondary consumers since they eat herbivores. Decomposers such as bacteria are not represented here. They are crucial to a food web due since they are responsible for breaking down organic matter and making it available to producers.

13. **The answer is d.** It was clear from Spemann's first experiment that the very young embryonic cells were not specialized. He then wanted to test whether older cells were specialized or not.

14. **The answer is a.** Since no effect was seen when Spemann reversed the position of the cells it was clear that these cells were not specialized yet.

15. **The answer is a.** The salamander eggs must have been fertilized as Spemann was studying embryonic development, which cannot occur without fertilization.

16. **The answer is c.** The variable is the characteristic that is measured in an experiment.

17. **The answer is c.** The optimal pH is approximately 8, and thus at lower and higher pH's, the activity declines. This creates a bell-shaped curve that shows activity increasing near the optimal pH and decreasing as the pH increases.

18. **The answer is c.** The cells shown in figure C are nerve cells, which are responsible for transmission of impulses throughout the body.

19. **The answer is a.** The cells in figure A are stratified (layered) epithelial cells. Stratified epithelium is usually found in areas that are subject to a great deal of friction like the lining of the cheek.

20. **The answer is s.** The cells in figure D are striated muscle cells, which respond to changes in body temperature by dilating and letting off heat or constricting and retaining heat. These muscle cells are also capable of promoting shivering.

21. **The answer is a.** Ribosomes are involved in protein synthesis; lysosomes in degradation of waste; mitochondria in energy production.

22. **The answer is c.** Protein digestion begins in the stomach and is completed in the small intestine.

23. **The answer is b.** The greatest portion of digestion occurs in the small intestine.

24. **The answer is d.** The semicircular canals in the inner ear are responsible for maintenance of dynamic balance.

25. **The answer is d.** As blood moves through the kidney, it is filtered at a microscopic level at the entrance to nephrons, which are the functional units of the kidney. Here, the fluid passes through a series of loops where reabsorption of water and ions occurs in such a manner that the urine is diluted or concentrated to meet the needs of the organism.

26. **The answer is d.** During cytokinesis (division of the cytoplasm) in plant cells, a cell plate divides the two new cells in half. In animal cells, the cytoplasm is pinched in half to form the two daughter cells.

27. **The answer is b.**

28. **The answer is d.** Thromboplastin is a clotting factor. Thus, release of excess amounts of this factor could promote the formation of a clot.

29. **The answer is b.** While tendons connect muscles to bones, ligaments are responsible for connection bone to bone.

30. **The answer is a.** The medulla controls many involuntary actions such as breathing and heart rate.

31. **The answer is a.** Monosaccharides make up polysaccharides, fatty acids make up lipids, and nucleic acids such as DNA and RNA are made up of nucleotides.

32. **The answer is a.** The specific gravity of a substance is a ratio of the mass of the substance to the mass of water of equal volume. Thus, it is not surprising that the specific gravity of water is 1. A substance that has a specific gravity of less than 1 is less dense than water and will float.

33. **The answer is c.** A catalyst increases the rate of a reaction by lowering the activation energy required for the reaction to proceed to completion.

34. **The answer is a.** Solids do not have a fixed shape and volume. Liquids do in fact have a fixed volume but take on the shape of whatever container they are in.

35. **The answer is b.** As a solution boils in this set up, the gas that forms flows into the long tube within a tube. In the outer portion, water is flowing to keep the tube cool. In the inner portion, gas flows and is condensed into a liquid due to the temperature decrease. Thus, a solution that contains alcohol and water can be separated since the two substances have different boiling points.

36. **The answer is b.** The balanced equation for the decomposition of water displays the ratio of gas produced to water decomposed.

$$2H2O \rightarrow 2H2 + O2$$

37. **The answer is a.** Tinctures are alcohol based.

38. **The answer is b.** AB represents melting, EF represents sublimation (solid changing directly to a gas), and KL does not represent a phase change.

39. **The answer is b.** A neutralization reaction is when a strong acid and a strong base react to produce a salt and water which are both neutral.

40. **The answer is a.** The mixing of A and B has clearly resulted in the formation of a new substance. However, the law of conservation of mass states that mass can neither be created nor destroyed. Thus, the mass of the reactants is equal to the mass of the products.

41. **The answer is d.** On the pH scale, a substance with a pH greater than 7 is basic. The strength of the base increases as the pH approaches 14.

42. **The answer is c.** The difference in electronegativities between K and Cl is greater than the other elements. Electronegativity refers to the ability of an atom to attract electrons to itself. Thus, Cl will pull an electron away from K and become negative while K becomes positive. The resulting opposite charges will allow the two atoms to bind.

43. **The answer is a.** The volume of an object is equal to the volume of water the object displaces when fully submerged. The millimeter marking of the bottom of the meniscus (curved part at surface of water), signifies the volume in ml. The marking changes from 18 mm to 32 mm. The volume is therefore 14 ml.

44. **The answer is c.** Water molecules naturally alternate between vapor and liquid form until the boiling temperature is reached. At this point, more liquid molecules enter the gas phase as boiling continues. The vapor pressure will be the highest in the container with the largest volume of water since there are more molecules of water available to become vapor.

45. **The answer is d.** A neutral atom has an equal number of protons and electrons. When an atom loses electrons it become a positively charged ion, or cation.

46. **The answer is b.** The half-life of a radioactive substance is the time it takes for half of the mass of the sample to disintegrate.

47. **The answer is d.** The energy emitted as an electron moves between two levels is the difference in the energy of the two energy levels.

48. **The answer is c.** At t = 5 seconds the velocity is constant at 20 m/sec. The acceleration is zero whenever velocity is constant.

49. **The answer is b.** The specific heat of a substance is the energy required to change the temperature of 1 kg of that substance by 1° Celsius. The boiling point of water is 100° Celsius. In order for the water in container A to boil the temperature of 1,000 ml of water must be raised 10° Celsius. In order for the water in container B to boil the temperature of 100 ml of water must be raised 10° celsius. In order for the water in container C to boil the temperature of 1,000 ml of water must be raised 5°. In order for the water in container D to boil the temperature of 100 ml of water must be raised 50°. Container B requires the least amount of heat for the water to reach a boil.

50. **The answer is d.** The force applied by the lever is proportional to the force itself and the distance away from the balance. The force applied at D is the greatest distance away, so less effort will be need here.

51. **The answer is b.** The wavelength of a wave is defined as the distance between crests of the wave.

52. **The answer is b.** Whenever a box moves along a surface with a coefficient of friction greater then zero, energy must be used to overcome the force of friction that is not needed when the box is simply lifted.

53. **The answer is a.** Alpha, beta, and gamma rays are all types of radiation. Ultraviolet rays are just a type of light, which the human eye can not detect.

54. **The answer is b.** A neutron is the only choice that does not carry any intrinsic charge. The other particles will be deflected because they will be attracted to the plate that has the opposite charge and repelled by the plate that has the same charge.

55. **The answer is d.** Any circuit with the same voltage across all resistors is a parallel circuit.

56. **The answer is b.** Whenever a wire is wrapped around a rod and connected across a power source like a battery, the device will act as an electromagnet.

57. **The answer is a.** Since the forces are in the opposite directions they are not added. The smaller force is subtracted from the stronger force, and the resultant force is in the same direction as the stronger force.

58. **The answer is a.** A freely falling object falls at a constant acceleration g = 9.8 m/s squared. The graph which shows velocity increasing at a constant rate is A.

59. **The answer is c.** The direction of the frictional force always points to oppose motion. In this case the motion is down the inclined plane, so the frictional force must point up the plane.

60. **The answer is a.** Resistance is proportional to length and inversely proportional to cross-sectional area.

Comprehensive Practice Test 3

Verbal Ability
Word Knowledge and Reading Comprehension

60 Minutes

WORD KNOWLEDGE: Read each sentence carefully. Then, *on the basis of what is stated in the sentence,* select the correct completion of the incomplete statement. The correct answers will be found at the end of this test.

1.   The artist cleansed the brushes with some paint.
     a. sediment.
     b. solvent.
     c. lacquer.
     d. antidote.

2.   After the accident, the investigators were searching for pieces of the fuselage.
     Fuselage refers to part of

     a. a ship.
     b. an airplane.
     c. a car.
     d. a train.

3.   Much of the monetary policy is set by the national government.
     Monetary refers to

     a. diplomacy.
     b. insurance.
     c. money.
     d. defense.

4.   One of the most famous recluses of the twentieth century was Howard Hughes.
     Recluse means

     a. agnostic.
     b. benefactor.
     c. atheist.
     d. hermit.

5.   The ancient burial ground was found under a knoll near the lake.
     Knoll means

     a. stone.
     b. mound.
     c. grove.
     d. glade.

6. The relationship eroded quickly when Helen went back to her old job.
   Eroded means
   a. ended.
   b. grew.
   c. deepened.
   d. diminished.

7. The lawyer succeeded in having the client's charge reduced by proving that the client acted
   a. in deference.
   b. with embellishment.
   c. under duress.
   d. foolishly.

8. After three years of work, we were successful in bringing our dream to
   a. dissidence.
   b. trepidation.
   c. gratuity.
   d. fruition.

9. It has been purported that an agreement will be reached before the deadline.
   Purported means
   a. published.
   b. discussed.
   c. rumored.
   d. considered.

10. The apathy during the campaign cost the politician the election.
    Apathy means
    a. corruption.
    b. indifference.
    c. resentment.
    d. obstacle.

11. I knew I could trust my friend with the secret because he had always been
    a. ingenious.
    b. trusting.
    c. discreet.
    d. callous.

12. Frank refused to listen to reason; he was just being perverse.
    Perverse means
    a. ignorant.
    b. contrary.
    c. silly.
    d. obtuse.

13. The differences between the two research study results were so small they were
    a. momentary.
    b. negligible.
    c. fragmented.
    d. critical.

14. With all of the sudden changes in the methods of childrearing, the society is definitely in a state of
    a. indiscretion.
    b. heresy.
    c. flux.
    d. secession.

15. The young man made several gibes while the politician was addressing the group.
    Gibes means

    a. gestures.
    b. taunts.
    c. applause.
    d. motions.

16. The terrorists left their hiding place to foray briefly into a local town.
    Foray means

    a. make a raid.
    b. take a chance.
    c. have a battle.
    d. carry a message.

READING COMPREHENSION: There are five reading passages in this section. Read each passage carefully. Then, *on the basis of what you have read in the passage*, select the correct answer for each question.

I

Zoologists have studied how cold-blooded insects go about their business all through winter, just as they have questioned how cold-blooded fish manage in the subfreezing water around Antarctica. Down to a certain temperature, winter insects can make do by absorbing sunlight; many are dark-colored so they can absorb as much heat as possible from the sun. Others absorb heat by basking on dark surfaces. Heavy layers of hair or scales slow the loss of heat generated or absorbed. Insects also beat their wings while at rest to warm themselves.

Many insect species adapt their behavior to cold. Southern or warm-climate species of black flies, for example, mate in the air, and females fly long distances for the blood meal necessary for the eggs to mature. But Arctic black flies mate on the ground when they are too cold to fly, and eggs are presupplied with nutrients.

Keeping active in the cold season is important; keeping alive—and unfrozen—is essential. When living tissue freezes, expanding ice crystals destroy cell membranes, causing irreversible and fatal damage. Death comes even before freezing is complete, when there is no longer enough liquid in the cell for the enzyme activity essential to life.

Insects survive subfreezing temperatures by supercooling, lowering the freezing point of their body fluids, and either by slowing ice formation or by being able to function even when their extracellular fluids have been frozen. Both groups use "antifreezes": the polyhydric alcohols sorbitol and glycerol (chemically similar to the glycerol used in automobiles) and the disaccharide trehalose.

Insects in the first group manage by reducing the chance that ice will form in their circulatory fluids. Ice tends to form rapidly around a nucleator, a tiny ice crystal or speck of dust that offers a solid frame for other molecules to attach themselves to. These insects purge their bodies of potential nucleators, principally by emptying their guts, and produce antifreezes, which lower the freezing point by raising the concentration of solutes in the body fluids (salt water has a lower freezing point than fresh water, for example). The antifreezes have multiple hydroxyl radicals in their molecules, which tend to bond with the hydrogen in the water molecules, thus greatly reducing their tendency to aggregate into ice crystals.

Excerpted from of *Science 83* Magazine, copyright the American Association for the Advancement of Science.

17.   Which of the following titles is best for this passage?
a.   "Insect Antifreeze"
b.   "Winter Adaptations by Insects"
c.   "Flies in Antarctica"
d.   "Cold Season Behaviors"

18.   It can be inferred that one means by which some insects lessen the likelihood of their body fluids freezing is
a.   drinking salt water.
b.   beating their wings.
c.   flying long distances.
d.   eliminating body wastes.

19.   The eggs of Arctic black flies contain
a.   trehalose.
b.   stored food.
c.   antifreeze.
d.   sorbitol.

20.   Which of these substances most likely reduces the ice formation in the insects' body fluids?
a.   protein
b.   acid
c.   alcohol
d.   lipid

21.   According to the passage, when living tissue freezes
a.   the cells lose fluid.
b.   the metabolic processes speed up.
c.   the cell structure is destroyed.
d.   the concentration of solutes increases.

22.   Within an insect's body fluids, the structure to which other molecules are attracted is referred to as
a.   antifreeze.
b.   glycol.
c.   trehalose.
d.   nucleator.

II

While toys have existed since ancient times, only in recent years have we come to understand their more extensive role and the meaning of play to a child's growth and development.

In more primitive, simple societies, children learned through play to familiarize themselves with their environment and to develop skills which would help them find food and provide shelter in order to survive. In an increasingly complex society, children today must learn more for survival. They must develop physically, mentally, emotionally and socially in order to cope.

This learning process begins for children through their play and toys are the educational tools to aid in this development. Though no toy can teach a child anything all by itself, with proper interaction between a child, his toys, and other people—and particularly with his parents—toys can teach many things.

Toys can help children in the development of specific skills such as walking, talking, reading, and generally, to develop confidence in the process of learning.

It is considerably more difficult for children today to mature from child to adult. Life patterns are more complex and a child is not always sure of his adult role. Toys are important in helping them prepare for adulthood by increasing their confidence, flexibility and self-expression. They help introduce children to modern technology and contemporary living by emulating current social trends, attitudes and interests.

Children gain a sense of values from their toys. As we said, toys by themselves cannot shape a child, but they can help to reinforce the lessons we teach them.

Toys help children get along better with others and to be more responsive to the needs of other people. Scientists refer to this as the development of interpersonal relationships.

Perhaps most important of all, toys teach children to love. They have traditionally provided companionship and security and served as objects of love for children. A favorite doll, a teddy bear or other special toy has helped many children cope with difficult moments in their young lives. Children have to learn to love and they learn partly from loving their toys.

Passage from *Toys Are Teaching Tools*, published by Toy Manufacturers of America, Inc., New York.

23. A good title for this passage would be
    a. "The Benefit of Toys"
    b. "The History of Toys"
    c. "The Study of Children's Play"
    d. "Children's Social Development"

24. It can be inferred from the passage that boys in primitive societies would most likely play with toy
    a. weapons.
    b. animals.
    c. musical instruments.
    d. money.

25. According to the passage, toys can serve as a means for a child to
     a. play independently.
     b. acquire intelligence.
     c. develop a role model.
     d. become grown-up.

26. The author suggests that a child should be expected to
     a. make use of each toy he owns.
     b. develop an attachment to a toy.
     c. require complex toys in a complex society.
     d. mature quickly because of play with toys.

27. The author emphasizes most the importance of a toy's
     a. responsiveness.
     b. technology.
     c. practicality.
     d. trends.

28. This passage would most likely have appeared in a
     a. weekly news magazine.
     b. toy catalogue.
     c. trade journal.
     d. child development text.

III

For the Jivaro Indians in the headwaters of the Amazon, beer is a greater necessity than solid food. Adult males drink from three to four gallons of it a day, adult females from one to two gallons, and a nine-year-old child will down half a gallon. Even though almost all of the protein in their diet must be obtained by going out to hunt, Jivaro hunters will often abandon the pursuit of prey and return to the settlement because the supply of beer is about to run out. Since women produce the beer, a man finds it desirable to acquire at least two wives so as to be able to entertain many guests and thus become known for his generosity. The Bemba also regard beer as equivalent to our notion of solid food; on days when beer is drunk, very little other food is eaten. The Bemba's high regard for beer as a major food is justified, because the sorghum from which it is made provides a number of B vitamins in which the rest of the diet is deficient, as well as a number of important minerals. A foreigner who sees Africans drinking beer, knowing that they are short of food, will usually condemn it—not realizing that beer is both a nutritional and a social necessity. If a man cannot give a beer party, even a small one, from time to time, he loses standing in his society. For the Bemba, providing beer is the most important way to repay social obligations, to honor kin, or to offer tribute to a chief. It rewards people who have given aid, and it is offered to deities. Tribal councils, marriages, and initiation ceremonies cannot take place without it. No wonder that the Bemba work hard at cultivating the land needed to produce enough grain for brewing.

Beer is similarly important in many modern societies; a pint of even a weak European beer provides nearly a tenth of the calcium and phosphorus needed daily, and about a fifth of the B vitamins, in addition to carbohydrates and several other vitamins and minerals—in effect serving as a liquid bread. In British villages and city neighborhoods, the pub is the focus for social life. It has long been the place for exchanging gossip, for the public airing and settlement of disputes, and for the reinforcement of friendships. A small village that loses its only pub loses much of what held the community together.

From *Consuming Passions* by Peter Farb and George Armelagos. Copyright © 1980 by the Estate of Peter Farb. Reprinted by permission of Houghton Mifflin Company.

29. Which of the following titles is best for this passage?
    a. "Beer: A Multipurpose Drink"
    b. "The Nutritional Significance of Beer"
    c. "The Beer: An International Drink"
    d. "The Social Influence of Beer"

30. The Bemba brew a beer from
    a. sorghum.
    b. corn.
    c. barley.
    d. malt.

31. The authors compare beer nutritionally to
    a. milk.
    b. soup.
    c. bread.
    d. protein.

32. A foreign visitor to the Bemba tribe is likely to regard their beer consumption as
    a. decadent.
    b. ceremonial.
    c. obligatory.
    d. nutritious.

33. For which of these reasons will the Jivaro men on the hunt return to the village when the supply of beer runs low?
    a. to make offerings to their deity
    b. to urge the women to produce beer
    c. to satisfy their appetite
    d. to harvest the grain for making beer

34. According to the passage, which of the following uses of beer in modern American society parallels a use of beer in the Bemba tribe?
    a. toasting the host at a party
    b. adding flavor to a sauce
    c. marking the end of the working day
    d. shampooing one's hair

IV

If housewives were left satisfied, amused, confused, irritated, frustrated, or bored by all the various information the different cookbooks pretended to give them, they were to be jounced right off their rocking chairs by the food faddists, whose numbers steadily grew as the 19th Century wore on. This strange group of men and women, with their even stranger ideas, were to have far-reaching effects on the American diet and eating habits. Sylvester Graham (1794–1851), whose last name is memorialized today on a sack of flour, can be looked upon as the first of these crusaders. When he launched his attack on the American diet, sometime around 1830, dyspepsia (severe indigestion) was so widespread as to seem a national disease. Thus his ideas for improving digestion (and elimination) fell on fertile ground. Imagine the housewife's consternation when he revealed to her that all the meat she so innocently served her husband and children actually inflamed tempers and induced sexual excesses. And what could her reaction have been when Sylvester Graham told her that condiments—the pepper and mustard she used to season her food, the bottle of catsup she placed so casually on the table— could induce insanity?

Graham saw health and salvation in bran, the outer portion of the wheat kernel, which was being sifted from flour by millers anxious to produce as purely white a product as possible. Dyspepsia could be cured, bodies purged and souls purified, he argued, if only bran were put back into flour. What he could not have known is that bran contained minerals and vitamins essential to health; what he did know is that as an irritant of the bowels it had a laxative effect. Graham bread, Graham crackers, Graham gems—all made with Graham flour containing a high percentage of bran—were his contribution to American cooking.

Foods of the World/American Cooking by Dale Brown and the Editors of Time-Life Books. © 1968 Time-Life Books Inc.

35. According to the passage, Graham was
    a. a diet faddist.
    b. a religious fanatic.
    c. a modern nutritionist.
    d. an industrial baker.

36. It can be inferred from the passage that Graham believed that sullenness and anger were induced by
    a. condiments.
    b. baked goods.
    c. vegetables.
    d. meat.

37. It can be inferred that bread baked with bran flour would be
    a. bitter.
    b. dark.
    c. hard.
    d. crusty.

38. Graham thought that bran contained
    a. irritating stimulants.
    b. chemical laxatives.
    c. natural enzymes.
    d. essential nutrients.

39. According to Graham, bran in the diet would do all of the following *EXCEPT*
    a. relieve indigestion.
    b. clean out the body.
    c. reduce insanity.
    d. care for the spirit.

40.   Much of the passage was written in a tone that could be described as
    a.   critical.
    b.   pedantic.
    c.   humorous.
    d.   argumentative.

V

An electro-mechanical artificial leg that accepts subconscious signals from the wearer has been developed at the Moss Rehabilitation Hospital for use by people with amputations above the knee.

Howard Hillstrom, senior research scientist for the project, said Thursday that the prosthesis was set in motion when the wearer consciously or subconsciously sent signals to remaining muscles about the knee and hip.

The hospital says research on the project began three years ago, under the direction of Dr. Gordon D. Moskowitz, after studies showed that muscles remained active after a limb was removed.

By analyzing muscular activity at the hip and thigh, the team of researchers determined a reliable pattern that upper leg muscles follow when the knee is willed to flex or extend, the hospital said.

Additional research revealed that a portion of the energy dissipated by the muscles could be recovered and used to create motion.

The research team then created a prototype of the electro-mechanical leg that has been successfully tested on an amputee, the hospital reported.

The prosthesis is controlled by an external minicomputer that receives impulses, causing the leg to react, Mr. Hillstrom said.

"It's feasible that the minicomputer will be contained within the leg as research on the project continues," he said.

Through subconscious signals, the wearer may walk with minimal effort while conscious signals permit him or her to avoid obstacles and stumbling, Mr. Hillstrom said.

The research team says it hopes to have a clinical model of the device, called the Drexel-Moss knee, ready in three to five years.

An ultralight plastic prosthetic material, also developed at the hospital, will provide a natural-looking enclosure for the knee, the researchers said.

Other principal researchers on the project are Donald Meyers of the National Bureau of Standards in Washington, and Ronald Triolo, a research scientist at the hospital's rehabilitation engineering center.

41.   The main topic of this passage is the
    a.   flow of brain waves to amputated limbs.
    b.   research in muscle movement.
    c.   energy produced by muscles.
    d.   development of an amputee's device.

42.   According to the passage, the development of the prosthesis has reached the
    a.   implementation stage.
    b.   production stage.
    c.   design stage.
    d.   pilot stage.

43.   Currently, the minicomputer is located
    a.   outside the body.
    b.   inside the artificial leg.
    c.   inside the amputee's stump.
    d.   inside the amputee's head.

44.   Research at the hospital has included work on artificial
    a.   cartilage.
    b.   ligaments.
    c.   skin.
    d.   nerves.

45.   Subconscious signals applied to the prosthesis control
    a.   sitting.
    b.   twisting.
    c.   stooping.
    d.   forward movement.

46.   The Drexel part of the name for the device most likely refers to
    a.   the name of the town.
    b.   a researcher in the field.
    c.   a donor to the research project.
    d.   a patient who has used the device.

47.   The negotiators broke off discussions because they had reached
    a.   an impasse.
    b.   a climax.
    c.   a concession.
    d.   a parley.

48.   The dealer suspected that the painting was bogus.
    Bogus means
    a.   copied.
    b.   original.
    c.   reproduced.
    d.   forged.

49.   The suspect implicated the young lawyer with his statement.
    Implicated means
    a.   involved.
    b.   convicted.
    c.   shocked.
    d.   charged.

50. A person who is difficult to please is said to be
    a. indignant.
    b. marked.
    c. notorious.
    d. fastidious.

55. The juvenile was behaving so defiantly that he could only be described as
    a. recalcitrant.
    b. taciturn.
    c. notorious.
    d. prohibitive.

56. The monarch issued several edicts before beginning the evening's entertainment.
    Edicts means

    a. proposals.
    b. commands.
    c. restrictions.
    d. retreats.

57. All of the shipping information was listed on the invoice.
    Invoice means

    a. bill.
    b. order.
    c. requisition.
    d. specifications.

58. The schism between the two families seemed irreparable.
    Schism means

    a. feud.
    b. separation.
    c. disagreement.
    d. relationship.

59. The young man's provincial attitude kept him from getting the job.
    Provincial means

    a. superior.
    b. belligerent.
    c. narrow.
    d. snobbish.

60. The knight threw down the gauntlet at the feet of his opponent to challenge him to fight.
    Gauntlet means

    a. sword.
    b. hat.
    c. glove.
    d. scarf.

Mathematics Comprehensive Practice Test 3

60 Minutes

Work each problem carefully. Use scrap paper to do your calculations. The correct answers will be found at the end of this test.

1. $0.206 \times 6.3 =$
    a. 1.2978
    b. 1.3608
    c. 1.5768
    d. 1.914

2. $(301 + 802) - (711 - 43) =$
    a. 349
    b. 435
    c. 1,761
    d. 1,771

3. If $A > 9$, A could equal
    a. 10.
    b. 9.
    c. 8.
    d. 0.

4. If a heart beats 27 times in 20 seconds, how many times does it beat in 1 minute?
    a. 108
    b. 98
    c. 81
    d. 71

5. If 1 kg equals 2.2 lb, how many kilograms will an 8.8 lb baby weigh?
    a. 19.36
    b. 11
    c. 6.6
    d. 4

6. A dieter consumed 1,550 calories on Monday, 1,630 on Tuesday, 1,420 on Wednesday, 1,725 on Thursday, and 1,500 calories on Friday. What was this person's average daily caloric intake?
    a. 7,825
    b. 1,565
    c. 1,500
    d. 1,145

7. $873.65 - 24.344 =$
    a. 630.21
    b. 849.306
    c. 849.314
    d. 859.31

8. A student spent $2.75 for lunch on Monday, $2.10 on Tuesday, and $3.25 on Wednesday. What was the average cost of lunch for the 3 days?
   a. $2.60
   b. $2.63
   c. $2.70
   d. $8.10

9. A piece of cloth is 15 ft long. If 2.1 ft at one end are damaged, how many feet of cloth remain undamaged?
   a. 12.9
   b. 13.1
   c. 13.9
   d. 17.1

10. $1\frac{3}{4} + 2\frac{5}{6} =$
    a. $4\frac{7}{12}$
    b. 4
    c. $3\frac{1}{5}$
    d. $2\frac{7}{24}$

11. 20% of the residents of a certain area are expected to become ill this year. If 25,000 people live in this area, how many are expected to become ill?
    a. 6,250
    b. 5,000
    c. 1,250
    d. 500

12. At 8 am, a patient's temperature was 99.4°F. At each of the next two readings, at 12 noon and again at 4 pm, the temperature had risen 0.4°F. What was the temperature at 4 pm?
    a. 98.6°F
    b. 99.8°F
    c. 100.2°F
    d. 100.6°F

13. What number is 29% of 150?
    a. 5.17
    b. 19.33
    c. 43.5
    d. 517.24

14. An income tax system requires that persons having a net income between $10,000 and $16,000 pay a tax of $800 plus 24% of that part of the income in excess of $10,000. How much tax should be paid on an income of $12,500?
    a. $600
    b. $1,400
    c. $3,000
    d. $3,840

15. If a regular pentagon has a perimeter of 15 cm, how long is each side?
    a. 3 cm
    b. 3.5 cm
    c. 3.75 cm
    d. 5 cm

16. What is the maximum number of 1½ inch strips of tape that can be cut from a 480 inch roll of tape?
    a. 160
    b. 240
    c. 320
    d. 720

17. A patient, who is supposed to get 2½ cups of low-fat milk per day, drinks ¾ cup at breakfast. If the remaining amount is to be equally divided, how much will she drink at each of two meals?
    a. ⅞ cup
    b. 1 cup
    c. 1½ cup
    d. 1¾ cup

18. 50.29 ÷ 0.47 =
    a. 1.07
    b. 1.7
    c. 17
    d. 107

19. The ratio of substance A to substance B in a mixture is 2:3. If the mixture contains 12 mg of substance A, how much is there of substance B?
    a. 18 mg
    b. 16 mg
    c. 9 mg
    d. 8 mg

20. A jogger travels x miles each morning. Which of these equations represents the number of days she will need to jog 200 miles?
    a. 200x = days
    b. 200 + x = days
    c. $\frac{x}{200}$ = days
    d. $\frac{200}{x}$ = days

21. 7½ − 4⅔ =
    a. 3
    b. 3⅓
    c. 2⅙
    d. 2⅚

22. An acute angle is best defined as one that is
    a. less than a right angle.
    b. greater than an obtuse angle.
    c. greater than a right angle.
    d. equal to an obtuse angle.

23. A man estimates that ⅕ of his salary is spent for taxes, ¼ for rent, and ⅒ for insurance. What fraction of his salary is left for other expenses and savings?
    a. ⁹⁄₂₀
    b. ¹¹⁄₂₀
    c. ³⁄₁₉
    d. ¹⁶⁄₁₉

24. What percentage of 200 is 250?
     a. 50
     b. 80
     c. 125
     d. 150

25. $2\sqrt{25} =$
     a. 7
     b. 10
     c. 25
     d. 50

26. Solve the following simultaneous equations:

     $$\begin{cases} 3x - 2y = 7 \\ x + 2y = 5 \end{cases}$$

     a. x = 5, y = 4
     b. x = 7, y = 5
     c. x = 1, y = -2
     d. x = 3, y = 1

27. 7 is 35% of what number?
     a. 245
     b. 20
     c. 5
     d. 2.45

28. Which of these decimals equals 3.7%?
     a. 3.70
     b. 0.37
     c. 0.037
     d. 0.0037

29. If ⅔ of x = 48, then ½ of x =
     a. 16
     b. 24
     c. 36
     d. 72

30. If x = 3 and y = 4, then $\dfrac{5x^2 + 2y}{3(x + y)} =$
     a. $233\!/\!21$
     b. $38\!/\!21$
     c. $53\!/\!13$
     d. $53\!/\!21$

31. Which of the following algebraic equations represents the statement shown below?

     8 less than 5 times a number (n) equals 30

     a. 8 − 5n = 30
     b. 5n − 8 = 30
     c. 5(n − 8) = 30
     d. 5n + 8 = 30

32. $3y^2 \times 2y^4 =$
  a. $5y^6$
  b. $6y^6$
  c. $5y^8$
  d. $6y^8$

33.   Which of these decimals is approximately equal to ⅜?
  a.   0.21
  b.   0.37
  c.   0.43
  d.   0.73

34.   If 33% of x = 99, x =
  a.   3
  b.   32.67
  c.   33.33
  d.   300

35. $176 - (-64) =$
  a.   112
  b.   240
  c.   11,264
  d. $-11,264$

36.   4½ × 3⅚ =
  a.   12 5/12
  b.   12⅝
  c.   13⅔
  d.   17¼

37.   If 75 ml of solution contain 30 ml of a specific medication, how much of that medication will be needed to provide 120 ml of the same solution?
  a.   18.75 ml
  b.   45 ml
  c.   48 ml
  d.   75 ml

38.   Barry has 4 more cards than Ken. Together, they have 44 cards. If x represents the number of cards Ken has, then which of these equations will represent the total number of cards?
  a. $x + 4 = 44$
  b. $2x - 4 = 44$
  c. $x + 4x = 44$
  d. $2x + 4 = 44$

39.   If 3/7 = 5/x, then x =
  a.   35/3
  b.   15/7
  c.   5/21
  d.   7/15

40.   If the monthly expenses for a family are represented by a circle graph, how many degrees of the circle will be needed to show that 20% of the expenses are used for clothes?
  a.   20°
  b.   36°
  c.   54°
  d.   72°

Science Comprehensive Practice Test 3

60 Minutes

Read each question carefully, and then select the best answer. The correct answers will be found at the end of this test.

1. A scientist is conducting an experiment using two beating frog hearts. Each heart is immersed in fluids, one heart in jar A and the second heart in jar B. The heart in jar A is stimulated and the heartbeat speeds up. Some of the fluid from jar A is placed around the heart in jar B. The heart in jar B also beats faster. The best explanation for this is
    a. the temperature of the fluid in jar A excites the heart in jar B.
    b. the nerve of the heart in jar A secreted into the fluid a chemical messenger that stimulates muscle movement.
    c. the increase in the rate of the heart in jar B was a coincidence.
    d. parts of the nerve from the heart in jar A broke off into the fluid.

2. The formula $C_{12}H_{22}O_{11}$ most probably represents a
    a. protein.
    b. lipid.
    c. carbohydrate.
    d. nucleic acid.

3. Which of these processes would be directly affected if a person's red blood cell count decreased significantly?
    a. oxygen transport
    b. phagocytosis
    c. immunologic reactions
    d. blood clotting

4. A short time after a drop of ink is placed in a glass of water, the water takes on a uniform color. This illustrates the process of
    a. osmosis.
    b. diffusion.
    c. active transport.
    d. pinocytosis.

5. Chloroplasts are found in which of these cell structures?
    a. the cytoplasm of a human liver cell
    b. the nucleus of a frog blood cell
    c. the cytoplasm of a bean leaf cell
    d. the nucleus of an onion skin cell

6. The graph below shows the electronegativities of the five halogens

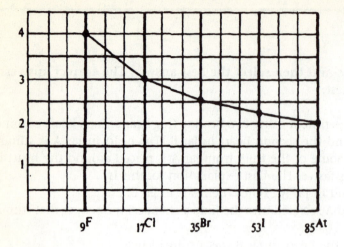

Which one has an electronegativity of 2.2?
a. Cl
b. Br
c. I
d. At

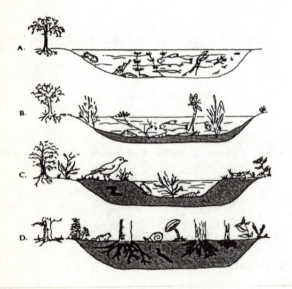

7. Which of these processes is most obviously represented by the diagrams above?
a. evolution
b. ecological succession
c. the formation of a marine biome
d. spontaneous generation

8. Which of these equations shows the synthesis of a compound?
a. $2Hg + O_2 \rightarrow 2HgO$
b. $2Na + Hg(NO_3)_2 \rightarrow 2NaNO_3 + Hg$
c. $HgBr_2 \rightarrow Hg + Br_2$
d. $2NaCl + Hg(NO_3)_2 \rightarrow 2NaNO_3 + HgCl_2$

9. Shivering to maintain a 98.6°F temperature in cold weather is an example of
    a. homeostasis.
    b. synthesis.
    c. hydrolysis.
    d. transpiration.

10. A plant cell is placed in a concentrated solution of salt water and subsequently shrinks. The shrinkage is most likely the result of
    a. salt leaving the cell.
    b. salt entering the cell.
    c. water leaving the cell.
    d. water entering the cell.

11. The atomic masses of Ca, O, and H are shown below.

    Ca = 40
    O = 16
    H = 1

    What is the molecular weight of $Ca(OH)_2$?
    a. 57
    b. 58
    c. 74
    d. 114

12. A common characteristic of the organic compounds synthesized by the cell is that they all contain
    a. hydrogen and oxygen atoms in a 2:1 ratio.
    b. monosaccharides.
    c. carbon, hydrogen, or oxygen.
    d. peptide bonds.

13. A student is observing a cell under a compound microscope. Which of these instruments would best remove the cell's nucleus?
    a. ultracentrifuge
    b. tissue forceps
    c. micrometer
    d. microdissection apparatus

14. The graph below shows the effect of heat added at a steady rate upon the temperature of a substance. The substance is a solid at 20°C.

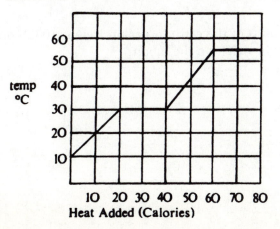

What is the melting point of the substance?
a. 0°C
b. 10°C
c. 30°C
d. 80°C

15. Organisms that reproduce sexually go through a stage of development called the blastula. The stage occurs during which part of the organism's development?
a. before conception
b. within several hours after conception
c. halfway through gestation
d. within several hours before birth

16. Finger-like projections in the small intestine that increase the surface area for absorption are called
a. cilia.
b. pseudopods.
c. tubules.
d. villi.

The next question refers to the diagram below.

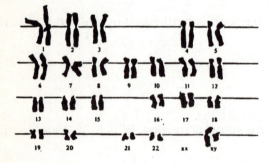

17. The diagram represents
a. a blood type.
b. a karyotype.
c. an X-ray.
d. an electron micrograph.

18. The moon has about one-seventh the mass of the earth. A person weighs 100 lb on earth. Approximately how much will this person weigh on the moon?
a. 7 lb
b. 14 lb
c. 86 lb
d. 700 lb

19. A negatively charged object has
a. only protons.
b. only electrons.
c. more protons than electrons.
d. more electrons than protons.

20. In which one of the following states of matter is the attraction between molecules strongest?
    a. solid
    b. liquid
    c. gas
    d. colloid

21. Burning and rusting of iron are similar processes in that they both
    a. require a flame for initiation.
    b. can use water as a catalyst.
    c. occur only above the kindling temperature.
    d. produce the same product.

22. Cellular respiration occurs in which of the following cell organelles?
    a. nucleus
    b. mitochondria
    c. ribosomes
    d. golgi bodies

23. Which of the following nuclear processes is illustrated by the following equation?

$$ {}_{1}^{1}H + {}_{1}^{3}H \rightarrow {}_{2}^{4}He $$

    a. alpha emission
    b. beta emission
    c. nuclear fusion
    d. nuclear fission

24. Two objects of different mass and temperature are in contact with one another. In which direction will heat flow?
    a. from the object of greater mass to the object of lesser mass
    b. from the object at higher temperature to the object at lower temperature
    c. from the object with less energy to the object with more energy
    d. from the object of greater density to the object of lesser density

25. Which one of the following acids would be described as a weak acid?
    a. hydrochloric acid
    b. sulfuric acid
    c. acetic acid
    d. nitric acid

26. An uncalibrated mercury thermometer is placed in an ice-water mixture, and the level of mercury is marked to indicate the temperature of the ice water. The thermometer is then placed in boiling water and the mercury rises 15 cm. If we wish to calibrate this thermometer for the Celsius scale, what would be the distance between each degree marking on the thermometer?
    a. 1.5 cm
    b. 0.15 cm
    c. 0.015 cm
    d. 0.0015 cm

27. An animal with a chitinous exoskeleton and jointed appendages would be classified in which of the following phyla?
    a. arthropoda
    b. chordata
    c. annelida
    d. protozoa

28. Which of these diagrams correctly represents the path of parallel light rays passing through the lens shown?

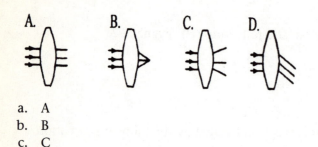

    a. A
    b. B
    c. C
    d. D

29. Which one of the following indicators would best be used to distinguish between a strong acid and a weak acid?
    a. litmus paper
    b. a pH meter
    c. limewater
    d. phenolphthalein

30. A risk group for the disease AIDS (acquired immunodeficiency syndrome) is intravenous drug users. To prevent further spread of the disease, which of these measures would be most effective for this group to take?
    a. undergo screening for the AIDS virus
    b. avoid sharing hypodermic needles with other drug users
    c. increase the fiber in their diets
    d. limit bodily contact with other drug users

31. A beaker contains a saturated solution of KNO_3 in water. Which one of the following actions will most likely increase the solubility of the KNO_3 in the water?
    a. increasing the temperature of the solution
    b. adding sodium chloride to the beaker
    c. adding KNO_3 to the beaker
    d. evaporating some water from the beaker

32. All the cells of the human body receive hormones as a direct result of the activity of which of these body systems?
    a. digestive
    b. reproductive
    c. respiratory
    d. circulatory

33. The chemical reactivity of an element is most closely related to the number of electrons in its
    a. nucleus.
    b. lowest energy level.
    c. valence shell.
    d. inner shells.

34. A true solution *CANNOT* be
    a. colored.
    b. dilute.
    c. heterogeneous.
    d. neutral.

35. Which of these compounds is an isomer of

$$\begin{array}{c} \text{H} \quad \text{H} \\ | \quad\ | \\ \text{H--C--C--O--H ?} \\ | \quad\ | \\ \text{H} \quad \text{H} \end{array}$$

    A.
$$\begin{array}{c} \text{H} \quad \text{H} \\ | \quad\ | \\ \text{H--O--C--C--H} \\ | \quad\ | \\ \text{H} \quad \text{H} \end{array}$$

    B.
$$\begin{array}{c} \text{H} \qquad\ \text{H} \\ | \qquad\ | \\ \text{H--C--O--C--H} \\ | \qquad\ | \\ \text{H} \qquad\ \text{H} \end{array}$$

    C.
$$\begin{array}{c} \text{H} \quad \text{H} \quad \text{H} \\ | \quad\ | \quad\ | \\ \text{H--C--C--C--O--H} \\ | \quad\ | \quad\ | \\ \text{H} \quad \text{H} \quad \text{H} \end{array}$$

    D.
$$\begin{array}{c} \text{H} \quad \text{O} \\ | \quad\ \| \\ \text{H--C--C--O--H} \\ | \quad\ | \\ \text{H} \quad \text{H} \end{array}$$

36. A drug that kills an organism by decreasing the enzyme activity needed for cellular respiration would initially affect which of these organelles?
    a. endoplasmic reticula
    b. lysosomes
    c. golgi apparatus
    d. mitochondria

37. A food substance is placed in blue Benedict's solution and heated. The color of the solution changes to brick red. This color change indicates the presence of
    a. fatty acids.
    b. glucose.
    c. protein.
    d. vitamin C.

38. If young tomato plants were grown under optimal conditions of temperature, soil, and light, the rate of photosynthesis would probably be increased by increasing the
    a. carbon dioxide content of the air.
    b. oxygen content of the air.
    c. glucose content of the soil.
    d. moisture content of the soil.

39. The part of the eye that contains light-sensitive receptor cells is the
    a. iris.
    b. retina.
    c. pupil.
    d. cornea.

40. A part of the human nervous system that controls both thought and sensory processes is the
    a. medulla.
    b. spinal cord.
    c. cerebral cortex.
    d. cerebellum.

41. Which of the following terms refers to a group of similar cells that are organized together to perform the same function?
    a. organ
    b. tissue
    c. organ system
    d. organism

42. The following data were obtained for the heating of a hydrate:

mass of empty crucible	15 g
mass of crucible + hydrate	22 g
mass of crucible + substance remaining after heating	18 g

    What was the mass of water in the hydrate?
    a. 3 g
    b. 4 g
    c. 7 g
    d. 22 g

43. By which one of the following processes will starch be converted to sugar?
    a. polymerization
    b. enzymatic hydrolysis
    c. protein synthesis
    d. neutralization

44. The caffeine that is found in coffee, tea, and colas is a
    a. food supplement.
    b. drug.
    c. preservative.
    d. food dye.

The next question refers to the following diagram of the human female reproductive system.

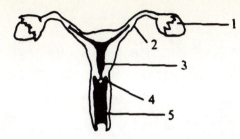

45.   Which of the structures shown above produces female sex hormones?
    a. 1
    b. 2
    c. 4
    d. 5

46.   Although there is a gap between two neurons, the nerve impulse is able to travel from one cell to another. This is because
    a. an electrical shock is produced across the gap.
    b. chemical substances from one neuron can stimulate an impulse in the other.
    c. axons carry the impulse between the neurons.
    d. the myelin sheath transports the impulse across the gap.

47.   In genetics, the physical appearance of a trait is called its
    a. phenotype.
    b. genotype.
    c. heterozygote.
    d. homozygote.

48.   Pieces of zinc are dropped into four different solutions of hydrochloric acid. The one that reacts most rapidly is probably
    a. most concentrated.
    b. most dilute.
    c. at the lowest temperature.
    d. freshest.

49.   Which one of the following actions will cause the greatest increase in the volume of one liter of a gas?
    a. heating the gas
    b. increasing the pressure on the gas
    c. heating the gas while increasing the pressure on it
    d. cooling the gas while increasing the pressure on it

50.   The production of lactic acid in the muscle cells of a runner who is completing a 20-mile race is due to
    a. hydrolysis.
    b. dehydration synthesis.
    c. aerobic respiration.
    d. anaerobic respiration.

51.   The table below indicates the ranges of wavelengths of different colors of light.

Color	Wavelength
violet	less than 4.5×10^{-7} m
blue	$4.5 - 5.0 \times 10^{-7}$ m
green	$5.0 - 5.7 \times 10^{-7}$ m
yellow	$5.7 - 5.9 \times 10^{-7}$ m
orange	$5.9 - 6.1 \times 10^{-7}$ m
red	greater than 6.1×10^{-7} m

What is the color of light having a wavelength of 5.6×10^{-7} m?
a.   blue
b.   green
c.   yellow
d.   orange

52.   If an object measures 5 millimeters in diameter, what is its diameter in microns (micrometers)?
a.   0.005
b.   50
c.   500
d.   5,000

53.   All motors get warm as they run. When doing the same work, motor X gets warmer than motor Y. Which of these statements is most likely to apply to motor X?
a.   It is running at a higher voltage than motor Y.
b.   It is more powerful than motor Y.
c.   It draws more current than motor Y.
d.   It is less efficient than motor Y.

54.   NaCl, KCl, and $CaCl_2$ are white, colorless salts. Which of the following procedures will best distinguish among them?
a.   Test to see whether they dissolve in water.
b.   Determine how quickly each burns.
c.   Determine how each affects the freezing point of water.
d.   Perform flame tests on each of them.

55.   An object is pulled along the ground at a steady velocity by a force of 10 newtons. This force is needed to
a.   overcome friction.
b.   overcome the object's inertia.
c.   give the object potential energy.
d.   overcome a moving object's natural tendency to stop.

56.   After viewing a paramecium under the high power of a compound microscope, a student switches back to low power. The image of the paramecium now becomes
a.   smaller and brighter.
b.   larger and brighter.
c.   smaller and darker.
d.   larger and darker.

57.　The rate at which a freely falling object accelerates is
　　a.　proportional to its weight.
　　b.　proportional to the distance.
　　c.　continually increasing.
　　d.　constant.

58.　The diagram below shows the paths taken by three rays of light from the flame of a candle as they pass through a lens.

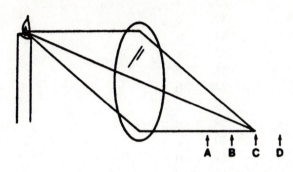

At which point should a screen be placed in order to get the sharpest image of the flame?
　　a.　A
　　b.　B
　　c.　C
　　d.　D

59.　Modern-day giraffes appear to have longer necks than their ancestors. Lamarck would explain this phenomenon by his theory of
　　a.　natural selection.
　　b.　mutation.
　　c.　survival of the fittest.
　　d.　use and disuse.

60.　The stimulant drugs sometimes referred to as "pep" pills belong to which of these classes of drugs?
　　a.　barbiturates
　　b.　hallucinogens
　　c.　narcotics
　　d.　amphetamines

Answers Comprehensive Practice Test 3

Verbal Ability: Word Knowledge and Comprehension

1.	b		31.	c
2.	b		32.	a
3.	c		33.	c
4.	d		34.	a
5.	b		35.	a
6.	d		36.	d
7.	c		37.	b
8.	d		38.	b
9.	c		39.	d
10.	b		40.	a
11.	c		41.	d
12.	b		42.	d
13.	b		43.	a
14.	c		44.	c
15.	b		45.	d
16.	a		46.	c
17.	b		47.	a
18.	d		48.	d
19.	b		49.	a
20.	c		50.	d
21.	c		51.	a
22.	d		52.	d
23.	a		53.	d
24.	a		54.	d
25.	d		55.	a
26.	b		56.	b
27.	c		57.	a
28.	c		58.	b
29.	a		59.	d
30.	a		60.	c

Mathematics

1. The answer is a.

$$
\begin{array}{r}
0.206 \quad \text{3 decimal places} \\
\times\ 6.3 \quad \text{1 decimal place} \\
\hline
618 \\
+\ 12360 \\
\hline
1.2978 \quad \text{4 decimal places}
\end{array}
$$

2.   **The answer is b.** Follow the order of operations to simplify this expression.

$$(301 + 802) - (711 - 43) =$$
$$1103 - 668 = 435$$

3.   **The answer is a.** If A > 9, it means all values of A are greater than 9. The only choice for A is 10.

4.   **The answer is c.** You may use a proportion to solve this problem. You will need to change 1 minute to 60 seconds. As always, make sure you align the units correctly: beats across from beats, and seconds across from seconds.

$$\frac{27\ beats}{20\ sec} = \frac{x}{60\ sec}$$ Rather than cross multiply in this case, examine the two fractions closely. Notice that $20 \cdot 3 = 60$. Because the two fractions are equal, you may multiply 27 by 3 to obtain the missing numerator: $27 \cdot 3 = 81$. Therefore, x = 81.

5.   **The answer is d.**

$$\frac{1\ kg}{2.2\ lbs} = \frac{x}{8.8\ lbs} \cdot 4 = 29$$ Rather than cross multiply in this case, examine the two fractions closely. Notice that $2.2 \cdot 4 = 8.8$. Because the two fractions are equal, you may multiply 1 by 4 to obtain the missing numerator: $1 \cdot 4 = 4$. Therefore, x = 4.

6.   **The answer is b.**

Total the five days of caloric intake: $1550 + 1630 + 1420 + 1725 + 1500 = 7825$
Divide this total by 5 to find the average: $7825 \div 5 = 1565$.

7.   **The answer is b.** Make sure you line up the decimal points when subtracting decimals.

```
  873.650
-  24.344
  849.306
```

8.   **The answer is c.** Total the amount of money spent on lunch over 3 days: $2.75 + $2.10 + $3.25 = $8.10
Divide this total by 3 to find the average: $8.10 \div 3 = 2.70

9.   **The answer is a.** Subtract the section of damaged cloth from the entire piece of cloth to find out how much remains undamaged.

```
  15.0   (It's ok to add this zero to the right of the decimal point.)
-  2.1
  12.9
```

10.   **The answer is a.** Find a common denominator and write equivalent fractions. The LCD is 12, because 4 and 6 are both factors of 12.

$$
\begin{aligned}
1\tfrac{3}{4} &= 1\tfrac{9}{12} \\
+\; 2\tfrac{5}{6} &= 2\tfrac{10}{12} \\
\hline
3\tfrac{19}{12} &= 4\tfrac{7}{12}
\end{aligned}
$$

11.   **The answer is b.** Find 20% of 25,000 by changing 20% to a decimal and multiplying it by 25,000.

$$20\% = 0.2$$

$$0.2 \cdot 25{,}000 = 5000$$

5000 = 20% of 25,000. Therefore, 5000 people are expected to become ill.

12.   **The answer is c.** The patient's temperature starts out at 99.4 degrees. It rises 0.4 degrees twice, ppfor a total of an 0.8 degree rise. To find the final temperature, add 0.8 to 99.4.

$$
\begin{aligned}
&99.4 \\
+\;&0.8 \\
\hline
&100.2 \quad \text{This is your answer.}
\end{aligned}
$$

13.   **The answer is c.** Turn the problem into an equation and solve for x: What number is 29% of 150?

$$
\begin{aligned}
x &= 29\% \cdot 150 \\
x &= 0.29 \cdot 150 \\
x &= 43.5
\end{aligned}
$$

14.   **The answer is b.** The tax to be paid will be $800 plus 24% of $2,500 (the income in excess of $10,000).

Calculate 24% of $2,500: 0.24 · $2500 = $600
Add $600 to $800 to obtain total taxes: $1,400.

15.   **The answer is a.** A regular pentagon is a pentagon (5 sided polygon) with all sides the same length. If the perimeter is 15 cm, then each side measures 15 ÷ 5 = 3 cm long.

16.   **The answer is c.** The question is really asking: "How many 1½'s are there in 480?" This is a division problem.

$$480 \div 1\frac{1}{2} \qquad \text{Change } 1\frac{1}{2} \text{ to an improper fraction.}$$

$$480 \div \frac{3}{2} \qquad \text{Invert the divisor and multiply.}$$

$$\frac{480}{1} \cdot \frac{2}{3} = \frac{960}{3} = 320 \quad \text{This is your answer.}$$

17.   **The answer is a.** Subtract the amount of milk already drunk $\left(\frac{3}{4}\right)$ from the total $\left(2\frac{1}{2}\right)$ to find out how much milk remains to be drunk.

$$2\frac{1}{2} = \frac{5}{2} = \frac{10}{4}$$
$$-\frac{3}{4} = \frac{3}{4} = \frac{3}{4}$$
$$\overline{\qquad\qquad \frac{7}{4}}$$

Divide ⅞ by 2 to find out how much the patient will drink at each meal.

$$\frac{7}{4} \div \frac{2}{1} =$$
$$\frac{7}{4} \cdot \frac{1}{2} = \frac{7}{8}$$

18.   **The answer is d.**

$$0.47\overline{)50.29} \quad \text{Multiply both the dividend and divisor by 100.}$$
$$\frac{107}{47\overline{)5029}} \quad 107 \text{ is your answer.}$$

Another way to solve this problem is by inspection. Once you've multiplied both the divisor and dividend by 100, inspect your answer choices. Of the four answers given, only "107" makes sense for this problem; all the others are too small. It is possible to answer this problem without dividing at all!

19.   **The answer is a.** You may use a proportion to solve this problem. You will need to recognize the ratio 2:3 as the same thing as ⅔. As always, be sure to align the units correctly: substance A across from substance A, and substance B across from substance B.

$$\frac{2}{3} = \frac{12}{x} \quad \text{Cross multiply.}$$
$$2x = 36 \quad \text{Divide both sides by 2 to solve for x.}$$
$$x = 18 \quad \text{This is your answer.}$$

20.   **The answer is d.** The rate of the jogger is x miles each morning, or x miles each day. To help you figure out the problem, let's pretend that x stands for 10 miles each day (I just made up that number). Plug that in to the equations and see if it makes any sense.

   a. $200 \cdot 10 = 2000$ days. 2000 days, at 20 miles each day? If this were right, the jogger would travel a total of 40,000 miles! *Try another choice.*

   b. $\dfrac{200}{10} = 20$ days, 20 days, at 10 miles each day, would allow the jogger to travel 200 miles. This is your answer!

21.   **The answer is d.** Find a common denominator and write equivalent fractions. The LCD is 6, because 2 and 3 are both factors of 12.

$$7\frac{1}{2} = 7\frac{3}{6} = 6\frac{9}{6}$$
$$-\ 4\frac{2}{3} = 4\frac{4}{6} = 4\frac{4}{6}$$
$$\rule{4cm}{0.4pt}$$
$$2\frac{5}{6}$$

22.   **The answer is a.** An acute angle is defined as an angle less than 90 degrees. A right angle is defined as angle equal to 90 degrees. Therefore, the best choice is A, which describes an acute angle as less than a right angle.

23.   **The answer is b.** Find the lowest common denominator (LCD) for all three fractions, and then change each of the fractions to an equivalent fraction with the new denominator. 4, 5, and 10 are all factors of 20, so 20 is the LCD. Add them together.

$$\frac{1}{4} = \frac{5}{20}$$
$$\frac{1}{5} = \frac{4}{20}$$
$$+\ \frac{1}{10} = \frac{2}{20}$$
$$\rule{3cm}{0.4pt}$$
$$\frac{9}{20}$$

If $\dfrac{9}{20}$ of the man's salary is spent already, then $\dfrac{11}{20}$ must remain. Why? Because the amount sent, plus the amount remaining must total the whole, or $\dfrac{20}{20}$.

24.   **The answer is c.** This is one of three types of common percent problems: finding the percent when you know the base and the percentage.
The problem again: What percent of 200 is 250?

$x\% \cdot 200 = 250$	Deal with "x" being a percent at the end of the problem.
$200x = 250$	Divide both sides by 200.
$x = 1.25$	Change 1.25 to a percent.
125%	is your answer.

25.   **The answer is b.**

26.   **The answer is d.**

27.   **The answer is b.** Turn the problem into an equation and solve for x.

7 is 35% of what number?

$7 = 35\% \cdot x$ Change 35% to a decimal.
$7 = 0.35x$ Divide both sides by 0.35 to solve for x.
$20 = x$ This is your answer.

28.   **The answer is c.** To change a percent to a decimal, divide the percent by 100 and drop the % symbol.

$3.7\% \div 100 = 0.037$

29.   **The answer is c.**

Solve the first equation for x. $\frac{2}{3}x = 48$

$x = 72$ Multiply both sides by $\frac{3}{2}$.

Now substitute 72 for x in the second equation: $\frac{1}{2} \cdot 72 =$ Simplify.

36 is your answer.

30.   **The answer is b.**

31.   **The answer is b.** You need to be familiar with certain words, and how they translate from word problems to equations.

Here is the problem again: 8 less than 5 times a number (n) equals 30.

"8 less than" means "-8"

"5 times a number (n)" means 5n

"equals 30" means "$= 30$".

Put this all together and you get: $5n - 8 = 30$

32.   **The answer is b.** Recall the rules for multiplying powers with similar bases: add the exponents. Therefore,

$3y^2 \cdot 2y^4 = 6y^{2+4} = 6y^6$

33.   **The answer is c.**

To convert $\frac{3}{7}$ to a decimal, divide 7 into 3: $7)\overline{.3000} \approx 0.43$ (quotient $.428$)

34. **The answer is d.** This is one of three types of common percent problems: finding the base when you know the percent and the percentage.
The problem again: 33% of x is 99?

$$0.33 \cdot x = 99$$
$0.33x = 99$ Divide both sides by 0.33 to solve for x.
$x = 300$ This is your answer.

35. **The answer is b.** Recall the rules for subtracting negative numbers: Subtracting a negative is like adding a positive. Therefore,

$$176 - (-64) = 176 + 64 = 240$$

36. **The answer is d.**

$4\frac{1}{2} \cdot 3\frac{5}{6} =$ Change each mixed number to an improper fraction.

$\frac{9}{2} \cdot \frac{23}{6} =$ Cross cancel between the 9 and the 6 (cancel out a 3).

$\frac{3}{2} \cdot \frac{23}{2} =$ Multiply.

$\frac{69}{4} = 17\frac{1}{4}$ This is your answer.

37. **The answer is c.** You may set up a proportion to solve this problem. As always, be sure to align the units correctly: ml of solution across from ml of solution, and ml of medication across from ml of medication.

$\frac{75}{30} = \frac{120}{x}$ Cross multiply.
$75\,x = 3600$ Divide both sides by 75 to solve for x.
$x = 48$ This is your answer.

38. **The answer is d.**

$x =$ Ken's cards
If Ben has four more cards than Ken, then Ben has $x + 4$ cards.
If their total number of cards is 44, then $x + x + 4 = 44$
$2x = 44$

39. **The answer is a.** By now, you are no doubt comforted by the familiar set up of a proportion!

$\frac{3}{7} = \frac{5}{x}$ Cross multiply.
$3x = 35$ Divide both sides by 3 to solve for x.
$x = \frac{35}{3}$ This is your answer.

40. **The answer is d.** Recall that there are 360 degrees in a circle. Once you know this, calculate 20% of 360: $0.2 \cdot 360 = 72$. 72 degrees represents 20% of the whole.

Science

1. **The answer is b.** Neurotransmitters serve as messengers between two neurons or a neuron and a target cell. Acetylcholine is a specific neurotransmitter which serves to stimulate muscle contractions.

2. **The answer is c.** Carbohydrates are composed of the elements carbon, hydrogen, and oxygen. The characteristic ratio of hydrogen to oxygen in carbohydrates is 2:1.

3. **The answer is a.** Red blood cells contain hemoglobin, which is a molecule that binds, transport, and deliver, oxygen.

4. **The answer is b.** Diffusion is the random dispersal of particles from areas of high particle concentration to areas of low particle concentration.

5. **The answer is c.** Chloroplasts are organelles found in plant cells that contain the pigment chlorophyll. This pigment serves to absorb light, which provides energy for the process of photosynthesis.

6. **The answer is c.** The graph indicates that I has an electronegativity of 2.2.

7. **The answer is b.** The diagrams represent ecological succession because the environment becomes progressively more complex.

8. **The answer is a.** A synthesis reaction involves the formation of one product from two or more reactants.

9. **The answer is a.** Shivering is the result of a number of small muscle contractions that serve to generate heat in order to maintain body temperature. Maintenance of a stable internal environment is referred to as homeostasis.

10. **The answer is c.** Water leaves the cell because water spontaneously flows from areas of low particle concentration to areas of high particle concentration by the process of osmosis.

11. **The answer is c.** The subscript 2 refers to all of the items inside the parenthesis. Thus, the mass of this molecule is:

    $$40 + 2 * (16 + 1) = 74$$

12. **The answer is a.** A compound with hydrogen and oxygen atoms in a two to one ratio is often a carbohydrate.

13. **The answer is a.** Centrifuges are means of separating out substances of different densities and masses. Thus, an ultracentrifuge could be used to extract different parts of a cell.

14. **The answer is c.** When a substance changes phase the temperature remains constant, even though the number of calories increases. This is due to the fact that all of the energy that is input during a phase change is used to break bonds to change a solid to a liquid or a liquid to a gas. Thus, at 20 calories and 30° Celsius, the substance is a solid while at 40 calories and 30° Celsius, the substance is a liquid.

15. **The answer is b.** In animals, rapid cell division begins a few hours after fertilization. These divisions are called cleavage and is divided into a number of stages: formation of the morula, blastulation, gastrulation, and neurulation. Cleavage is an early developmental process.

16. **The answer is d.** Cilia and pseudopods are structures that are involved with cell locomotion while tubules often lend structural support to a cell.

17. **The answer is b.** A karyotype is a printed array of a person's chromosomal make-up. As seen in the diagram, there are 23 pairs of chromosomes present, thus 46 chromosomes. Often karyotyping is done to check for chromosomal abnormalities such as Down's syndrome which is characterized by an extra copy of chromosome 21.

18. **The answer is b.** Since the mass of the moon is approximately one-seventh the mass of the earth, the weight of the person on the moon is approximately one-seventh of the person's weight on earth. $100/_7$ is approximately 14 lbs.

19. **The answer is d.** Electrons are negatively charged subatomic particles while protons are positively charged subatomic particles. When the number of protons is equal to the number of electrons, the atom is neutral. If, however, the number of protons exceeds the number of electrons, an atom with a positive charge is formed, a cation. If the number of electrons is greater than the number of protons, an atom with a negative charge is formed, anion.

20. **The answer is a.** As a substance changes phase from a gas to a liquid to a solid the attraction between the molecules in the substance increases.

21. **The answer is d.** The processes of burning and rusting both involve reactions with oxygen and in the case of iron, both produce iron oxide as a product.

22. **The answer is b.** The nucleus is the control center of the cell; the ribosomes are the sites of protein synthesis; the golgi bodies are involved with transport and modification of synthesized proteins.

23. **The answer is c.** The combination of the subatomic particles of two nuclei is seen in nuclear fusion. This particular reaction occurs in the sun and releases a great deal of energy.

24. **The answer is b.** Heat between two bodies that are in contact with each other is transferred by conduction. Heat always transfers from the warmer molecules to the cooler molecules.

25. **The answer is c.** Hydrochloric, sulfuric, and nitric acids are strong acids due to the fact that almost 100% of the associated hydrogens dissociate, in solution. In acetic acid, only approximately 5% of the hydrogens dissociate, and thus acetic acid is a weak acid. In general, the amount of hydrogen dissociation determines the strength of an acid, and the amount of hydroxide dissociation (OH^-) determines the strength of a base.

26. **The answer is b.** Water freezes at 0 degrees Celsius and boils at 100 degrees Celsius. Thus, if 15 cm represents this difference, then .15 cm must represent 1 degree Celsius.

27. **The answer is a.** An example of an arthropod is a lobster.

28. **The answer is b.** Parallel light waves passing through a convex lens would bend at the center and converge at the focal point as represented in diagram B.

29. **The answer is b.** All of the methods shown are methods that can be used to distinguish between an acid and a base. However, a pH meter allows for a much more accurate measure of pH and thus would be the most useful in distinguishing between a strong and weak acid.

30. **The answer is b.** The human immunodeficiency virus (HIV), which causes acquired immuno-deficiency syndrome (AIDS) is carried in the blood stream. Thus, intravenous drug users who share hypodermic needles are at a high risk for HIV. Using clean needles is a preventive measure taken against exposure to HIV. Limiting bodily or sexual contact is a preventive

measure as well, however, this would not be the most effective measure in a intravenous drug using population.

31.   **The answer is a.** Increasing the temperature of a solution increases the ability of a solute to be dissolved in a solvent. This ability is referred to as the solubility of a solution.

32.   **The answer is d.** Hormones travel via the circulatory system to their target organs.

33.   **The answer is c.** The valence shell, or outer shell, of an atom contains electrons that are most often involved in chemical reactions.

34.   **The answer is c.** A true solution must be uniform throughout, or homogeneous.

35.   **The answer is b.** Isomers are compounds with the same mass and composition of elements but different structures.

36.   **The answer is d.** Cellular respiration occurs in the mitochondria.

37.   **The answer is b.** Benedict's test indicates the presence of monosaccharides, i.e. glucose.

38.   **The answer is d.** Oxygen and glucose are products of photosynthesis, while carbon dioxide and water are the reactants. Carbon dioxide is readily available in the air; it is more likely that water is the limiting factor in this case.

39.   **The answer is b.** The retina contains photoreceptor cells, which are sensitive to light.

40.   **The answer is c.** The medulla is responsible for controlling involuntary activities such as heart rate, while the cerebellum is involved with balance and coordination.

41.   **The answer is b.** Tissues are groups of cells that are organized as organs. An organism is made up of groups of organ systems.

42.   **The answer is b.** Heating the substance causes the water to evaporate leaving a dehydrated product. Since the mass of the hydrated substance was 7 grams and after heating 3 grams remain, 4 grams of water were lost.

43.   **The answer is b.** Enzymes aid in the process of hydrolysis, which refers to the way in which starches are broken down. The name arises from the fact that a water molecule is added during this process. Thus, enzymatic hydrolysis is the means by which starches are converted to simple sugars.

44.   **The answer is b.** Caffeine is a central nervous system stimulant. A substance does not have to be taken in pill form to be considered a drug.

45.   **The answer is a.** The ovaries produce estrogen and progesterone. #2 is pointing at the fallopian tubes along which the egg travels and is fertilized. #3 is pointing at the uterus where the fertilized egg implants. #4 is pointing at the cervix, which is the opening to the uterus. #5 is pointing at the vaginal canal, or birthing canal.

46.   **The answer is b.** A nerve impulse causes neurotransmitters to be released from the end of one neuron. These chemicals travel to the next neuron and thus propogate the message or impulse.

47.   **The answer is a.** The genotype refers to the genetic make-up rather than the physical appearance. If the trait is homozygous, it means that there are two copies of either the dominant or recessive allele. If the trait is heterozygous, one allele is dominant while the other is recessive.

48.   **The answer is a.** The most concentrated HCl provides the most Cl^- ions to react with the zinc to form $ZnCl_2$ and H_2 gas.

49. **The answer is a.** Charles's Law states the volume and temperature change proportionally. Thus as temperature increases, volume increases as well. Boyle's Law states that pressure and volume are inversely related; an increase in pressure causes a decrease in volume. Finally, Gay-Lussac's Law states that pressure and temperature are related proportionally. Thus, when temperature increases, pressure increases as well.

50. **The answer is d.** Anaerobic respiration breaks down glucose into lactic acid. This occurs in the absence of oxygen in the cell, for instance, in a runner who has exhausted her supply of oxygen in a 20-mile race.

51. **The answer is b.** According to the table green light has a wavelength range of $5.0 - 5.7 \times 10^{-7}$ m. The wavelength of 5.6×10^{-7} m fits into the green light range.

52. **The answer is d.** 1000 microns = 1 millimeter.

53. **The answer is d.** Efficiency = work done/energy used. Since motor Y gets warmer than motor X, motor Y uses more energy for the same amount of work and is therefore less efficient.

54. **The answer is d.** Elements of the first two groups of the periodic table are metals, which are characterized by easily excitable outer electrons. In a flame, these electrons are easily excited (jump to a higher energy level) and as they return to their normal level, emit energy in the form of visible light. Each metal has a characteristic color emitted in such a "flame test" and this process can be used to identify substances.

55. **The answer is a.** Velocity is speed in a given direction. Friction opposes the motion of an object. The force is needed to overcome friction between the object and the ground and maintain the steady velocity of the object.

56. **The answer is a.** Lower power means less magnification, and thus the image will appear smaller. Since the image is now not taking up as much of the field, more light will be seen by the viewer.

57. **The answer is d.** A freely falling object accelerates down at the constant rate of g = 9.8 m/s squared.

58. **The answer is c.** The screen should be placed at point c on the diagram. Point c is at the focal point where the light rays converge. This point would provide the sharpest image on the screen.

59. **The answer is d.** Lamarck believed that physical characteristics that were useful in an organism's ability to survive in its environment became stronger, while those that were not useful became weaker. This was his theory of use and disuse. He also believed that these traits could be passed on to an organism's offspring, and this was his theory of acquired characteristics.

60. **The answer is d.** Amphetamines are central nervous system stimulants; they cause wakefulness and euphoria.

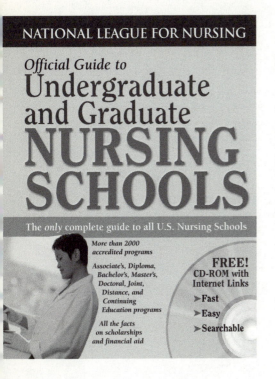